Immunodiagnosis For Clinicians:
Interpretation Of Immunoassays

Immunodiagnosis For Clinicians:
Interpretation Of Immunoassays

MICHAEL H. GRIECO, M.D.
Professor of Clinical Medicine
Columbia University
College of Physicians and Surgeons
R.A. Cooke Institute of Allergy
St. Luke's-Roosevelt Hospital Center
New York, New York

and

DAVID K. MERINEY, M.D.
Assistant Clinical Professor of Medicine
Columbia University
College of Physicians and Surgeons
R.A. Cooke Institute of Allergy
St. Luke's-Roosevelt Hospital Center
New York, New York

YEAR BOOK MEDICAL PUBLISHERS, INC.
CHICAGO • LONDON

Library of Congress Cataloging in Publication Data
Main entry under title:

Immunodiagnosis for clinicians.

    Includes index.
    1. Immunologic diseases—Diagnosis.   2.   Immunodiagnosis.
3. Immunoassay.   I. Grieco, Michael H.   II. Meriney,
David K.   [DNLM: 1. Immunoassay.   2.   Immunologic technics.
3. Immunologic diseases—Diagnosis. QW 570 G848i]
RC582.2.I45   1983   616.07'56   83-3567
ISBN 0-8151-4003-7

To Kenneth P. Mathews, M.D.
and
William B. Sherman, M.D. (deceased),
for their contributions to Allergy
and Clinical Immunology and
for their stimulation of our interest
in this field.

Contributors

JOHN J. CONDEMI, M.D.
Professor of Medicine, University of Rochester, School of Medicine and Dentistry, Rochester, New York

C. CUNNINGHAM-RUNDLES, M.D., Ph.D.
Associate, Sloan Kettering Institute; Assistant Professor of Biochemistry and Immunology, Cornell University Medical College, New York, New York

W.F. CUNNINGHAM-RUNDLES, M.D.
Adjunct Assistant Attending in Immunology, Sloan Kettering Institute, New York, New York

DICKSON D. DESPOMMIER, Ph.D.
Professor of Public Health and Microbiology (Parasitology), Division of Tropical Medicine, School of Public Health, College of Physicians & Surgeons, Columbia University, New York, New York

RICHARD EVANS III, M.D., COL. M.C.
Associate Professor, Departments of Medicine and Pediatrics, Uniformed Services University of the Health Sciences; Consultant in Allergy and Immunology to the Surgeon General of the Army, Walter Reed Army Medical Center, Washington, D.C.

PETER D. GOREVIC, M.D.
Associate Professor of Medicine and Pathology, Division of Allergy, Rheumatology and Clinical Immunology, State University of New York, Stony Brook, New York

MICHAEL H. GRIECO, M.D.
Professor of Clinical Medicine, Columbia University, College of Physicians and Surgeons, New York, New York, Director, R. A. Cooke Institute of Allergy, St. Luke's-Roosevelt Hospital Center, New York, New York

PETER A. GROSS, M.D.
Professor of Medicine, New Jersey College of Medicine and Surgery, Hackensack Medical Center, Hackensack, New Jersey

SUDHIR GUPTA, M.D.
Professor of Medicine, Chief, Division of Basic and Clinical Immunology, Department of Medicine, University of California at Irvine, Irvine, California

MICHAEL LANGE, M.D.

Assistant Professor of Clinical Medicine, Columbia University College of Physicians and Surgeons; Assistant Chief, Division of Infectious Diseases and Epidemiology, St. Luke's-Roosevelt Hospital Center, New York, New York

STEPHEN D. LITWIN, M.D.

Scientific Director, Guthrie Foundation for Medical Research, Sayre, Pennsylvania; Visiting Professor, Department of Microbiology, New York College of Veterinary Medicine, Cornell University, Ithaca, New York

KLAUS MAYER, M.D.

Associate Chairman of Clinical Laboratories, Department of Medicine; Director of Blood Bank and Hematology Laboratories, Memorial Sloan Kettering Cancer Center; Professor of Clinical Medicine, Cornell University Medical Center, New York, New York

DAVID K. MERINEY, M.D.

Assistant Clinical Professor of Medicine, Columbia University College of Physicians and Surgeons, New York, New York, Assistant Chief, Division of Allergy and Clinical Immunology, St. Luke's-Roosevelt Hospital Center, New York, New York

STEPHEN I. ROSENFELD, M.D.

Associate Professor of Medicine, University of Rochester School of Medicine and Dentistry, Rochester, New York

MICHAEL W. RYTEL, M.D.

Professor of Medicine; Head, Division of Infectious Disease, Department of Medicine, Medical College of Wisconsin, Milwaukee, Wisconsin

RICHARD J. SUMMERS, M.D., LT.C. M.C.

Associate Professor, Department of Medicine and Pediatrics, Uniformed Services University of the Health Sciences; Chief, Allergy-Clinical Immunology Service, Walter Reed Army Medical Center, Washington, D.C.

Contents

Preface

THE DISCIPLINES of basic and clinical immunology have developed rapidly over the past few decades. As a result, immunologic assays have been increasingly utilized by clinical laboratories. Clinicians are now required to interpret many tests based on immunologic principles. We feel, therefore, that it would be helpful to bring together information relating to the interpretation of immunologic assays in clinical medicine. This book is not a comprehensive text in immunology, nor is it an immunology laboratory manual. Rather, it is designed for use by clinicians, not necessarily immunologically oriented, in day-to-day practice.

The first three chapters in Part I give background information on basic immunology and methodology. These chapters may be consulted to help clarify discussions of the assays discussed in subsequent chapters. The 12 chapters in Part II deal with the interpretation of immunoassays grouped according to clinical disorders. Some overlap is inescapable, and the index may be consulted to determine when clinical entities are discussed in more than one chapter.

Some of the assays discussed are not available in the routine clinical laboratory but have been included because they are available in commercial reference or referral center laboratories or may soon become so. No attempt has been made to describe assays that are purely of investigative interest.

We wish to express our gratitude to the contributing authors for their hard work and cooperation. We also wish to express special appreciation to Ms. Yolanda Sandoval for her extensive effort in typing and correcting manuscripts, and to Mr. Daniel Doody of Year Book Medical Publishers for guidance in organizing and editing this project.

MICHAEL H. GRIECO, M.D.
DAVID K. MERINEY, M.D.

PART I

Concepts and Methods
in Immunology

1

Fundamentals of Immunology

David K. Meriney, M.D.

Michael H. Grieco, M.D.

IMMUNE RESPONSES

The Humoral Immune Response

THREE CELL types are involved in the humoral immune response. Two of these, T and B cells, are varieties of lymphocytes. The third type is the monocyte-derived macrophage.

The lymphocytes involved develop from bone marrow lymphocyte precursors along two pathways.[1] Precursors that develop via a pathway known as the "bursal equivalent" are known as B cells. (The term "bursal" derives from the bursa of Fabricius in birds, an organ known to be involved in B cell development. The identity of an analogous organ in mammals is uncertain, and the pathway is therefore referred to as the bursal equivalent.) B cells are the precursors of plasma cells, which in turn are the producers of immunoglobulins (humoral antibody). Precursor lymphocytes that differentiate in the thymus are called T cells. T cells mediate cellular immunity and are also important in regulating the humoral immune response. After differentiation, T and B cells localize in the spleen and lymph nodes, the major sites of humoral antibody production.

Monocyte-derived macrophages also participate in the regulation of the immune response.[2, 3] They are necessary for the response of T cells to antigen. Monocytes and macrophages are phagocytic cells, and both derive from bone marrow stem cells. Monocytes circulate in the blood, whereas macrophages are more mature cells that have settled in tissues.

The initial step in the immune response is the uptake and processing of antigen by the macrophage. The macrophage metabolizes antigen and presents antigenic determinants to the T lymphocyte. The cell presenting the antigen to the T lymphocyte must be syngeneic for T cell–dependent antigenic responses, because initial cellular interaction depends on recognition by the T lymphocyte of both antigen and a gene product on the surface of the antigen-presenting cell. Antigen presentation by the macrophage may also involve processing of antigen to make it immunogenic. The macrophage produces a soluble factor, interleukin-1, which promotes the development of helper T cells (see below), as well as a factor that augments the B cell response (Fig 1–1).

Following the interaction of macrophages and T cells, there arises a subset of cells called helper T cells that aid the B cell in producing antibody-secreting plasma cells. The growth of the helper T cell population is promoted by secretion of a soluble factor from the T cells that is initially stimulated by macrophages. The mechanism by which helper T cells aid the response of B lymphocytes to various antigens is unclear but may involve factors secreted by the helper T cell (helper factors) that are related to immune response gene products.[4]

The B lymphocyte has surface receptors that bind antigen as a first step in the process of development into an antibody-producing cell. This process is aided by the helper T cell. A few structurally simple antigens can elicit an antibody response without helper T cells; they are known as T cell–independent antigens. The majority of antigens are T cell–dependent. Following activation, B lymphocytes are transformed into lymphoblasts and

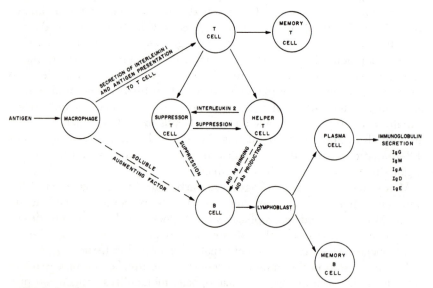

Fig 1–1.—Humoral immune response. The interrelationships of macrophages, B cells, and T cells are shown. *Ag,* antigen; *Ab,* antibody.

plasma cells, go through several divisions, and subsequently secrete immunoglobulins. Many immunoglobulin-producing cells appear morphologically as plasma cells, although others appear as medium to large lymphocytes or lymphoblasts. All the immunoglobulins produced by a given cell are of the same antigenic specificity. Usually antibody of a single class is produced, although in some instances more than one type may be produced (e.g., IgM and IgG).

Another regulatory subset of T cells, suppressor T cells, proliferate along with B cells at the onset of the immune response but probably in a second phase. The activation of T suppressor cells is facilitated by interleukin-2. Suppressor T cells suppress the immune response largely via soluble factors. Suppressor factors, like helper factors, have antigenic determinants encoded by the immune response gene. Suppressor factors probably act largely on helper T cells, although evidence suggests direct action on B cells in some cases (see Fig 1–1).

It is likely that there are additional subsets of both helper and suppressor T cells that would make the details of the immune response more complex than described above. In any case, such details are subject to revision pending ongoing research.

The initial exposure of an organism to an antigen results in what is termed the "primary response." Following an induction period of 3–14 days, during which the antigen is processed and cellular proliferation and differentiation occur, circulating antibodies can be detected.[5] Peak antibody levels are reached a few days to 3 months after initiation of the primary response, depending on the type of antigen. Antibodies formed early in the primary response are predominantly of the IgM class and of low affinity for the antigen. Antibodies formed later in the primary response are usually of the IgG class and of much higher affinity.

A second exposure to the same antigen evokes a much more rapid appearance of circulating antibody. This is termed the "secondary response" or "anemnestic response." Peak antibody levels are higher and persist longer; the antibodies formed are usually of the IgG class and are of high affinity. Differences between the primary and secondary response can be largely attributed to the formation of B and T memory cells at the time of the primary response. At the time of secondary antigenic stimulation, the antigen-sensitive memory cells present result in a greater pool of antibody-forming cells, and therefore a greater amount of antibody is produced. The amount of antigen required to initiate a secondary response is much less than that needed for a primary response.

The cellular events involved in humoral immune responses are shown in Figure 1–1.

Cell-Mediated Immune Response

Another function of the T lymphocyte is the expression of the cell-mediated immune response. This process does not involve B cells or the production of circulating immunoglobulin. Introduction of antigen is followed by its recognition by a T lymphocyte precommitted to such recognition. Antigen may be bound directly by the T lymphocyte or presented by macrophages. A proliferative phase follows, resulting in cells that morphologically resemble lymphoblasts. The macrophage may be required for this proliferative phase.

Activated T cells are generated as a result of the proliferative phase. Activated T cells can elaborate effector molecules, called lymphokines, which mediate a number of responses leading to the recruitment and activation of cells participating in cellular immunity. Another subpopulation of activated lymphocytes is directly cytotoxic. Most cells participating in the cell-mediated immune response are not specifically committed lymphocytes but rather non-antigen-specific cells recruited by lymphokines. Memory T cells are produced as well as suppressor T cells that may have a modulating effect on effector cell activity. Other than direct cytotoxicity, the host defense responses of cell-mediated immunity are effected by phagocytosis and lysosomal enzyme release of macrophages activated by lymphokines. The cell-mediated immune response is summarized in Figure 1–2.

GENETIC REGULATION OF IMMUNE RESPONSE

In addition to regulation of the immune response by the interactions of T cells, B cells, and macrophages, as described above, further regulation at another level is provided by the gene products of a set of genes that determines the structure of the major transplantation antigens.[6] The designation of these gene products as transplantation antigens refers to their initial identification as major antigenic barriers to transplantation between members of the same species. The corresponding closely linked group of genes that produces these products has been designated the major histocompatibility complex (MHC). MHC antigens in humans were first identified on lymphocytes and are therefore called human leukocyte antigens (HLA); the system is called the HLA system. The genes of the HLA system are closely linked on human chromosome 6. They are designated A, B, C, and D (Fig 1–3). The HLA antigens are glycopeptides. Antigens A, B, and C are found on all nucleated cells and platelets. Lymphocyte-determined HLA-D antigens and serologically determined HLA-DR antigens are found on the surface of B lymphocytes, some T lymphocytes, antigen-presenting macrophages, and some other macrophages (see Chap. 3).

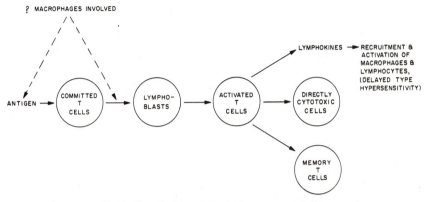

Fig 1–2.—Cell-mediated immune response.

In the mouse, genes affecting the immune response to a number of antigens are found in a region analogous to the HLA-D region in humans. These genes in the mouse have been designated immune response genes. Gene products in humans have subsequently been designated immune response–associated antigens and are identified with an area of the HLA-D region. Near the HLA-B area are genes for the second and fourth components of complement and properdin factors of the alternative complement pathway.

Information on the regulatory functions of HLA antigens has been obtained in studies on humans and by extrapolating from studies on MHC in other species. Antigens A, B, and C determine the number and specificity of cytotoxic killer T cells produced in response to immunization with a given antigen.[6] HLA-D antigens regulate the efficiency of interaction between T cells and macrophages, between T cells and B cells, and possibly between B cells and macrophages.[6] They also play an important role in delayed-type hypersensitivity.

STRUCTURE AND FUNCTION OF IMMUNOGLOBULINS

There are five classes of immunoglobulins secreted by plasma cells: IgG (four subclasses), IgM, IgA (two subclasses), IgD, and IgE. The overall molecular structure of a prototype IgG molecule is illustrated in Figure 1–4. Each immunoglobulin class possesses two basic areas of structure and function. The Fab region contains the antigen-binding sites represented by the six to eight linear amino acid sequences in the hypervariable regions in the V_H and V_L domains.[7] Binding of antigen by noncovalent linkages to the Fab region of an antibody permits expression of biologic function by the Fc region. A partial listing of such functions includes complement fixation,

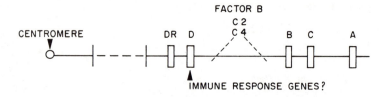

CHROMOSOME 6

Fig 1–3.—Genes of the HLA system.

fixation to Fc receptors for IgG on cells such as polymorphonuclear leukocytes, monocytes, lymphocytes, and platelets, fixation to skin, placental transfer, and interaction with staphylococcal protein A. The C_H2 region of IgG appears to contain the site for classic complement activation via C1q binding, while the site for binding to Fc IgG receptors on monocyte is present in the C_H3 region. Thus, IgG molecules may attach to opsonizing cells via either generated C3b or directly by attachment of the Fc region to cell membrane receptors.

Pentameric 19S IgM also activates the classic complement pathway, while IgA appears to be able to initiate alternative complement activity (at least in vitro) so that both may initiate phagocytosis via heat-labile C3b opsonins. Neither functions as a heat-stable opsonin, but IgM is capable of direct complement-induced cytotoxicity, as reflected in bactericidal activity. Both 19S IgM and dimeric IgA, when found in external secretions,

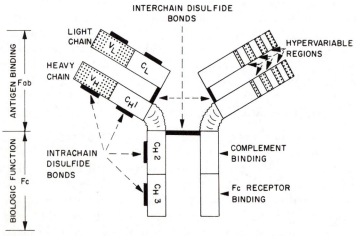

Fig 1–4.—Overall molecular structure of prototype IgG molecule composed of two light chains and two heavy chains.

have a J chain polypeptide incorporated into the structure prior to secretion by plasma cells.

IgD exists exclusively as a monomer unit with no polymerizing capabilities; it may play a critical role in B cell differentiation but does not appear to have significant effector functions. Human serum contains IgE in extremely small amounts. The IgE molecule has a strong affinity for mast cells and basophils of the species in which it is produced and is therefore termed the homocytotropic antibody. It is this property of IgE that leads to its role in type I (immediate) hypersensitivity.

CLASSIFICATION OF HYPERSENSITIVITY REACTIONS

It is apparent that some reactions of the immune system may be damaging to the host rather than protective; it is also apparent that immune tissue damage can be mediated in a number of ways. In an attempt to clarify the relations between immune system activities and host, two British immunologists, Gell and Coombs, more than a decade ago devised a classification of hypersensitivity reactions, graded as types I through IV. This classification system will be used as the basis for the following discussion. It should be noted, however, that some immune reactions do not fit well into the Gell-Coombs classification; they will be mentioned separately. It should also be kept in mind that a given disease entity with immunologic features may involve more than one type of reaction.

Type I Reaction

Type I reactions are related to the so-called reaginic or homocytotropic antibody. This antibody is usually of the IgE class, although occasionally a subtype of IgG, IgG4, is involved. Reaginic antibody has an affinity for Fc receptors on mast cells and basophils. Accordingly, large numbers of IgE molecules may be found on such cells that have been passively sensitized with antiserum (about 30,000–100,000 IgE molecules per cell). To initiate a type I reaction, antigens against which these antibodies are directed cross link with several IgE molecules (a process called bridging), which results in the activation of enzymes in the cell membrane. Bridging results in the release of preformed chemical mediators stored in intracellular granules, as well as in the formation and release of mediators that are not preformed (Fig 1–5). The released mediators affect smooth muscle and blood vessels to produce the manifestations of the reaction. The type I reaction is potentially reversible and does not result in permanent tissue damage unless combined with another of the reaction types.

The release of mediators from the mast cell or basophil is modulated by the intracellular cyclic nucleotides: cyclic adenosine monophosphate

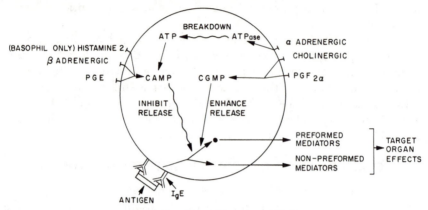

Fig 1–5.—Type I hypersensitivity.

(cAMP) and cyclic guanosine monophosphate (cGMP). These nucleotides in turn are affected by a number of cell surface receptors which, when activated, promote or inhibit their formation (see Fig 1–5). Increasing intracellular levels of cAMP are associated with inhibition of mediator release, and increasing levels of cGMP are associated with stimulation of mediator release. The rise and fall of intracellular levels of these nucleotides is usually reciprocal.

The preformed mediators are histamine, eosinophil chemotactic factors of anaphylaxis (ECF-A), and neutrophil chemotactic factor of anaphylaxis. They are listed in Table 1–1, along with their characteristics and modes of action. The nonpreformed mediators are slow-reactive substance of anaphylaxis (SRS-A; leukotrienes), prostaglandins (PG), platelet-activating factor (PAF), and basophil kallikrein (see Table 1–1). Among the nonpreformed mediators, the relationships of products of the arachadonic acid pathway (SRS-A, PG, and related compounds) have recently been clarified (Fig 1–6).[8, 9]

Clinical entities that may be considered as type I reactions include acute anaphylaxis, allergic rhinitis, and some cases of urticaria and bronchial asthma. The type I reaction is summarized in Figure 1–5.

Type II Reaction

Type II reactions involve the binding of antibody via the antigen-specific Fab portion of immunoglobulin with antigen that is part of or intimately attached to a cell surface. The immunoglobulins involved are of the IgG or IgM class. Cell destruction may occur subsequently by one of two mechanisms: phagocytosis after coating of the cell surface by antibody, or via complement-mediated cell damage. The complement-mediated pathoge-

TABLE 1-1.—MEDIATORS OF TYPE I SENSITIVITY

MEDIATOR	CHARACTERISTICS	MODE OF ACTION
	Preformed	
Histamine	Low molecular weight amine	Smooth muscle contraction, increased vascular permeability, increased goblet mucus, etc.
Eosinophil chemotactic factor of anaphylaxis (ECF-A)	At least two acidic tetrapeptides	Eosinophil chemotaxis; prevents egress of eosinophils from site of inflammation
Neutrophil chemotactic factor	Not well characterized	Neutrophil chemotaxis
Serotonin	5-hydroxytryptamine	Increased vascular permeability (not clearly implicated in human type I reactions)
	Not Preformed	
Slow-reacting substance of anaphylaxis (SRS-A, leukotrienes)	Arachadonic acid metabolites— lipoxygenase pathway	Smooth muscle contraction; increased vascular permeability
HETE (hydroxy-eicosatetraenoic acid)		Regulation of eosinophil and neutrophil function
Prostaglandins (D, F, I_2)	Arachadonic acid metabolites— cyclo-oxygenase pathway	Smooth muscle contraction; vasodilation
HHT (hydroxy-heptadecatrienoic acid)		Chemotaxis
Thromboxanes		Smooth muscle contraction
Platelet-activating factor (PAF)	Not well characterized	Aggregates platelets; releases vasoactive ammines, including histamine, from platelets
Basophil kallikrein	Not well characterized	Kinin-generating enzyme (not clearly implicated in human type I reactions)

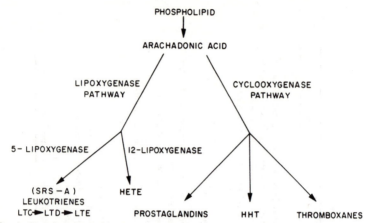

Fig 1–6.—Arachadonic acid metabolites. *LT,* leukotriene; *HETE,* hydroxy-eicosatetraenoic acids; *HHT,* hydroxy-heptadecatrienoic acid; (see also Table 1–1).

netic sequence is similar to that occurring in type III reactions (see below). Clinical examples of type II reactions include autoimmune hemolytic anemia, transfusion reaction and Goodpasture's syndrome. In Goodpasture's syndrome, cross-reactive antigens of pulmonary and glomerular basement membranes react with anti-basement membrane antibodies to activate complement. Complement-mediated tissue damage ensues. The type II reaction is summarized in Figure 1–7.

Type III Reaction

In type III reactions, soluble antigen-antibody complexes (also called toxic complexes or immune complexes) are formed in moderate antigen excess. The immunoglobulin class involved is usually IgG. Soluble immune complexes are formed in the circulation or locally, and subsequently are deposited in vessel walls, tissue spaces, or on cell surfaces. Complement is

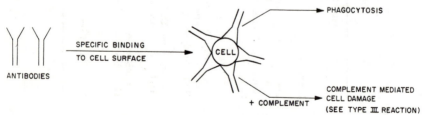

Fig 1–7.—Type II hypersensitivity.

then bound by the immune complex, which causes activation of the classic complement pathway. Three chemotactic factors, C3a, C5a, and C567, are formed in this process. C5a is by far the most important of the chemotactic factors. It causes the attraction of polymorphonuclear leukocytes and monocytes, which in turn initiate an inflammatory response. C3a, C4a, and C5a also function as anaphylatoxins, causing release of mediators from mast cells (see discussion of type I reactions). The resultant increase in vascular permeability permits further trapping of immune complexes along vascular membranes as well as an additional influx of cells involved in the inflammatory response. Polymorphonuclear leukocytes and monocytes, which have receptors for C3 and the Fc area of IgG, adhere to immune complexes deposited in tissue. The ensuing phagocytic or nonphagocytic release of lysosomal enzymes from these cells results in tissue damage.

Clinical examples of type III reactions include serum sickness, the renal disease of systemic lupus erythematosus, and some other types of glomerulonephritis. The type III reaction is summarized in Figure 1–8.

Type IV Reaction

Type IV reactions are the result of specifically sensitized T lymphocytes reacting with antigens deposited locally in tissues. This reaction leads to lymphocyte transformation and the release of biologically active mediators known as lymphokines. Subsequently, additional lymphocytes as well as macrophages are recruited to the tissue site and an inflammatory response ensues. Lymphokines have many actions, including the attraction of macrophages to the inflammatory site, the modification of behavior of lymphocytes and macrophages, and a direct cytotoxic effect on cells (Table 1–2). Cell damage in the type IV reaction can be due to (1) direct cytotoxicity of activated T cells, (2) release of lymphokines injurious to cells, or (3) release of lymphokines, leading to recruitment and activation of macrophages.

Basophil infiltration is a prominent feature of some varieties of type IV

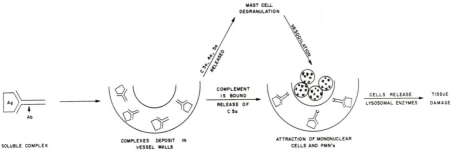

Fig 1–8.—Type III hypersensitivity. *C*, component of complement.

TABLE 1–2.—LYMPHOKINES

LYMPHOKINE	ACTION*	COMMENT
Mitogenic factor	Promotes cell division in lymphocytes; may affect helper T cell function	Modification of lymphocyte behavior
Lymphocyte inhibitory factor (LIF)	May affect suppressor T cell function	
Migration inhibition factor (MIF)	Inhibits migration of normal macrophages, allowing accumulation at site of inflammation	
Macrophage activating factor (MAF)	Increases ability to kill intracellular organisms	Modification of macrophage behavior
Chemotactic factor (CF)	Attracts macrophages toward chemotactic stimulus	
Lymphotoxin (LT)	Destroys target cells	Kills cells
Interferon	Inhibits viral replication	May be secondarily released from macrophages

*Some of the biologic effects may represent different activities of the same molecule. For a detailed discussion of lymphokine activity, see Parker.[4]

reactions such as contact skin sensitivities. This type of reaction is known as cutaneous basophil hypersensitivity.

Clinical examples of type IV reactions include aspects of tissue graft rejection and contact dermatitis. The type IV reaction is summarized in Figure 1–9.

Other Types of Immune Response

Two types of immune tissue damage have been recently described that do not fit easily into the Gell-Coombs classification and they are therefore described separately. These are (1) antibody-dependent cell-mediated cytotoxicity (ADCC), and (2) antireceptor-antibody reactions.

ADCC

A subpopulation of lymphocytes has been described in which the lymphocytes do not carry markers for T lymphocytes, are not B cells, but do have surface receptors for the Fc portion of the IgG molecule. These lymphocytes have been variously termed third population cells, killer (K) cells, or null cells. They represent about 10% of peripheral circulating lymphocytes. It has been found that target cells coated with specific IgG antibody are subject to lysis by K cells. It is not necessary for K cells to be specifically sensitized to antigens on the target cell for this reaction to take place. The effector cells in ADCC are therefore "nonimmune," as opposed to cytotoxic effector T lymphocytes in type IV reactions or the cells involved in specific interactions of the type II response. Polymorphonuclear leukocytes and macrophages have also been described as effector cells in some ADCC reactions.

Clinical examples of ADCC are less well delineated than other types of hypersensitivity reactions. There is fairly good evidence that lymphocyte-mediated ADCC is significantly involved in the pathogenesis of disorders such as Hashimoto's thyroiditis.

Antireceptor Antibodies

Antireceptor antibodies have been identified in Graves' disease, some cases of insulin-resistant diabetes, and myasthenia gravis.[10] Such antibodies interfere with normal physiologic organ function. An IgG antibody to a thyroid follicular cell receptor (thyroid-stimulating immunoglobulin) is found in Graves' disease. This antibody performs the same function as thyroid-stimulating hormone, thereby increasing thyroid activity. On the other hand, antireceptor antibodies in insulin-resistant diabetes and myasthenia gravis interfere with the activities of insulin and acetylcholine, re-

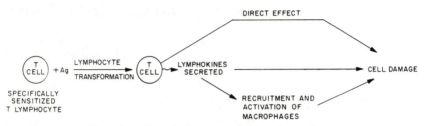

Fig 1–9.—Type IV hypersensitivity. *Ag,* antigen.

spectively, and so are probably involved with the pathogenesis of these diseases. Antireceptor antibody reactions have been designated type V, stimulatory hypersensitivity, by Roitt.[11]

HOST DEFENSE MECHANISMS

Effector immunologic mechanisms that in some instances subserve the pathogenesis of clinical diseases are also involved in host defense against microbes. These defenses include protective mechanisms operating at epithelial and mucosal surfaces, antibodies, serum proteins (complement, kinins, clotting factors, and fibrinolysin), and cellular responses.

Protective Mechanisms at Epithelial Surfaces

The principal mechanisms operative in the skin are desquamation, dehydration, maintenance of an acid pH, and production of bacteriostatic lactic and fatty acids from sebum. On the mucosal surfaces, microorganisms unable to adhere to host epithelial receptors are swept away by fluid flow, propulsive organ motility, or cell shedding. The mucociliary clearance apparatus in the lower respiratory tract is an important example of a mechanical defense mechanism. Additional protective elements include lysozyme, α_1-antitrypsin, lactoferrin, secretory IgA, and interferon.

Microbe-Specific Antibodies

Acute and chronic infectious disorders are often reflected in plasma protein changes involving many of the more than 100 individual proteins in the circulation. The most specific of these changes is the production of antibodies specific for antigenic components of invading microbes. Following the binding of multivalent antigenic determinants (epitopes) to the Fab combining sites of immunoglobulins, structural changes occur in the Fc regions to facilitate cytophilia and complement activation. Some of these activities are summarized in Table 1–3.

TABLE 1–3.—ANTIBODY FUNCTIONS ASSOCIATED WITH
HOST RESISTANCE

FUNCTION	IMMUNOGLOBULIN CLASS*
Interference with adherence	SIgA
Neutralizing activity	SIgA, IgG, IgM
Bactericidal and virocidal activity	IgG, IgM
Immune adherence and phagocytosis	IgG, IgM
Antibody-dependent cellular cytotoxicity	IgG

*S, secretory.

Cellular Responses

Neutrophils and monocytes are effector cells involved in both antibody and cell-mediated immunologic responses. In addition, T cells are effector cells in delayed-type protective immune responses and cell-mediated direct cytotoxicity.

Lymphokines released from T cells and, to some extent, from B cells include various mediators that influence antibody synthesis, are cytotoxic and cytostatic, and attract macrophages, neutrophils, eosinophils, basophils, and other lymphocytes. Delayed-type hypersensitivity reactions are characterized by recruitment of various nonspecific cells by factors elaborated when T lymphocytes are specifically triggered by antigen. The recruited cells constitute 95% of the infiltrate and comprise principally monocytes and, in smaller numbers, neutrophils and basophils. Macrophage inhibitory, activating, chemotactic, aggregating, fusing, and growth factors are presumed to be responsible for the recruitment and stimulation of activated macrophages. Released interferon inhibits viral multiplication in host cells while lymphotoxin inhibits cell growth. HLA-H2 restriction to delayed-type hypersensitivity appears to be located within the D region of the HLA complex.

T cell–mediated cytotoxicity is probably restricted by the A and B loci. Presumably the membrane virus-related and modified A and B antigens allow recognition of both nonphagocytically and phagocytically modified self cells by cytotoxic T cells. This type of HLA restriction has been detected in murine infections with lymphocytic choriomeningitis virus, vaccinia virus, and influenza.

REFERENCES

1. Broder S., Waldmann T.A.: The suppressor cell network in cancer.: Part I. *N. Engl. J. Med.* 299:1281, 1978.
2. Rosenthal A.S.: Regulation of the immune response: Role of the macrophage. *N. Engl. J. Med.* 303:1153, 1980.

3. Unanue E.R.: Cooperation between mononuclear phagocytes and lymphocytes in immunity. *N. Engl. J. Med.* 303:977, 1980.
4. Paul W.E.: Lymphocyte Biology, in Parker C.W. (ed.): *Clinical Immunology.* Philadelphia, W.B. Saunders Co., 1980, p. 1438.
5. Herscowitz H.B.: Immunophysiology: Cell Function and cellular interactions, in Bellanti J. (ed.): *Immunology,* ed. 2. Philadelphia, W.B. Saunders Co., 1978, pp. 151–202.
6. McDevitt H.O.: Regulation of the immune response by the major histocompatibility system. *N. Engl. J. Med.* 303:1514, 1980.
7. Capra J.D., Kehoe J.M.: Hypervariable regions, idiotypy and antibody-combining sites. *Adv. Immunol.* 20:1, 1974.
8. Goetzl E.J.: Mediators of immediate hypersensitivity derived from arachadonic acid. *N. Engl. J. Med.* 303:822, 1980.
9. Ramwell P.W.: Biologic importance of arachadonic acid. *Arch. Intern. Med.* 141:275, 1981.
10. Stobo J.D.: Autoimmune antireceptor diseases. *Hosp. Pract.* March, 1981, 16:49.
11. Roitt I.M.: *Essential Immunology.* Boston, Blackwell Scientific Publications, 1980, p. 358.

2

Methodology of Immunologic Assays Relating to Humoral Components

David K. Meriney, M.D.

THIS CHAPTER discusses the methods used to measure humoral elements in clinical immunoassays. Most of this methodology focuses on the measurement of antigen-antibody interaction or the measurement of one of the potential components of this interaction. These observations usually depend on phenomena occurring as a result of the formation of antigen-antibody complexes rather than on the direct observation of primary antigen-antibody interaction. Such phenomena are termed secondary reactions.

Secondary reactions include precipitation, agglutination, lysis, and complement fixation (CF). These secondary effects are named by the antiserum involved, e.g., precipitin, agglutinin. This does not imply exclusive functional properties of the antibody but rather is a convenience in describing the conditions of the reaction. For example, a precipitating antibody might also be an agglutinating antibody or might participate in complement fixation under suitable conditions.

Agglutination, turbidimetric, nephelometric, and neutralization assays will be discussed initially, followed by an explanation of precipitation and electrophoretic techniques as well as methods that combine these two principles. Finally, radioimmunoassays, enzyme immunoassays, immunofluorescence, and assays relating to serum complement will be described.

AGGLUTINATION ASSAYS

Agglutination reactions consist of clumping of particulate matter, such as cells, by antibodies. The reaction takes place on the surface of particles such as erythrocytes, bacteria, or latex, with antigen located in such a manner as to be available to specific binding sites on antibodies. Eight kinds of agglutination assays are described below.

Direct agglutination involves the clumping of cells or particulate antigen by specific antibody molecules that link the particles in suspension (Fig 2–1, A). Methods designed to decrease ionic strength or to increase fluid viscosity can aid in demonstrating agglutination. Cells and bacteria can be rendered more agglutinable by enzyme treatment.

Indirect (passive) agglutination consists of agglutination by antibodies of cells or particles coated with soluble antigen. Conversely, antibody may be bound to the particles. The particles act as passive carriers of antigen or antibody and serve as vehicles to demonstrate the reaction (Fig 2–1, B). Indirect agglutination systems have been developed using various inert particles as carriers. Two frequently used carriers are bentonite (potters clay) and latex (a polystyrene polymer). Bentonite clay, a kind of aluminum silicate, and latex particles are used for adsorption of several types of proteins and thereby serve as a source of particulate antigen.

Indirect hemagglutination (IHA) is a type of indirect agglutination in which human or animal erythrocytes are used (passive hemagglutination). Adsorption of some protein antigens occurs spontaneously on the surface of erythrocytes; adsorption of others occurs only after the erythrocytes have been exposed to tannic acid or other reagent. Alternatively, antigens may be covalently linked to the red blood cell (RBC) surface, e.g., with *bis*-diazobenzidine.

Agglutination inhibition (HI) reactions are used to assess specificity and titer of antibody based on competition of particulate and soluble antigen for combining sites. Antibody and soluble antigen are first allowed to react together. Antibodies in the medium (e.g., serum) that react with soluble antigen form soluble antigen-antibody complexes and will not react with antigen-coated particles subsequently added. Agglutination will therefore be inhibited (Fig 2–1, C). Inhibition methods can be applied to a wide variety of agglutination techniques, including hemagglutination and direct agglutination of viruses to erythrocyte membranes (virus hemagglutination inhibition).

Immuno-electron microscopy is a specialized method of observing the effects of antigen-antibody aggregation. Serum to be tested for antibody is mixed with antigen, e.g., a viral suspension. After incubation and centrifugation, the sediment is examined by electron microscopy. The amount of antibody-coated aggregate or single particles is determined. This technique is useful for detection of certain viral antibodies (Fig 2–1, D).

Immune adherence hemagglutination (IAHA) is used to detect antibody that has reacted with test antigen and complement to form immune complexes. IAHA detects immune complexes by hemagglutination resulting from immune complexes binding C3b receptors on erythrocytes. Serum to be tested is first inactivated by heating. Antigen and complement are added, with appropriate incubation. An erythrocyte suspension is added

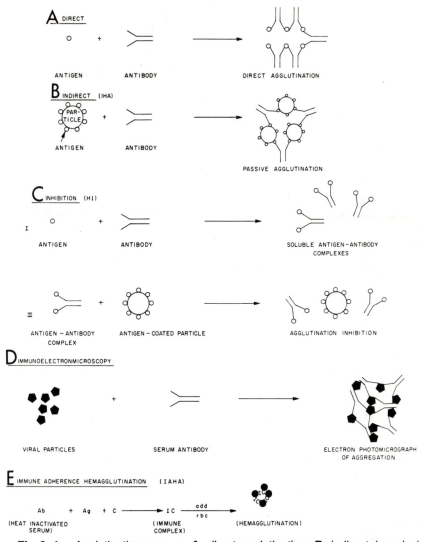

Fig 2–1.—Agglutination assays. **A,** direct agglutination. **B,** indirect (passive) agglutination. **C,** agglutination inhibition. **D,** immuno-electron microscopy. **E,** immune adherence agglutination.

and subsequent hemagglutination patterns are interpreted. The IAHA test is considered to be more sensitive than the CF test (Fig 2–1, E).

Coagglutination (COAG) is a method that has been used for the detection of some microbial antigens. COAG takes advantage of the fact that some strains of staphylococci will bind IgG class antibody via the Fc area, leaving the antibody combining site free. Suspensions of appropriate *Staphylococcus* strains are mixed with antibody directed against the organism to be detected (e.g., *Pneumococcus*). When the appropriate organism is added, coagglutination occurs with the antibody-coated staphylococci.

The antiglobulin test, or *Coombs test* (AGT), is an agglutination method used to detect RBC-associated (direct AGT) or serum (indirect AGT) antibodies in patients with autoimmune hemolytic anemia and other disorders (see Chap. 7). In the direct AGT, erythrocytes, presumably with antibody attached, are incubated with antiserum to IgG and C3d. The resulting agglutination is determined. In the indirect AGT, the patient's serum is mixed with donor erythrocytes. Antibody present in the patient's serum will coat the erythrocytes. Antiglobulin serum is then added, as in the direct AGT, and agglutination is assayed.

Agglutination reactions have several disadvantages.[1] The method is only semiquantitative. Results of antibody titers from run to run with the same sample can vary fourfold. If a specimen contains only IgG antibodies, the agglutination reaction may not be completed. IgM antibodies are much more efficient in agglutination reactions.

If antigen or antibody is present in excess, the agglutination reaction may not occur because of improper equilibrium conditions. This is known as the *prozone phenomenon*. The prozone phenomenon can also occur in the presence of excessive extraneous colloid material and can be induced by the heating of protein antigens. Despite their disadvantages, agglutination assays are widely used because of their broad applicability, simplicity, and high sensitivity.

TURBIDIMETRIC AND NEPHELOMETRIC ASSAYS

Turbidimetry is a measure of the reduction in the transmittance of light (that is, absorbence) through a solution due to light scattering. Such observations are made with a spectrophotometer. Nephelometry is a measure of the light scattered from a solution at a specific angle. This procedure requires the use of an instrument called a nephelometer, which can determine concentration or particle size of suspensions by means of transmitted or reflected light. Turbidimetry and nephelometry can be used to measure protein antigens quantitatively because a relationship can be established between the concentration of a protein antigen and absorbance or light scattering during antigen-antibody interaction.[1] Turbidimetric and nephelometric methods have been developed for measuring antibodies such as IgG and IgM and antigens such as haptoglobin, and for determining antiserum titers.

Nephelometric and turbidimetric determinations can be either "quasi-equilibrium" or kinetic in type. Quasi-equilibrium methods use a single measurement of light scattering at a time when the rate of change in scattering due to antigen-antibody interaction is very small. In determining serum immunoglobulin levels by these techniques, unknown sera are mixed with specific antiserum of the immunoglobulin to be tested. Antigen-antibody interaction proceeds during subsequent incubation (Fig 2–2). Light scattering or absorbance is then measured at an appropriate time. A reference curve is used to determine the concentration of the protein in question.

Kinetic methods of nephelometry and turbidimetry monitor the rate of formation of antigen-antibody complexes. After antigen and antibody are mixed, the reaction is followed over time, and the results are related to a known reference sample. Kinetic assays can be performed more quickly and also eliminate variations in measurements found between cuvettes in the quasi-equilibrium techniques.

NEUTRALIZATION ASSAYS

Neutralization refers to the loss in infectivity of a microorganism (virus) or loss of toxicity of a product of a microorganism (a toxin) after interaction with a specific antibody. One can therefore speak of viral neutralization or toxin neutralization. Viral neutralization assays can be used to determine levels of antibody production after infection or immunization. Serum is mixed with virus and incubated in a susceptible host system in which the presence of unneutralized virus may be detected (e.g., inoculated cell cultures) (Fig 2–3). The level of serum-neutralizing antibody to a given viral agent can be determined by using a constant amount of virus and varying the concentrations of serum. Viral neutralization tests are expensive and time-consuming and may be difficult to interpret because of variability in end-point titration and possible nonspecificity of neutralization.

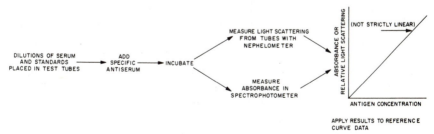

Fig 2–2.—Quasi-equilibrium nephelometry or turbidimetry.

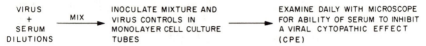

Fig 2–3.—Viral neutralization.

PRECIPITATION ASSAYS

Because of the physical properties of many antibodies and antigens that relate to numbers of binding sites, it is possible, using proper proportions of each, to cause linkage of antigen and antibody in a lattice formation. Under these circumstances, large conglomerates can form which become insoluble. Visible precipitates will therefore form when appropriate amounts of antigen and antibody are mixed.[2] This phenomenon is the basis for several immunologic assays. Currently the most useful methods for demonstrating antigen-antibody precipitation involve the use of an agar gel.

The *capillary precipitation test,* or *interfacial ring test,* is a rapid means of detecting soluble antigen or antibody. A solution containing antigen is layered over a solution containing antibody. This can be done in a test tube or a capillary tube. As the antigen diffuses into the solution containing antibody, a precipitin band will form when it reaches the area of optimum antigen-antibody ratio. Alternatively, the antigen and antibody solutions can be mixed, in which case the precipitate will settle to the bottom of the tube. The size of the precipitin band or the amount of precipitate may be graded semiquantitatively.

Double Diffusion (Ouchterlony Technique)

Molten agar is poured onto glass slides or into Petri dishes and allowed to harden. Small wells are then punched out of the agar a few millimeters apart. Samples of antigen and antibody are placed in opposing wells and allowed to diffuse toward one another for 24 hours. The resultant precipitin lines, representing antigen-antibody complexes, are analyzed visually in indirect light with the aid of a magnifying lens. Double diffusion is commonly performed by placing the antigen and antibody wells at various angles for comparative purposes. The number of precipitin bands observed when an antigen mixture reacts with an antiserum directed against all of the mixture's components is an approximate indication of the number of antigenic constituents in the mixture. If two antigen mixtures in different wells diffuse simultaneously against the same antiserum, similarities and differences between the antigens can be analyzed. Three common patterns are shown in Figure 2–4.

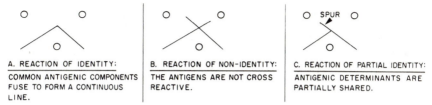

A. REACTION OF IDENTITY: COMMON ANTIGENIC COMPONENTS FUSE TO FORM A CONTINUOUS LINE.

B. REACTION OF NON-IDENTITY: THE ANTIGENS ARE NOT CROSS REACTIVE.

C. REACTION OF PARTIAL IDENTITY: ANTIGENIC DETERMINANTS ARE PARTIALLY SHARED.

Fig 2–4.—Double diffusion assay.

Rheophoresis is a double diffusion technique that provides increased sensitivity roughly equivalent to counterimmunoelectrophoresis (CIE). An agar gel diffusion dish with a surrounding moat and a cover containing a central hole is used. The moat is fulled with trisaminomethane buffer. Antibody is placed in a center well and antigens are placed in surrounding peripheral wells. Under proper test conditions, the antigens migrate rapidly toward the center well as the buffer evaporates through the central hole in the dish cover. This test has been used to detect hepatitis B virus markers.

Radial Immunodiffusion (RID)

RID was introduced in 1965 by Mancini. One of two reactants, usually antibody, is uniformly distributed in a layer of agar or agarose gel. The other reactant (usually antigen) is placed in circular holes punched in the gel. The antigen diffuses radially into the gel-antibody mixture, forming a visible ring of precipitate (Fig 2–5). A quantitative relationship exists between the diameter of the precipitin ring and the concentration of antigen such that the logarithm of the antigen concentration is proportional to the diameter of the ring. A standard curve is experimentally determined with known antigen standards. This curve can be used for determination of antigen concentrations corresponding to any diameter size.

ELECTROPHORESIS

Electrophoresis is a method for separation of proteins in an electric field. Originally the technique was developed for use in a liquid-phase medium. The development of a stabilizing porous support (zone electrophoresis) allowed the technique to be used in clinical medicine. The most widely used support matrixes today are cellulose acetate, starch, acrylamide, agar, and agarose. The support matrix usually used in the clinical laboratory is cellulose acetate. Its advantages over paper and other support media include minimal absorption of proteins, uniform pore size, short time of separation (60–90 minutes), and the requirement of very small quantities of sample.

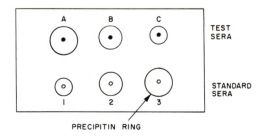

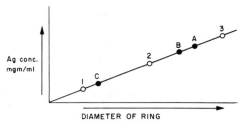

Fig 2–5.—Radial immunodiffusion assay. *Ag,* antigen.

The major clinical application of electrophoresis is to separate constituents of serum and other body fluids.

In zone electrophoresis (see Fig 4–1), proteins are separated on the basis of surface charge. Proteins to be separated move in a buffer of fixed pH. The main role of the buffer is to maintain pH and conduct electricity. At a given pH the net charge of the protein molecule depends on the content of amino acids with ionizable side chains. At its isoelectric point, a molecule has no electrophoretic mobility and will remain at its point of origin. Electrophoretic mobility therefore depends on how different the pH of the buffer is from the pH of the protein's isoelectric point. The greater the difference, the farther and faster a molecule will move in a constant electric field. Proteins usually have minimal solubility at their isoelectric point and may precipitate out of solution. Also, at neutrality, a mixture of proteins may move partly to the negative pole, partly to the positive pole, or remain stationary. Therefore, in routine serum electrophoresis an alkaline buffer is used so that all molecules will be negatively charged and move to the positive pole. Under these conditions, the highest mobility will be of prealbumin and albumin and the lowest will be of γ-globulin (see Fig 4–1).

After electrophoresis, the matrix is stained with a fixative dye solution. Dyed cellulose membranes can then be scanned in a densitometer, which traces the pattern of fractions on graph paper, permitting visual analysis of the pattern. In the densitometer, the stained strip is passed through a light beam. Variable absorption due to different serum protein concentrations is detected by a photoelectric cell and reproduced by an analog recorder as a tracing. Scanning converts the band pattern into peaks and permits quantitation of the major peaks.

A variant of zone electrophoresis, *immunofixation,* allows the immobilization of one reactant of an antigen-antibody system in or on gels or paper.[1] For example, a dilute solution of antigen is electrophoresed in thin-layer agarose gel. An antiserum-saturated cellulose acetate strip is then laid over the gel. The antigen is fixed by the antibody diffusing into the gel, washed free of unreacted protein, and stained for identification. Another variant of the electrophoretic procedure, *isotachophoresis,* allows the ultraviolet detection of complex proteins. Non-ultraviolet-absorbing proteins that have mobilities in the same range are used as "spacers."

ASSAYS COMBINING ELECTROPHORESIS AND PRECIPITATION

Immunoelectrophoresis

Immunoelectrophoresis (IEP) combines the principles of zone electrophoresis with antigen-antibody reaction in gel. IEP is a two-step procedure. Step 1 involves separating a mixture of proteins by zone electrophoresis; step 2 involves the interaction of groups of proteins separated by their electrophoretic mobility with specific antisera to allow development of precipitation arcs.[3]

A glass slide is covered with molten agar in buffer. An antigen well and an antibody trough are cut with a template cutting device. A serum sample (antigen) is placed in the well and separated in an electric field for 30–60 minutes (see Fig 4–2). Antiserum is then placed in the trough, and both separated serum components and antibodies are allowed to diffuse for 18–24 hours. The resulting precipitation lines are then analyzed and may be compared against patterns of normal sera.

Electroimmunodiffusion

ONE-DIMENSIONAL SINGLE ELECTROIMMUNODIFFUSION (Laurell's rocket technique).—This is a rapid, quantitative method for determination of immunoglobulin levels. It requires 4–5 hours. The technique combines IEP analysis and RID.[4] Antiserum to the particular antigen one wishes to quantitate is incorporated into a support matrix such as agarose or cellulose acetate. The specimen containing antigen is placed in agarose wells or spotted on cellulose acetate. Electrophoresis of the antigen into the antibody-containing matrix results in the appearance of rocket-shaped precipitin arcs

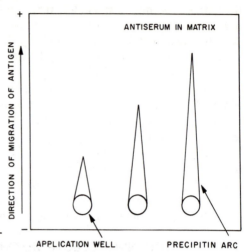

Fig 2–6.—Electroimmunodiffusion.

(Fig 2–6). The distance from the well to the tip of the "rocket" is proportional to the concentration of antigen originally added to the well. This permits construction of a standard curve similar to that used for RID. Compared with RID, electroimmunodiffusion has the advantage of more rapid results and increased sensitivity. On the other hand, it is technically more difficult and more expensive to set up than radial immunodiffusion, and so is less often used.

ONE-DIMENSIONAL DOUBLE ELECTROIMMUNODIFFUSION (counterimmunoelectrophoresis; CIE).—In this technique, antigen and antibody are placed in opposing wells and driven together with an electric current, re-

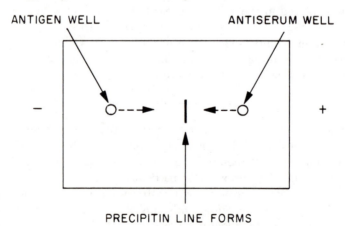

Fig 2–7.—Counterimmunoelectrophoresis.

sulting in the formation of a precipitin line (Fig 2–7). Since antigen and antibody migrate toward each other during electrophoresis, they must have different electrophoretic mobilities. The technique is only semiquantitative, but its speed and sensitivity have made it popular for the clinical analysis of some antigens, particularly those of certain bacteria and fungi.

Crossed Immunoelectrophoresis

Crossed immunoelectrophoresis is a modification of conventional immunoelectrophoresis. Serum is first separated by zone electrophoresis in one direction and then by electrophoresis at right angles to the first direction into a gel containing antiserum (Fig 2–8). This procedure can be performed on a glass slide, about 50 by 75 mm, covered by agar gel. The second separation results in a precipitation pattern of multiple peaks. The patterns are usually quite complex. The plates can be washed, dried, and stained for long-term preservation.

RADIOIMMUNOASSAYS AND ENZYME IMMUNOASSAYS

Radioimmunoassays

Radioimmunoassay (RIA) was initially developed for quantitation of plasma insulin levels. It has since been extended and modified for use in determining the levels of other hormones, certain drugs, and a variety of

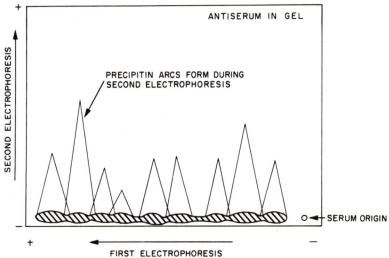

Fig 2–8.—Crossed immunoelectrophoresis.

antigens.[5] The principle has also been adapted to measure antigen-specific antibody (RAST). The general method of RIA (competitive type) is as follows. Antibody is reacted with a radiolabeled antigen under conditions that result in complete precipitation of the antigen (Fig 2–9, A). In a second reaction, excess unlabeled antigen is included in the reaction mixture, and under these conditions, much less labeled antigen is found in the precipitate (Fig 2–9, B). By varying the amount of unlabeled antigen added to a mixture, a quantitative relation can be obtained between the amount of antigen present and the amount of radioactivity in the precipitate and supernatant. A standard graph can then be constructed by plotting the percent of label in the precipitate (or supernatant) against the amount of unlabeled antigen added (Fig 2–9, C). The amount of antigen in an unknown material can then be found by determining the effect of the addition of unknown on the antibody-labeled antigen system. Amounts of antibody and labeled antigen are kept constant.

The standard RIA technique can be used to measure many substances, including several hormones, some viruses, hepatitis B–associated antigen, and tumor-associated antigens.

A quantitative noncompetitive RIA has been found useful for measuring antibody and immunoglobulin levels. In contrast to competitive RIA, no radiolabeled antigen is used in the first step. Proteins are made insoluble by binding to a solid phase (cellulose, polystyrene tubes, etc.). These proteins can be purified antigens if detection of specific antibodies is desired, or they may be specific antisera if immunogobulins are to be quantitated. After formation of the solid phase, serum or other fluid to be assayed is added. Antibodies or immunoglobulins are bound specifically and then quantitated by addition of a specific radiolabeled antibody. The binding of the radiolabeled antibody is directly related to the antigen content. Two examples are given below.

The radioimmunosorbent test (RIST) is a modification of the radioimmunoassay used for determination of total serum IgE levels. Reference or unknown serum is incubated with insolubilized anti-IgE (e.g., anti-IgE attached to filter paper disks). IgE present in the serum will combine with the IgE-particle complex (Fig 2–10). The insoluble antigen particles are then washed and incubated with radiolabeled anti-IgE. Binding of radiolabeled anti-IgE is directly related to the IgE content of the test serum.

The radioallergosorbent test (RAST) is a method for the in vitro determination of allergen-specific antibody. An allergen is coupled to a cyanogen bromide–activated carrier, usually sepharose, filter paper disks, or fine cellulose particles. After washing, the insoluble antigen particle complexes are incubated with the serum to be analyzed (Fig 2–11). Antibody in the serum directed toward the allergen will react with the conjugate. Unbound serum

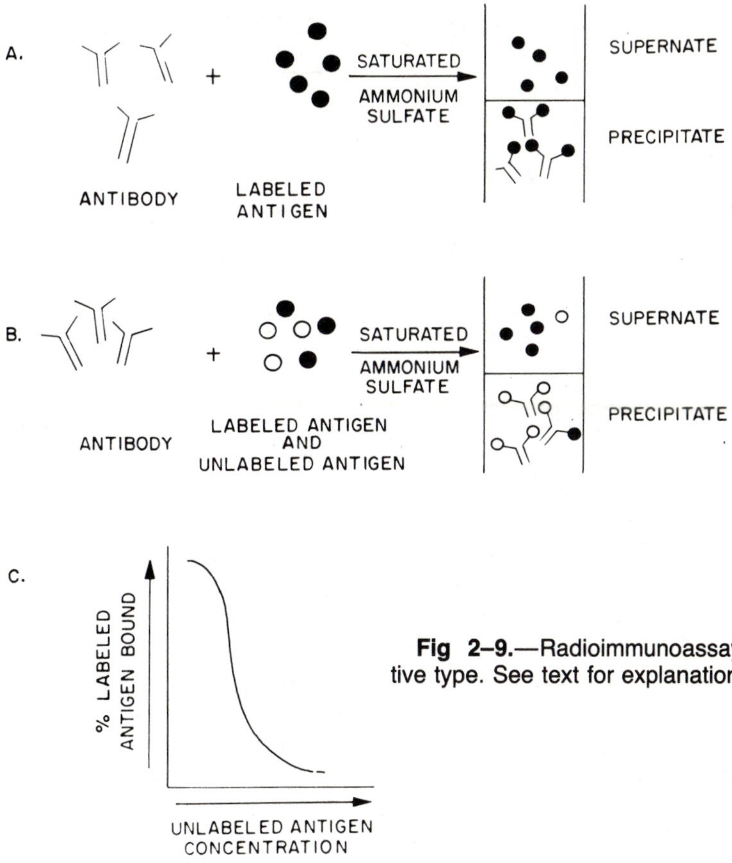

A.   ANTIBODY   LABELED ANTIGEN   +   SATURATED AMMONIUM SULFATE   →   SUPERNATE   PRECIPITATE

B.   ANTIBODY   +   LABELED ANTIGEN AND UNLABELED ANTIGEN   SATURATED AMMONIUM SULFATE   →   SUPERNATE   PRECIPITATE

C.   % LABELED ANTIGEN BOUND   /   UNLABELED ANTIGEN CONCENTRATION

Fig 2–9.—Radioimmunoassay, competitive type. See text for explanation.

components are then washed off the particles and ^{125}I-labeled anti-IgE is added. The radiolabeled anti-IgE will bind to IgE antibody present on the particles. After washing again, uptake of labeled anti-IgE is measured in terms of radioactivity in a gamma counter. The resulting count is proportional to the amount of allergen-specific IgE present.

The double antibody RIA is very precise and reproducible. After completion of a competitive binding incubation, a second antibody is added as a precipitating antiserum (Fig 2–12). This assay takes 2 days to complete and can be expensive. It is useful as an investigative method.

Enzyme Immunoassays

The enzyme-linked immunosorbent assay (ELISA) is a quantitative technique for the detection of antigens and antibodies. Enzymes are linked to

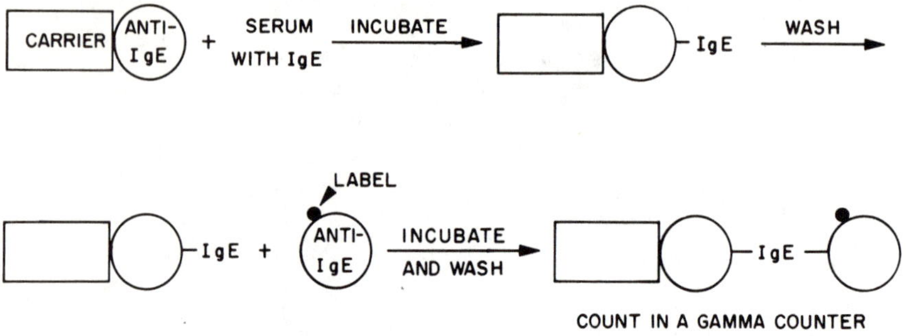

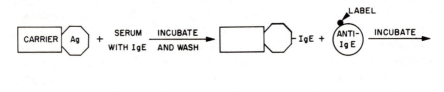

Fig 2–10.—Radioimmunosorbent test (RIST), a noncompetitive radioimmunoassay.

either antigen or antibody as a label which can be detected by measurement of enzyme activity. This assay is similar to RIA. Several different ELISA methods are available. The indirect method for antibody uses an antigen attached to a solid support, such as cellulose. This is incubated with an enzyme-labeled antiglobulin (Fig 2–13, A). Enzyme substrate is then added and the amount of enzyme activity adherent to the solid phase is measured. Such activity is related to the amount of antibody bound.

An ELISA inhibition method for antigen uses a reference antigen linked to a solid-phase carrier (Fig 2–13, B). Enzyme-labeled specific antibody is added and activity adherent to the solid-phase carrier is determined, as described above. In a second step the antigen and labeled antibody are mixed with test serum, incubated, and washed, and enzymatic activity is then determined. The difference in substrate degradations between test serum with reference conjugate and reference conjugate alone is proportional to the amount of antigen in the test sample.

A competitive ELISA may be used to detect antigen. Enzyme-labeled antigen is mixed with test serum, incubated, and then added to insoluble

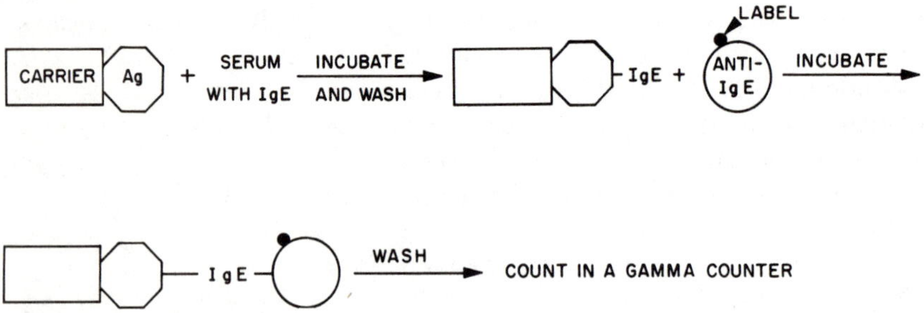

Fig 2–11.—Radioallergosorbent test (RAST), a noncompetitive radioimmunoassay.

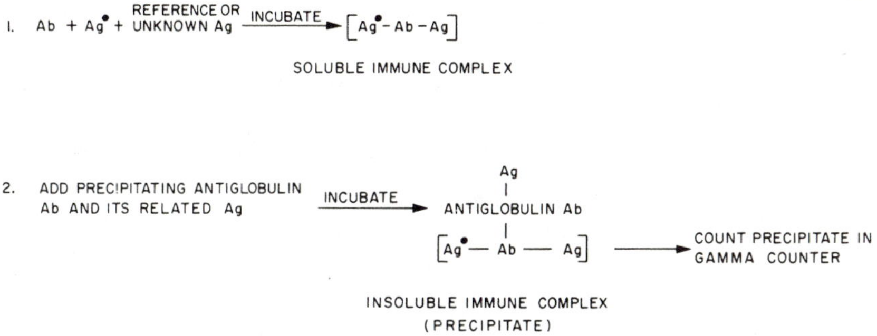

1.   Ab + Ag* + REFERENCE OR UNKNOWN Ag —INCUBATE→ [Ag*– Ab –Ag]

SOLUBLE IMMUNE COMPLEX

2.   ADD PRECIPITATING ANTIGLOBULIN Ab AND ITS RELATED Ag —INCUBATE→

Ag
|
ANTIGLOBULIN Ab
|
[Ag*— Ab —— Ag] ——→ COUNT PRECIPITATE IN GAMMA COUNTER

INSOLUBLE IMMUNE COMPLEX
(PRECIPITATE)

Fig 2–12.—Double antibody radioimmunoassay. *Ab,* antibody; *Ag,* antigen; *=radiolabeled.

antibody. Enzyme substrate is then added (Fig 2–13, C). In a reference assay insoluble antibody and enzyme-labeled antigen are added together without the test serum. Differences in substrate degradation between the two assays are compared. The more antigen in the test serum, the less the substrate will be hydrolyzed and the greater the difference will be between the two assays.

Another ELISA for antigen detection is the double antibody sandwich technique. The test sample is added to insoluble antibody. After incubation and washing, the same antibody, labeled with enzyme, is added (Fig 2–13, D). Substrate is subsequently added, and hydrolysis is proportional to the amount of antigen in the test sample.

In the enzyme-multiplied immunoassay technique (EMIT), an enzyme is chemically bound to an antigen or hapten in such a way that binding occurs near the active site of the enzyme. The subsequent binding of added antibody to the antigen inhibits action of the enzyme on the substrate by sterically hindering substrate binding. High concentrations of antigen in test samples will displace the enzyme–antigen from the antibody. The resultant change in spectrophotometric absorbance is measured. There is a direct correlation between a change in absorbance and antigen concentration in a test sample. A high concentration of antigen will bind most antibody, freeing the enzyme-linked antigen to react with substrate. The use of EMIT is limited to the assay of low molecular weight antigens, such as drugs and some bacterial antigens.

IMMUNOFLUORESCENCE

Immunofluorescence is a histochemical or cytochemical technique for detection and localization of antigens. The tracer used in this technique is a specific antibody conjugated with a fluorescent compound. The antibody,

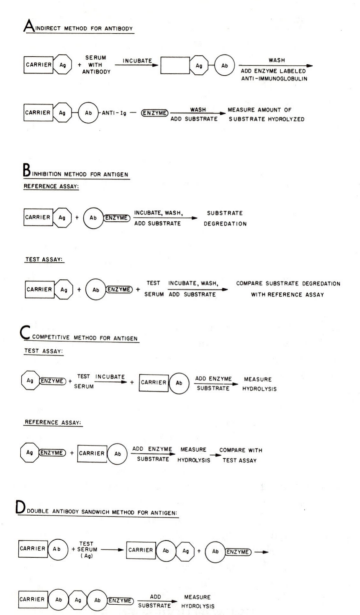

Fig 2–13.—Enzyme-linked immunosorbent assays (ELISA). *A,* indirect method for detection of antibody. *B,* inhibition method for detection of antigen. *Ag,* antigen; *Ab,* antibody; *Ig,* immunoglobulin. *C,* competitive method for detection of antigen. *D,* double antibody sandwich method for detection of antigen. *Ag,* antigen; *Ab,* antibody.

usually in the form of antiserum, is added to cells or tissues and becomes fixed to the antigen. Nonantibody proteins are then removed by washing and the preparation is observed under a fluorescence microscope against a dark background. The fluorescence microscope contains a light source producing wavelengths capable of fluorescence activation. Antigens bound to fluorescent antibody are detected by the bright color of the antibody. Four different immunofluorescent techniques are described below.

In the direct immunofluorescence technique, conjugated antiserum is added directly to a tissue section or cell suspension. This makes possible the detection of antigens present in tissue (Fig 2–14, A).

The indirect immunofluorescence technique can be used to detect antibody in serum. Test serum dilutions are placed on microscope slides containing tissue sections. After incubation and rinsing, the sections are treated with antiserum labeled with fluorescein or rhodamine isothiocyanate. After further rinsing the slides are mounted and examined under the fluorescence microscope (Fig 2–14, B).

A variant of the indirect technique is fluorescence microscopy of antibody directed against membrane antigen (FAMA). FAMA is used to determine susceptibility to varicella. Human embryonic lung fibroblasts are infected with varicella zoster–infected cells. The infected cell suspension is mixed with test serum, incubated, and centrifuged. The resultant cell pellet is washed. Fluorescein-labeled antiglobulin is added and suspended cell pellets are examined under a fluorescence microscope. If the test serum contains antibody, a ring of fluorescence is seen around varicella zoster–infected cells.

The sandwich technique is used to identify antibody in tissue sections. Antigen is added to tissue and is bound by specific antibody in the tissue. Specific fluorescein-labeled antibody is added and reacts to antigen fixed to the tissue (Fig 2–14, C). The complement technique depends on the fact that complement is usually fixed during an antigen-antibody reaction if it is present while the reaction takes place. The presence of complement is then detected by the addition of fluorescein-labeled antibody to complement (Fig 2–14, D).

COMPLEMENT ASSAYS

Functional assays.—Hemolysis of sensitized erythrocytes requires the presence of all primary complement pathway factors. The hemolytic assay is suitably convenient and quantitative and is therefore the functional complement assay of greatest value. The assay quantifies the dilution of serum required to lyse a given proportion of indicator cells under standard conditions. A common assay (Mayer's) bases the hemolytic unit on the dilution

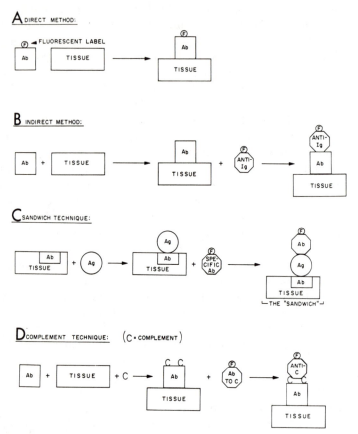

Fig 2–14.—Fluorescent antibody techniques. *A,* direct method. *B,* indirect method. *Ag,* antigen; *Ab,* antibody; *Ig,* immunoglobulin. *C,* sandwich technique. *D,* complement technique. *Ab,* antibody; *Ag,* antigen; *C,* complement.

of test serum which will lyse 50% of indicator erythrocytes (Fig 2–15). This is designated the CH_{50}.

Precipitation assays.—Components of complement pathways can be assayed by single RID utilizing monospecific antisera. This assay has been commonly adapted for C4 and C3 determinations and, to a lesser extent, for C1q, C1 esterase inhibitor, properdin, and factor B. Electroimmuno-diffusion and immunofluorescence techniques have also been used for complement assays.

CF.—CF is used for the determination of antibody, antigen, or both. The test is done in two stages. In the first stage, antigen and antibody react in the presence of a known amount of complement (Fig 2–16). Comple-

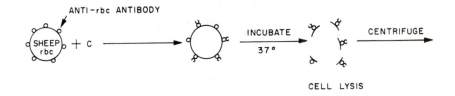

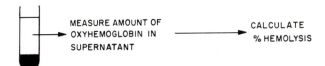

Fig 2–15.—Hemolytic complement assay. *C*, complement.

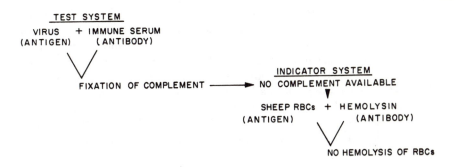

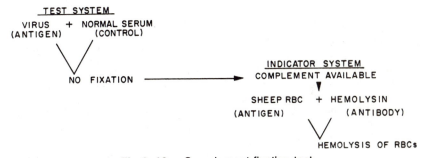

Fig 2–16.—Complement fixation test.

TABLE 2–1.—SENSITIVITIES OF
IMMUNOASSAYS*

IMMUNOASSAY	SENSITIVITY (per dl)
Serum protein electrophoresis	100 mg
Immunoelectrophoresis	5–10 mg
Radial immunodiffusion	<1–2 mg
Counterimmunoelectrophoresis	<1 mg
Electroimmunodiffusion	<0.5 mg
Double diffusion in agar	<0.1 mg
Nephelometry	0.1 mg
Complement fixation	1 μg
Agglutination	1 μg
Enzyme immunoassay	<1 μg
Quantitative immunofluorescence	<1 pg
Radioimmunoassay	<1 pg
Viral neutralization	<1 pg

*Modified from Fudenberg et al.,[3] p. 373.

ment is consumed (fixed). In the second stage, residual hemolytic complement activity is measured by an indicator system to determine the amount of complement fixed in stage 1, and thus the amount of antigen or antibody present in the initial stage. The amount of complement activity remaining is titrated and the results are expressed as the highest serum dilution showing fixation of complement. Each dilution of serum giving hemolysis equal to or less than 30% is considered positive for antibody. On occasion, factors in a given serum (e.g., some lipids) will interfere with the CF test. Such sera are designated "anticomplementary," and test results must be interpreted with caution.

RELATIVE SENSITIVITY OF IMMUNOASSAYS

The relative sensitivities of the various humoral immunoassays are listed in Table 2–1.

REFERENCES

1. Nichol W.S., Nakamura R.M.: Agglutination and agglutination inhibition assays, in Rose N.R., Friedman H. (eds.): *Manual of Clinical Immunology*, ed. 2. Washington D.C., American Society for Microbiology, 1980, pp. 15–22.
2. Sell S.: *Immunology, Immunopathology and Immunity*. Hagerstown, Md., Harper & Row, Publishers, 1975, pp. 87–109, 284.
3. Stites D.P.: Clinical laboratory methods for detection of antigens and antibodies, in Fudenberg H.H., Stites D., Caldwell J.L., et al. (eds.): *Basic and Clinical Immunology*, ed. 2. Los Altos, Calif., Lange Medical Publishers, 1978, pp. 237–374.
4. Daniels J.C.: Practical applications of gel diffusion tests, in Nakamura R.M.,

Dito W.R., and Tucker E.S. III (eds.): *Immunoassays in the Clinical Laboratory.* New York, Allen R. Liss, Inc., 1979, pp. 23–61.

5. Martin J.B.: Immunoassays in clinical medicine, in Freedman S.O., Gold P. (eds.): *Clinical Immunology.* Hagerstown, Md., Harper & Row, Publishers, 1976, pp. 590–599.

3

Immunologic Assays of Cellular Function

Michael H. Grieco, M.D.

ASSAYS FOR CELLULAR COMPONENTS OF IMMUNOLOGIC RESPONSES

Lymphocyte Subpopulation Surface Markers

THE ABILITY to distinguish subsets of circulating and tissue lymphocytes represents an extremely important advance in immunology. Table 3–1 summarizes distinguishing characteristics of B cells, T cells, and third population (TP) cells.

Preparation of Cell Suspensions

Human peripheral blood for all types of lymphocyte studies can be collected by venipuncture and either heparinized or defibrinated. Mononuclear cells can be obtained by centrifuging whole blood on Ficoll-Hypaque gradients, as described by Böyum.[1] Mononuclear lymphocytes and monocytes are recovered at the Ficoll-Hypaque-plasma interface and washed, while erythrocytes and neutrophils pass to below the Ficoll-Hypaque layer[2] (Fig 3–1). Premixed commercial preparations are available for this purpose. In addition, it is possible to separate unique human lymphocyte subpopulations using cellular immunoabsorbent chromatography to isolate surface immunoglobulin (SIg)-negative cells from SIg-positive cells, and then to fractionate these populations using rosetting techniques.[3] These two procedures permit isolation of SIg-positive, E rosette–positive and SIg-negative, E rosette–negative cells that correspond in general to B, T, and TP lymphocytes.

TABLE 3–1.—DISTINGUISHING CHARACTERISTICS OF B CELLS, T CELLS, AND
THIRD POPULATION (TP) CELLS

	B CELLS	T CELLS	TP CELLS
Peripheral blood	10%–15%	80%–85%	5%–10%
Assays involving rosette formation:			
Spontaneous E rosette assay (E)			
Sheep		+	
Rhesus		+	
Mouse	+		
Fc region of Ig (EA)			
IgG	+	On subset (Tγ)	+
IgM	+	On subset (Tμ)	+
IgA	+	+	+
IgE	On subset	On subset	
Complement (EAC)			
CR$_1$ and CR$_2$	+		
CR$_1$ alone	+	+	
Fluorescence microscopy			
mIg	+		
IgG Fc	+	+ in subset (Tγ)	+
Ia-like antigens	+	+ in activated cells	+ in 20%
Helix pomatia		+	
Peanut agglutinin		+ on pre-T cells	
EBV	+		+ in subset
T cell antigens		OKT$_3$: all T cells OKT$_4$: helper/inducer cells OKT$_8$: T suppressor/cytotoxic cells	
Microcytotoxicity			
HLA-A, -B, -C	+	+	+
HLA-DR	+		
Enzymatic markers			
TdT		pre-T cells	
Affinity columns			
H$_2$ receptors		T suppressor cells	
Lymphocyte culture			
MLC	+		

Assays Involving Rosette Formation[4]

SPONTANEOUS ERYTHROCYTE ROSETTE ASSAY (E).—Sheep erythrocytes adhere in a delicate fashion to T lymphocytes during incubation, at 4 C, of a mixture of 0.1 ml of 0.5% sheep RBC suspension and 0.1 ml of balanced salt solution containing 1×10^6 mononuclear cells with sheep RBC-absorbed, heat-inactivated human AB serum or fetal calf serum. A lymphocyte is scored as rosette-forming if 3 or more erythrocytes adhere, as observed in a hemocytometer chamber. Cells taking up trypan blue are excluded from the count, as are monocytes containing latex polystyrene

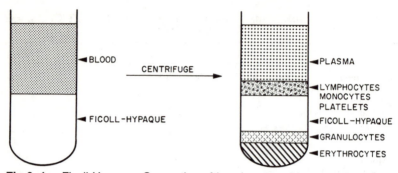

Fig 3–1.—Ficoll-Hypaque Separation of lymphocytes. After centrifugation, the lymphocyte layer is drawn off, washed in a clean tube, centrifuged, and resuspended in an appropriate medium.

particles, indicating phagocytosis. E rosette–forming T cells account for 80%–85% of lymphocytes in peripheral blood. Use of serum in the rosette reaction or modification of the erythrocyte surface, as with neuraminidase treatment, stabilizes the rosettes. Some peripheral lymphocytes have relatively stronger binding to sheep RBCs that occurs rapidly and at warmer temperatures and leads to stable E rosette formation. Most lymphocytes have weaker rosette formations so that values for E rosettes vary considerably, depending on laboratory methodology. Gentle resuspension is essential to permit maximal labeling of T lymphocytes.

Rhesus monkey RBCs form rosettes with T cells, while mouse RBCs form spontaneous rosettes with a subpopulation of B lymphocytes. It should be noted that the inability of ox RBCs to form spontaneous rosettes allows them to be used as carriers for IgM, IgA, and IgG to permit detection of Tμ, Tα, and Tγ cells with a rosetting assay.

RECEPTORS FOR FC REGION OF IMMUNOGLOBULINS (EA).—Four immunoglobulin Fc receptors have been identified. Methods of detecting them are described below.

IgG Fc receptors.—There are at least six different Fc receptor test systems, with varying ability to detect Fc receptors on lymphocyte subpopulations. In some EA rosette systems using human RBCs coated with either human or rabbit IgG antibodies, the coated RBCs have been reported to adhere to B cells, TP cells, and a small subset of T cells with a range of 5%–10% of peripheral blood lymphocytes.

Easily dissociable complexes are formed between IgG-coated ox RBCs and lymphocytes bearing Fcγ receptors. The mixture is incubated for 2 hours or more at 4 C prior to resuspension and counting. T cells isolated by sheep RBC adherence and centrifugation can be examined selectively for the presence of Fc receptors. Tγ cells appear to function as suppressor and cytotoxic cells. Fc receptors on TP and T cells are essential for antibody-dependent cell-mediated cytotoxicity.

IgM Fc receptors.—These receptors are detected using erythrocyte-antibody (EA) systems with IgM antibodies to sensitize the erythrocytes. Monomeric or pentameric IgM Fc is capable of binding to the IgM Fc receptor on T cells (Tμ). These receptors are present as well on B and TP cells. Tμ cells appear to function as helper cells for antibody synthesis and for delayed-type hypersensitivity.

IgA Fc receptors.—These receptors have been detected on B, T, and TP lymphoid cells.[5] The IgA Fc receptor is detected by employing either anti-ox RBC antibody of the IgA class to sensitize ox RBCs or trinitrophenol (TNP)-coated ox RBCs treated with a mouse IgA myeloma (MOPC-315) that has anti-TNP specificity.

IgE Fc receptors.—IgE Fc receptors are detected with IgE myeloma attached to RBCs. IgE Fc receptors have been demonstrated on a small subset of B and T lymphocytes.

RECEPTORS FOR COMPLEMENT (EAC).—Receptors for complement components are detected by sheep erythrocyte antibody complement (EAC) complexes adhering to two different types of C receptors, CR_1 (C4b-C3b) and CR_2 (C3d). The two complement receptors are structurally distinct and located separately on the lymphocyte membrane. EAC 1, 4b or EAC 1, 4, 2, 3b complexes form rosettes only with cells bearing CR_1, whereas EAC 3d complexes form rosettes only with cells bearing CR_2. Some peripheral blood lymphocytes have only CR_1 receptors, while others have both types. Unlike E rosettes, EAC rosettes form readily with lymphocytes in suspension and are stable and difficult to disrupt, so that a slide and coverslip may be used instead of a counting chamber. Incubation for 20 minutes at 37 C minimizes spontaneous sheep RBC adherence.

Fluorescence Microscopy

MEMBRANE IMMUNOGLOBULIN (MIG).—IgM and IgD are the predominant SIg classes on B lymphocytes, while IgA and IgG account for less than 10% of the mIg-positive cells. The presence of Fc receptors for IgG must be taken into consideration since immune complexes in residual serum or aggregates present in the antiserum preparation will be nonspecifically taken up and produce false positive staining. The Fc regions of the anti-immunoglobulin antibodies are removed by pepsin digestion and then conjugated with fluorochrome. A screening mixture composed of a pool of $F(ab^1)_2$ reagents specific for IgG, IgA, IgM, and IgD or with specificity to κ and λ determinants can be used. Detection of the binding of antibody tagged with fluorochrome requires the use of incident fluorescent illumination-epi-illumination. Cells with homogenous cytoplasmic staining due to early cell death are not counted. Normal individuals have been reported to have a mean of 11.4% mIg-positive lymphocytes.[4]

IgG Fc RECEPTORS.—These receptors can be detected using soluble immune fluorochrome-conjugated complexes of IgG antibody and antigen (direct method), or soluble aggregates of Cohn fraction II IgG that have been denatured by heating. In the latter assay these aggregates are bound to Fc receptor–bearing cells and the bound complexes are detected by anti-human IgG antibodies conjugated with fluorescein (indirect method). Some immune complex systems preferentially bind to Fcγ receptors on T and TP cells, while others preferentially bind to B cell Fcγ receptors. Aggregates formed by heat denaturation of IgG tend to have a broader range of specificity.

DRw ANTIGENS (IA).—Ia antigens are detectable by alloantisera used in indirect fluorescence, radioimmunoassay, or cytotoxicity assays. The use of heteroantiserum in direct fluorescence obviates the precise selection of an alloantiserum. At present, the relationship between the HLA-D (D) and HLA-DR (DR) antigens and Ia-like molecules is not completely understood. The D antigens were originally defined as human B cell alloantigens that stimulate the mixed lymphocyte response. These antigens are under the genetic control of the HLA-D locus of the human major histocompatibility complex (MHC) on chromosome 6. The DR antigens are defined serologically and are controlled by a locus that is near the D locus and may be identical to it. However, there appears to be definite but incomplete correspondence between HLA-D and HLA-DR. DR and probably D antigens are carried on polymorphic allotypic Ia-like molecules composed of two glycoproteins of 34,000 and 28,000 dalton molecular weight. Heterogeneity among the human Ia-like molecules is suggested by studies with monoclonal antibodies.[6] A new monoclonal antibody, OKIa$_1$,* has been shown to react with the DR framework of the Ia antigens and identifies 90% of B lymphocytes, 20% of null cells, activated T lymphocytes, and some monocytes. Fluorescent goat antimouse Ig is used for visualization. Control subjects have been reported to have 9.3% ± 3.0% (SD) OKIa$_1$– positive lymphoid cells.[7]

DR alloantigens are usually determined by the microcytotoxicity typing assay using the patient's B lymphocytes and test sera of known DR specificity. DRw specificities 1 to 7 have been defined by the Seventh International Histocompatibility Workshop (see Chap. 15).[8]

HELIX POMATIA RECEPTOR.—Receptors for a hemagglutinin derived from Helix pomatia (HP), an edible land snail, have been reported on 70%

---

*Ortho Pharmaceutical Corporation, Raritan, N.J.

of peripheral blood lymphocytes, predominantly T cells, and are easily detected by immunofluorescence when neuraminidase-treated lymphocytes are incubated with fluorescein isothiocyanate–labeled HP. HP receptors on B lymphocytes form a weaker bond than that formed between HP and T lymphocytes.[9]

PEANUT AGGLUTININ RECEPTORS.—Fluorescein-labeled peanut agglutinin adheres to receptors on pre-T cells in a very early stage of differentiation but has also been noted on cells from sera of patients with B cell Burkitt's lymphoma and acute myeloid leukemia.[10]

EPSTEIN-BARR VIRUS (EBV) RECEPTORS.—In man, EBV is lymphotrophic for B cells and a subset of TP cells that are presumably of B cell lineage. Supernates containing EBV are added to lymphocytes, incubated for one hour at 37 C, exposed to fluorescein-conjugated antimembrane antigen for 30 minutes at room temperature, and examined by fluorescence microscopy under oil immersion for membrane fluorescence.[11]

T CELL DIFFERENTIATION ANTIGEN.—Monoclonal mouse antisera prepared by the hybridoma method of Kohler and Milstein[12] are now available for indirect fluorescence detection of T cell differentiation antigens. Reinherz and Schlossman[13] have developed monoclonal antibodies to OKT_3 that identify T cell human peripheral lymphocytes (81.1% of lymphocytes), OKT_4 on T helper/inducer cells (52.1% of lymphocytes), and OKT_8 on T suppressor/cytotoxic cells (32.5% of lymphocytes).[7] These antisera are commercially available* and make possible the precise delineation of T cell subpopulations. Monoclonal antihuman Leu-1 is also available† as a purified antibody, biotin conjugate, and fluorescein conjugate with specificity for an antigen found on all peripheral T cells but not on B cells, monocytes, or granulocytes.[14] Fluorescein conjugates are used for direct fluorescence and for fluorescence-activated cell sorter analysis.

Microcytotoxicity

HLA alloantigens controlled by the A, B, and C loci are detectable on the cell membranes of all nucleated cells and platelets. The NIH technique developed by Terasaki and the Amos technique are widely used cytotoxicity procedures.[15] Lymphocytes to be typed are incubated with human sera containing HLA antibodies of known specificity, exposed to complement, and then exposed to vital dyes; cells bearing antigens recognized by the HLA test antibodies will suffer membrane damage, as indicated by uptake of the dye. The HLA-A, -B and -C antigens are serologically defined, while

---

*Ortho Pharmaceutical Corp., Raritan, N.J.
†Becton Dickinson, Sunnyvale, Calif.

HLA-D antigens are detected by the mixed lymphocyte culture (MLC). HLA-DR antigens are also detectable by microtoxicity on B cells separated by depletion of T cells through sheep RBC rosetting and adherence and subsequent elution of B cells from nylon wool columns, and by the adsorption and elution of B cells from goat anti-Hu $F(ab^1)_2$-coated tissue culture flasks.

Enzymatic Markers

Terminal deoxynucleotidyl transferase (TdT) is detectable in pre-T cells and in cells from patients with acute lymphoblastic leukemia and from some patients with pre-B cell leukemia and acute B cell leukemia.

Affinity Columns

Histamine-2 receptors

H_2 receptors for histamine are present on suppressor T cells and are detectable using affinity columns that contain insolubilized conjugates of histamine and rabbit serum albumin.[16]

In Vitro Tests of Lymphocyte Function

Lymphocyte Transformation to Mitogen, Antigen, and Allogeneic Cells (Fig 3–2)

In 1960 Nowell[17] reported that phytohemagglutinin (PHA), a lectin from kidney beans, transformed small lymphocytes into proliferating lymphoblasts in tissue culture. This discovery was followed by the development of useful assays to assess lymphocyte responsiveness to mitogens, antigens, and allogeneic cells. Isolated mononuclear cells are cultured in medium containing 15%–20% autologous or pooled homologous plasma or serum. Adequate nutritional support is provided by media such as Eagle minimal essential and enriched RPMI 1640. The assays can be performed by both macroculture and microculture techniques.[2] Assays of DNA synthesis and protein synthesis and morphological evaluation may be used to evaluate lymphocyte transformation. It takes 2–4 days of incubation for optimal DNA synthesis to occur in response to mitogens, whereas optimal lymphocyte reactions to antigenic stimulants take 4.5–7 days. The incorporation of tritiated thymidine-labeled TdR, 0.5 μCi per well (specific activity,

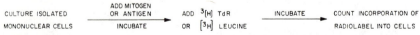

Fig 3–2.—Lymphocyte transformation using radiolabeled thymidine or leucine.

2 Ci/mmole) is commonly used to evaluate DNA synthesis in S phase. The assay of DNA synthesis, although slower than assay of protein synthesis as determined by radiolabeled leucine incorporation, is more sensitive and requires fewer lymphocytes. Lymphocytes from adults and neonates have receptors to mitogens such as PHA, concanavalin A (Con A) and pokeweed mitogen (PWM) and respond without prior sensitization. In contrast, prior sensitization is required for transformation with specific antigens such as purified protein derivative, candida, mumps, tetanus toxoid, and strepto-kinase. The stimulation index in normal subjects (ratio of mean counts per minute in stimulated cultures divided by mean counts per minute in unstim-ulated cultures) is usually greater than 10 for mitogens and 3 for allergens. It is important to control for technical variability by testing age-matched normal controls simultaneously with the subject. In addition, one should use multiple doses of a stimulant, since only the reaction to suboptional doses may be abnormal.

The MLC assay does not depend on prior sensitization. Allogeneic lym-phocytes from two unrelated donors are mixed and primary sensitization occurs in vitro as each donor responds to the HLA-D region antigens in the B lymphocytes and monocytes of the other. The MLC assay can be used to type the HLA-D antigens in a oneway reaction in which donor cells are inactivated by mitomycin. The primary clinical use of MLC assay is in the selection of a compatible donor for organ transplantation; the assay represents the in vitro equivalent of the afferent or sensitization phase of cellular immunity.

Direct Lymphocyte-Mediated Cytotoxicity[18]

Cell-mediated lympholysis using release of ^{51}Cr or ^{111}In is thought to mimic in vitro the efferent or cell destruction phase of HLA-A and HLA-B target antigens. Cytotoxic T lymphocytes have antigen specificity derived from prior immunization, as in an MLC reaction. Specific lysis greater than 5% of maximal release, and corrected for spontaneous release, is consid-ered a positive result.

Antibody-Dependent, Cell-Mediated Cytotoxicity (ADCC)[18]

In this test, nonimmune killer (K) cells recognize and interact with anti-body molecules that coat the surface of target cells. Macrophage-depleted, Ficoll-Hypaque-depleted nonimmune human lymphocytes are mixed with ^{51}Cr-labeled lymphocytes, RBCs, or tumor cells in the presence of heat-inactivated (56 C for 45 minutes) antitarget antibody. Following incubation, the amount of specific ^{51}Cr released is determined after subtracting the amount of ^{51}Cr released in cultures without effector lymphocytes. TP and Tγ cells have this cytotoxic property. The antibody class active in ADCC has been predominantly reported to be IgG.

Natural Killer[18]

Natural killer (NK) lymphocytes lyse a variety of malignant or virus-infected target cells. NK cells are surface immunoglobulin–positive, about one third bear complement receptors, most bear Fc receptors, and they are nonadherent and nonphagocytic. Most studies indicate that NK cells have low-affinity receptors for sheep RBCs and are lysed by anti-T antibody and complement, suggesting T cell lineage. Sample target cells include myeloid cell line K-562 and measles-infected HeLa cell line. Calculations and interpretations are similar to those for the lymphocyte-mediated cytotoxicity and ADCC assays. Experimental data make it unlikely that ADCC or Fc receptors are involved in NK activity, although there is suggestive evidence the K and NK cells may be the same. Apparently the cells mediate two kinds of cytotoxic activities by different receptors, K activity via Fc receptors and NK activity via receptors for NK-related antigens.

Lymphokine Assays

A variety of lymphokines are released from lymphocytes following stimulation by antigens, mitogens, MLC reactions, and activation of certain membrane receptors, including C3, Fc, and surface immunoglobulin. Release of lymphokines does not depend on concomitant lymphocyte transformation.

MACROPHAGE MIGRATION INHIBITORY FACTOR (MIF).—Macrophage MIF is distinct from the factor responsible for neutrophil migration inhibition. Production of macrophage MIF in vitro by specific antigen correlates with delayed-type hypersensitivity skin testing. There are two methods available for the assay of human MIF.[19] In the one-step direct assay, sensitized lymphocytes are mixed with guinea pig or human monocytes in a capillary tube, specific antigen is added, and inhibition of migration is assayed over 24 hours. In the two-step indirect assay, sensitized lymphocytes are cultured with antigen to produce MIF over 24 to 48 hours. Then cell-free supernatant is assayed on nonimmune guinea pig or human monocytes. The main advantage of the indirect method is that it permits examination of each component of the lymphocyte-macrophage interaction. Human MIF has the properties of a protein of 23,000-dalton molecular weight.[20] The results are expressed as a percentage of inhibition and are calculated by dividing the test area by control supernatant fluid area migration. In general, greater than 20% inhibition of migration is considered to be a positive MIF response. Both B and T cells elaborate macrophage MIF.

LEUKOCYTE MIGRATION INHIBITORY FACTOR (LMIF).—LMIF may be produced by T and B lymphocytes and has a molecular weight of approximately 85,000 daltons. LMIF can also be assayed by a direct one-step method, using capillary tube and macroagarose assays, or by an indirect two-step method, using capillary tube and agarose microdroplet assays.[21] The inhibition of migration is calculated and interpreted as for macrophage MIF.

LYMPHOCYTE CHEMOTACTIC FACTOR.—Lymphocyte-derived chemotactic factors are assayed utilizing upper and lower chambers separated by a micropore filter. Polymorphonuclear leukocytes are placed in the upper chamber and lymphocyte-derived chemo-attractant is placed in the lower chamber. Active supernatant fluid will usually increase the cell count five to ten times above that seen with control supernatant fluid.

OTHER LYMPHOKINES.—Assays are available to permit detection of lymphotoxins (LTs), interferon, and lymphocyte mitogenic factor (LMF). Lymphotoxins are glycoproteins that are released and expressed on the surface of activated lymphocytes that kill cells or inhibit their growth. Lymphotoxins may serve as effectors of tissue destruction by lymphocytes. LT molecules are more complex than originally thought. The smaller α, β, and γ LT classes are only weakly lytic and cause lysis of certain cells such as L-929. The larger C_X and α-$_H$ classes cause nonspecific cytolysis of a wide range of allogeneic targets, while specific cytolysis results only from the C_X class derived from alloimmune activated lymphocytes. LMF, or blastogenic factor, is a soluble product of lymphocytes stimulated by antigens, mitogens, or allogeneic cells. Its activity is detected by the assays described above for lymphocyte transformation. T lymphocytes produce LMF but require monocyte cooperation to respond to antigenic stimulation. The assay for LMF uses B lymphocytes that are unresponsive to antigen in this assay.

SUPPRESSOR CELL ASSAYS.—T cells, monocytes, and B cells have been shown to be suppressive in different in vitro systems. Suppressor T cells have usually been identified as nonadherent sheep RBC rosetting lymphocytes with surface $Fc\gamma$ receptors and OKT_8 antigens. Assays for unfractionated spontaneously occurring or Con A–inducible suppressor cells usually involve co-cultivation with autologous or allogeneic responder mononuclear cell suspensions.[22] The co-culture test systems in which the suppressor cells are assayed may reflect a wide variety of in vitro functions. One can use PWM-induced B cell function and observe intracytoplasmic immunoglobulin, supernatant immunoglobulin, hemolytic plaque-forming cells (PFC), or blastogenesis of B cells. Alternatively, one can assay for T cell blastogenic responses induced by Con A, PHA, or MLC. Cultures are incubated at 37 C in 5% CO_2 in air and 100% humidity for up to 5 days to assay for T cell blastogenic responses, 6–7 days for PFC and intracytoplasmic immunoglobulin, and 10–12 days for supernatant immunoglobulin.

Delayed-Type Hypersensitivity (DTH) Skin Testing

DTH skin testing reflects the release of lymphokines by sensitized lymphocytes following exposure to antigen and the subsequent inflammatory response, which is characteristically monocytic. Tests for preexisting immunity are extremely valuable for the clinical assessment of cell-mediated immunity. The standard procedure is to inject 0.1 ml of an allergenic extract intradermally into the volar aspect of the forearm. Readings should be made at 24 and 48 hours and should be graded as follows: 0, less than 5 mm induration; 1+, 5–10 mm induration; 2+, 10–20 mm induration, 3+, more than 20 mm induration and 4+, accompanying necrosis. A separate, sterile, 1-ml tuberculin syringe with a 27-gauge needle should be used for each injection. A screening panel for anergy may include mumps (1 mg/ml), PPD stabilized solution (5 tuberculin units (TU)/0.1 ml), *Trichophyton* sp. (1:300), *Candida albicans* (1:1,000), streptokinase-streptodornase (SK-SD, 40 and 10 U/ml), mixed respiratory vaccine (1:5) and *Staphylococcus* phage lysate (1:5). SK-SD is not commercially available in the United States at this time. Current lots of mumps antigen have not been standardized for skin test reactivity (as they were previously) and may not yield consistent results. Second-strength antigens are then applied if the 24-hour or 48-hour readings are negative for the intermediate strength antigens. Second-strength antigens include PPD (250 TU/0.1 ml), *Trichophyton* sp. (1:30), *Candida albicans* (1:100 and 1:10), and SK-SD (400 and 100 U/ml followed by 1,000 and 250 U/ml). The intradermal response to 1-µg and 5-µg test doses of purified PHA may also be used to assess cellular immunity. Patients with suspected active tuberculosis should be tested with initial 1-TU doses of PPD to avoid occasional necrotic reactions accompanied by systemic symptoms. DTH sensitivity response is considered to be diminished if the individual responds to fewer than two antigens in the allergy test panel. A positive response consists of 10 mm or more of induration.

Dinitrochlorobenzene sensitization can be used to assess primary sensitization. Sensitization is induced with 0.2 ml of a concentration of 10 mg/ml in acetone applied to the skin and followed in 14 days by 0.2 ml of test concentrations of 500, 250, 150, and 50 µg/ml. The test sites are examined 2, 4, and 6 days after application of the test doses. If the 2-week readings are negative the test concentrations are reapplied and reading is repeated 2 weeks later. The nonspecific inflammatory response can be evaluated with dermal application of 10 µg/ml of sodium lauryl sulfate. The patch test is the only practical test available for demonstrating contact-type allergy. The test substance is applied to a piece of cloth or soft paper which is then placed on intact skin, covered with an impermeable substance, and affixed to the skin with tape. After either 24 or 48 hours, the test material is removed and the underlying skin is examined. The midportion of the upper back or the upper outer arm is preferred. The AL-Test is manufactured in Sweden and consists of a round disk of cellulose affixed to polyethylene-coated aluminum paper. In the United States the virtually nonsensitizing Dermicel tape is preferred. Most test substances require dilution to be nonirritating under patch test conditions. White petrolatum is the preferred diluent.

EVALUATION OF POLYMORPHONUCLEAR LEUKOCYTES AND MONONUCLEAR PHAGOCYTES

Random Migration and Chemotaxis

Random migration of leukocytes by the capillary tube method: buffy coat leukocytes and plasma are centrifuged in the tube, set upright and incubated at room temperature. The migration of leukocytes is measured at the junction of the cell sediment and plasma interface by light microscopy.

The chemotactic response of leukocytes isolated by Dextran-induced sedimentation and of monocytes isolated with a Ficoll-Hypaque gradient is measured in vitro by one of two techniques: the micropore method[23] or the "under agarose" technique.[24] The former is the method of choice because of its increased sensitivity. In the micropore method, leukocytes or monocytes are placed in an upper chamber and migrate toward a chemoattractant placed below a 13-mm-diameter micropore filter. Stainless steel and clear acrylic chambers are available. An optional incubation period allows the fastest migrating cells to reach more than halfway but not completely through the thickness of the filter. Chemotactic preparations for neutrophils include culture supernatants of *Escherichia coli*, zymosan-activated serum, and a synthetic, *N*-formyl-methionyl-leucyl-phenylalanine. For monocytes, zymosan-activated serum or the lymphocyte-derived monocyte chemotactic factor are used as attractants. Cells that migrate to the distal region of the filter paper can be counted by microscopy. Alternative methods of assessment include the "leading front" technique, which measures the distance traveled by the faster cells, and the "cell distance" technique, which measures the distance each cell has traveled from the proximal surface cell monolayer.

Chemiluminescence

Elicitation of chemiluminescence by a phagocytosable particle depends on both cellular activation and intracellular metabolism.[25] Combined Ficoll-Hypaque and Dextran sedimentation yields granulocyte-rich leukocyte preparations. Removal of residual erythrocyte contaminants is important, since colored solutions quench the light emission. Allen et al.[26] first described chemiluminescence in neutrophils phagocytosing opsonized bacteria, and subsequent reports have established polymorphonuclear leukocyte chemiluminescence using opsonized zymosan. The reaction mixtures contain opsonized zymosan and cell suspensions providing a ratio of 100 zymosan particles to one neutrophil. Light emission peaks at 20–30 minutes and is counted in out-of-coincidence mode in a scintillation counter and expressed in counts per minute. An amplified system using the chemiluminescent compound luminol produces enough light so that almost any instrument equipped with a photomultiplier tube can be used. Deficient chemiluminescence responses do not distinguish abnormalities of phagocytosis or intracellular killing. However, the assay appears to be the best screening test available for disorders of phagocytosis or intracellular killing.

Nitroblue Tetrazolium Reduction Test

This assay is simple but very limited in usefulness. Normal neutrophils and mononuclear cells are stimulated, and a yellow redox compound is internalized and then reduced by superoxide ions to a purple insoluble formazan that can be measured quantitatively by spectrophotometry or semiquantitatively by microscopy. Stimulation of phagocytes by particles, chemicals, or bacterial products such as endotoxin leads to the formation of formazan deposits in more than 80% of cells. Phagocytes unable to generate NADPH oxidase in patients with chronic granulomatous disease, lipochrome histiocytosis, or complete absence of G6PD fail to reduce the NBT dye.

Evaluation of Phagocytosis and Bactericidal Activity

Since reduced chemiluminescence may be related to abnormalities of phagocytosis or bactericidal activity, abnormal chemiluminescence results must be followed up by specific assays. For evaluation of the ingestion process it is preferable to measure the accumulation of particles within cells rather than the disappearance of particles from the extracellular medium. The former permits use of saturation quantities of particles and shorter incubation periods. There is marked variation in test results because of the many factors that are involved. Measurement of the extracellular release of β-glucuronidase can be used to assay degranulation. Bactericidal assays are difficult to perform. The method of Maaløe[27] with modifications is usually employed. The test requires prolonged incubation since the disappearance of viability is determined under nonsaturating conditions. Agglutination of phagocytes and bacteria on phagocytes may occur and confuse separation of ingestion from nonspecific adherence. Studies with *Staphylococcus aureus* are facilitated by the availability of lysostaphylin to selectively eliminate extracellular organisms.

Assessment of Phagocyte Mobilization

Epinephrine stimulation, cortisone stimulation, and the Rebuck skin window are available for assessment of phagocytic mobilization in vivo. Epinephrine is administered subcutaneously, 0.4 mg/sq m of body surface, in a 1:1,000 dilution. In normal subjects the total neutrophil count will increase more than 40% above baseline. Intravenous injection of 100 mg of hydrocortisone hemisuccinate should be followed by an increase in the neutrophil count by 2,000/cu mm. Migration of phagocytes into a skin abrasion (Rebuck skin window) permits examination of the acute and chronic inflammatory cell reaction over 24 hours.

EVALUATION OF MAST CELLS AND BASOPHILS

Although mast cells and basophils differ in origin, they have several features in common and are critical for immediate hypersensitivity reactions. Clinically useful tests involve function and not enumeration of these cells.

Skin Testing for Immediate Hypersensitivity

Epicutaneous testing techniques are relatively simple and consist of scratch, prick, and multiple puncture techniques.[28] Usually 1:5 to 1:100 w/v commercial perennial and 1:20 w/v pollen antigens are used. Only a small amount of antigen reaches the surface; therefore, reaction sizes are small and test sensitivity is low. In the scratch testing technique the skin is abraded mechanically and a drop of glycerinated antigen is applied. In the prick puncture technique a drop of glycerinated antigen is applied to the skin and the skin is pricked through the drop with a hypodermic needle or other sharp device. A multiple puncture device is available* that permits the simultaneous application of eight test materials.

Intracutaneous testing techniques are widely used for evaluation of immediate hypersensitivity.[29] They are sensitive, have a high degree of re-

---

*Multi-test; Lincoln Laboratories, Decatur, Ill.

producibility, and require sterile, disposable, plastic 1-ml tuberculin syringes with 26- or 28-gauge needles. Approximately 0.01–0.02 ml of antigen diluted in buffered saline is injected with the syringe bevel down to achieve an initial minimally discernible wheal. Saline and histamine injections are used as controls. Although the antigen used in intracutaneous testing is more diluted than in epicutaneous testing, a much larger volume is inoculated. Intracutaneous testing is 100 to 1,000 times more sensitive than epicutaneous testing against a variety of seasonal and perennial antigens. Sites are read 15–20 minutes after placement of various test substances. The diameter of the wheals and erythema at each site should be measured. Grading has not been standardized but is usually on a scale of 0 to 4+, with grade 0 indicating a wheal of less than 5 mm and grade 4 a wheal of 15 mm or more and with multiple pseudopods.

In *serial dilution end point titration* techniques, serial dilutions of antigens in aqueous buffer are injected intracutaneously in adjacent sites. The dilution that produces the first increment in size of induration is the end point of the test. This method appears to be more precise than conventional skin testing but is too time-consuming for routine clinical use.

Histamine Assay

Histamine is a primary amine with an imidazole ring. It is preformed in mast cells and basophils and released by both allergic and nonallergic stimuli into tissue and blood. While leukocyte histamine release is a research procedure, the measurement of the mediator in serum or blood is useful in some clinical disorders, as discussed in Chapter 8. Histamine can be assayed by several techniques. Bioassay, such as guinea pig ileum contraction, is the classic technique.[30] The fluorometric assay requires multiple extractions and chemical coupling to a fluorophase o-phthalaldehyde[31] and has recently been automated.[32] Double and single isotope assays utilize enzymatic methylation of histamine to N-(3)-methyl-^{14}C-histamine.[33,34] This technique is sensitive to 0.1 ng/ml in normals[35] but higher values of 1–4 ng/ml have been reported by Atkins et al.[36] High-pressure liquid chromatography can be used in a fluorometric assay.[37] A method for measuring urine histamine has been developed based on cation-exchange chromatography, organic solvent extraction, o-phthalaldehyde condensation, and measurement of fluorescence.[38]

Neutrophil Chemotactic Factor Assay

Neutrophil chemotactic factor can be detected in plasma after cold challenge of patients with cold urticaria, following provocation of cholinergic and solar urticaria and in association with antigen bronchial challenge.[39]

The neutrophil-specific factor for cold urticaria has a molecular weight in excess of 750,000 daltons and a neutral isoelectric point. The neutrophil chemotaxis assay is performed using a Boyden chamber.[40] Chemotaxis is quantitated by counting the number of neutrophils migrating to the most distant layer from the cellular surface in five high power fields and is reported as the mean number of cells per ten high power fields.

REFERENCES

1. Böyum A.: Ficoll-Hypaque Method for Separating Mononuclear Cells and Granulocytes from Human Blood. *Scand. J. Clin. Lab. Suppl.*, 1966, p. 77.
2. Oppenheim J.J., Schechter B.: Lymphocyte transformation, in Rose N.R., Friedman H. (eds.): *Manual of Clinical Immunology*, ed. 2. Washington, D.C., American Society for Microbiology, 1980, chap. 28, pp. 233–245.
3. Chess L., Schlossman S.F.: Methods for the separation of unique human lymphocyte subpopulations, in Rose N.R., Friedman H. (eds.): *Manual of Clinical Immunology*, ed. 2. Washington, D.C., American Society for Microbiology, 1980, chap. 27, pp. 229–237.
4. Ross G.D., Winchester R.J.: Methods for enumerating lymphocyte populations, in Rose N.R., Friedman H. (eds.): *Manual of Clinical Immunology*, ed. 2. Washington, D.C., 1980, chap. 26, pp. 213-228.
5. Gupta S., Winchester R.J., Good R.A.: General orientation of human lymphocyte subpopulations. *Clin. Immunol. Immunopathol.* 4:1, 1980.
6. Lampson L.A., Levy R.: Two populations of Ia-like molecules on a human B cell line. *J. Immunol.* 125:293, 1980.
7. De Waele M., Thielemans C., Van Camp B.K.G.: Characterization of immunoregulatory T cells in EBV-induced infectious mononucleosis by monoclonal antibodies. *N. Engl. J. Med.* 304:460, 1981.
8. Bodmer W.F., Bodmer J. (eds.): *Histocompatibility Testing 1977: Proceedings of the Seventh International Histocompatibility Workshop.* Copenhagen, Munksgaard, 1978.
9. Hammerstrom S., Hellstrom U., Perlman P.: A new surface marker on T lymphocytes of human peripheral blood. *J. Exp. Med.* 133:1270, 1973.
10. Raisner Y., Biniaminor M., Rosenthal E.: Interaction of peanut agglutinin with normal human lymphocytes and leukemic cells. *Proc. Natl. Acad. Sci. USA* 76:447, 1979.
11. Einhorm L., Steinitz M., Yefenof E., et al.: Epstein-Barr virus (EVB) receptors, complement receptors, and EBV infectibility of different lymphocyte fractions of human peripheral blood: II. Epstein-Barr virus studies. *Cell. Immunol.* 35:43, 1978.
12. Kohler G., Milstein C.: Continuous culture of fused cells secreting antibody of pre-defined specificity. *Nature* 256:495, 1975.
13. Reinherz R.L., Schlossman S.F.: The differentiation and function of human T lymphocytes. *Cell* 19:821, 1980.
14. Engleman E.G., Levy R.: Immunologic studies of a human T lymphocyte antigen recognized by a monoclonal antibody. *Clin. Res.* 28:511-A, 1980.
15. Amos, D.B., Pool P., Grier J.: HLA-A, HLA-B, HLA-C, and HLA-DR, in Rose N.R., Friedman H. (eds.): *Manual of Clinical Immunology*, ed. 2. Washington, D.C., American Society for Microbiology, 1980, chap. 129, pp. 979–986.

16. Rocklin R.E., Greineder D.K., Lithman B.H., et al.: Modulation of cellular immune function in vitro by histamine receptor-bearing lymphocytes: Mechanism of action. *Cell. Immunol.* 37:162, 1978.
17. Nowell P.C.: Phytohemagglutinin: An inhibitor of mitosis in cultures of normal human leukocytes. *Cancer Res.* 20:462, 1960.
18. Garovoy M.R., Carpenter C.B.: Lymphocyte-mediated cytotoxicity, in Rose N.R., Friedman H. (eds.): *Manual of Clinical Immunology*, ed. 2. Washington, D.C., American Society for Microbiology, 1980, chap. 35, pp. 290–296.
19. Rocklin R.E.: Production and assay of macrophage migration inhibitory factor, in Rose N.R., Friedman H. (eds.): *Manual of Clinical Immunology*, ed. 2. Washington, D.C., American Society for Microbiology, 1980, pp. 246–251.
20. Rocklin R.E., Remold H.G., David J.R.: Characterization of human migration inhibitory factor (MIF) from antigen-stimulated lymphocytes. *Cell. Immunol.* 5:436, 1972.
21. McKoy J.L., Maluish A., Halliday W.J., et al.: Leukocyte migration inhibitory factor and leukocyte adherence inhibition assays, in Rose N.R., Friedman H. (eds.): *Manual of Clinical Immunology*, ed. 2. Washington, D.C., American Society for Microbiology, 1980, pp. 252–260.
22. Fauci A.S.: Assays for suppressor cells, in Rose N.R., Friedman H. (eds.): *Manual of Clinical Immunology*, ed. 2. Washington, D.C., American Society for Microbiology, 1980, pp. 297–303.
23. Maderazo E.G., Woronick C.L.: Micropore filter assay of human granulocyte locomotion: Problems and solutions. *Clin. Immunol. Immunopathol.* 11:196, 1978.
24. Nelson R.D., Quie P.G., Simmons R.L.: Chemotaxis under agarose: A new and simple method for measuring chemotaxis and spontaneous migration of human polymorphonuclear leukocytes and monocytes. *J. Immunol.* 115:1650, 1975.
25. Trush M.A., Wilson M.E., Van Dyke K.: The generation of chemiluminescence (CL) by phagocytic cells. *Methods Enzymol.* 63:462, 1978.
26. Allen R.C., Stjernholm R., Steele R.: Evidence for the generation of an electronic excitation state (S) in human polymorphonuclear leukocytes and its participation in bactericidal activity. *Biochem. Biophys. Res. Commun.* 47:679, 1972.
27. Maaløe O.: *On the Relation Between Alexin and Opsonin.* Copenhagen, Munksgaard, 1946.
28. Kniker W.T., Hales S.W., Les L.K.: Diagnostic methods to demonstrate IgE antibodies: Skin testing techniques. *Bull. NY Acad. Med.* 57:524, 1981.
29. Norman P.S.: In vivo methods of study of allergy, skin, and mucosal tests and interpretation, in Middleton E. Sr., Reed C.E., Ellis E.F. (eds.): *Allergy Principles and Practice.* St. Louis, C.V. Mosby Co., 1978, chap. 16, p. 256.
30. Austen K.E.: Assay of histamine, in Williams C.A., Chase M.W. (eds.): *Methods in Immunology and Immunochemistry.* New York, Academic Press, 1976, vol. 5, p. 126.
31. Shore P.A., Burkhalter A., Cohn V.H. Jr.: A method for the fluorometric assay of histamine in tissues. *J. Pharmacol. Exp. Ther.* 127:182, 1959.
32. Siraganian R.P.: Refinements in the automated fluorometric histamine analysis system. *J. Immunol. Methods* 7:283, 1975.
33. Snyder S.H., Baldessarini R.J., Axelrod J.: A sensitive and specific enzymatic isotopic assay for tissue histamine. *J. Pharmacol. Exp. Ther.* 153:544, 1966.

34. Beaven M.A., Horakova Z.: The enzymatic isotopic assay of histamine, in Rocha E., Silva M. (eds.): *Handbook of Experimental Pharmacology.* Berlin, Springer-Verlag, 1978, vol. 18/2, p. 151.
35. Kaliner M., Shelhamer J.H., Ottesen E.A.: Effects of infused histamine: Correlation of plasma histamine level and symptoms. *J. Allergy Clin. Immunol.* 69:283, 1982.
36. Atkins P.C., Valenzano M., Zweiman B.: Plasma concentrations of histamine measured by radioenzymatic assay: Effects of histaminase incubations. *J. Allergy Clin. Immunol.* 69:39, 1982.
37. Mall L.D. Jr., Hawkins R.N., Thompson R.S.: Fluorometric determination of histamine in biological fluids and tissues by high-performance liquid chromatography. *J. Liquid Chromatogr.* 2:1393, 1979.
38. Myers G., Donlon M., Kaliner M.: Measurement of urinary histamine: Development of methodology and normal values. *J. Allergy Clin. Immunol.* 67:305, 1981.
39. Wasserman S.I., Center D.M.: The relevance of neutrophil chemotactic factors to allergic disease. *J. Allergy Clin. Immunol.* 64:231, 1979.
40. Atkins P.C., Norman M., Weiner H., et al.: Release of neutrophil chemotactic activity during immediate hypersensitivity reactions in humans. *Ann. Intern. Med.* 86:415, 1977.

PART II

Interpretation
of Immunologic
Laboratory Assays

4

Assessment of Immunoglobulins and Other Serum Proteins: Gammopathies

Peter D. Gorevic, M.D.

INTERPRETATION OF THE SERUM PROTEIN ELECTROPHORESIS[1-3]

Methodology

ELECTROPHORETIC TECHNIQUES utilize the charge characteristics of serum proteins to effect separation at various pHs. The method was first introduced in 1937 by Tiselius, who employed an entirely fluid medium, and was able to divide serum proteins into four main fractions, namely, albumin and α-, β-, and γ-globulins.[4] Greater resolution was achieved than with earlier techniques, which had used differential solubility properties for crude fractionations.

Beginning with the use of filter paper by Konig in 1937, and continuing with the introduction of starch block and cellulose acetate in the 1950s, the technique of zone electrophoresis, in which separation is effected on inert solid carriers, permitted even greater resolution of serum proteins, with the further definition of α_1 and α_2 fractions.[5, 6] Utilizing current methodology, serum protein electrophoresis may be done on 10–25 λ (0.1–0.25 μl) serum, i.e., about 7–16 μg protein, and the procedure completed within 1–2 hours.

Cellulose acetate electrophoresis is run in low ionic strength buffer (usually barbital) at a pH of 8.6. The slightly alkaline pH produces a net negative charge on most proteins, causing them to migrate toward the anode (positive electrode). Under these conditions, five distinct bands become apparent, with albumin being most anodal and γ-globulins being slightly cathodal. The position of the latter is due to intrinsic slight positive charge and to streaming with water molecules, which, because of the intrinsic negative charge of the supporting media, develop a positive charge and migrate to the cathode (electro-endosmosis). The five bands may then be fixed in dilute acid, developed with protein-binding dyes such as Ponceaus or Coomassie, the background reduced with a clearing agent, and the electrophoretogram scanned by densitometry to yield a typical tracing. A variety of colorimetric and turbidimetric methods are available for the quantitation of total serum protein. Since the area under each curve of the densitometry tracing is proportional to the amount of protein in this fraction, the tracing may be combined with the total serum protein to yield a calculation of the percent relative contribution, as well as the absolute amount, of each of the five components of normal serum. Results are then compared with normal values established in the particular reference laboratory.

Serum protein electrophoresis (SPEP) (Fig 4–1) provides a scanning overview of the more than 100 known serum proteins but will rarely provide a definitive diagnosis (Table 4–1). Each band represents a composite

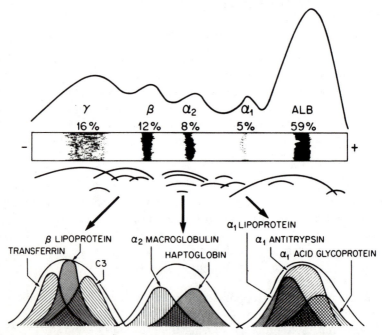

Fig 4–1.—Serum protein electrophoresis. *Top,* cellulose acetate and corresponding densitometry tracing of normal human serum, showing relative contributions of albumin *(Alb),* α_1, α_2, β, and γ bands. Further resolution is seen as multiple precipitin arcs of the corresponding immunoelectrophoresis, run against anti-normal human serum. *Bottom,* major proteins comprising the α_1, α_2, and β bands, showing relative contribution to the total protein content of each band.

TABLE 4–1.—CHARACTERISTICS OF SELECTED SERUM PROTEINS*

PROTEIN	ELECTROPHORETIC MOBILITY	MOLECULAR WEIGHT	CONCENTRATION (MG/DL)	FUNCTION
Prealbumin	Prealbumin	54,980	25	Transport
α_1-Acid glycoprotein		44,100	90	Acute-phase reactant
α_1-Antitrypsin		54,000	290	Acute-phase reactant Protease inhibitor
Transcortin	α_1	55,700	4	Transport protein
α_1-Antichymotrypsin		68,000	45	Protease inhibitor
α_1-Lipoprotein		. . .	40–90 (HDL2) 225 (HDL3)	. . .
9.5S α_1-glycoprotein		308,000	5.5	Acute-phase reactant
Thyroxine-binding globulin		60,700	1.5	Transport protein
Antithrombin III		65,000	29	Protease inhibitor
Zn α_2-glycoprotein	α_1/α_2	41,000	5	Acute-phase reactant
Ceruloplasmin		132,000	35	Transport protein Acute-phase reactant
Inter-α-trypsin inhibitor		160,000	45	Protease inhibitor
Haptoglobin		100,000	170–235	Transport protein Acute-phase reactant
α_2-HS glycoprotein	α_2	49,000	60	Acute-phase reactant
α_2-Macroglobulin		820,000	240–290	Protease-inhibitor
Hemopexin		57,000	80	Transport protein
β-Lipoprotein		. . .	350 (LDL)	. . .
Transferrin		80,000	295	Transport protein
C3		185,000	110	. . .
C4		240,000	30	. . .
Fibronectin	β	350,000	33	. . .
Transcobalamin II		53,900	Trace	Transport protein
Plasminogen		81,000	12	
Fibrinogen		341,000	300	Acute-phase reactant
C1 inhibitor		104,000	24	Protease inhibitor

*Adapted in part from Putnam.[3]

of a number of different constituents, as well as polymorphic variants of a number of these proteins (for example, there are 23 electrophoretically distinct variants of albumin). The amount of each fraction reflects in turn a balance of synthesis and catabolism/loss of the contributing serum proteins, with abnormalities being masked by, or reflecting changes in, each of these parameters. Clinical correlation is of paramount importance, as inconsistencies may reflect only laboratory error or improper handling of serum. For example, if plasma rather than serum is used, fibrinogen may appear as a monoclonal spike at the application point (β-γ region); hemolyzed specimens give artifactual α_2-globulin fractions due to the presence of complexes of haptoglobin-hemoglobin; sera allowed to stand for prolonged periods of time have artifactually low α_1-globulin fractions which could be mistaken for α_1-antitrypsin deficiency. Despite these limitations, however, the SPEP is as essential a part of the initial patient screen as is the blood count.

Immunoelectrophoretic Analysis

Immunoelectrophoresis (IEP) combines electrophoretic separation with immunodiffusion against monospecific antisera.[7–9] The most commonly employed system is that described by Grabar and Williams in 1953, involving diffusion in a gel medium, usually 1%–2% agar or agarose.[10] Five microliters of serum electrophoresed for 2–3 hours and diffused against a polyvalent antiserum to normal human serum will resolve at least 20–30 species of molecules apparent as multiple precipitin arcs. This method clearly reflects the complexity of the α- and β-globulin bands of the SPEP and may be used to define the mobility of specific proteins when compared to arcs obtained with monospecific antisera.

The major value of IEP is in the corroboration and further definition of abnormalities in the γ-globulin region, i.e., gammopathies. Serum is run against a polyvalent anti-immunoglobulin (anti-Ig) and monovalent antisera to all three major Ig classes (IgG, IgA, IgM) as well as to κ and λ determinants of light chains. The configuration of the precipitin line is a function of the concentration of the antigen, its electrophoretic mobility, heterogeneity, and the avidity of the antibody utilized (Fig 4–2). The method can be enhanced by specific stains or labeling techniques and requires only 5 μl of serum, urine, or spinal fluid (concentrated 50- to 100-fold). The

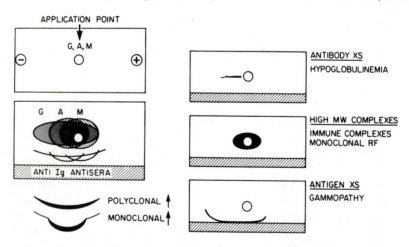

IMMUNOELECTROPHORESIS

Fig 4–2.—Immunoelectrophoresis. Relative electrophoretic mobilities of IgG, IgA, and IgM classes. Different configurations of precipitin arcs are seen in polyclonal and monoclonal hyperimmunoglobulinemia. Artifacts may result from conditions of antibody or antigen excess, and in the sera of some patients with immune complex diseases.

length of the precipitin arc, as well as its position in relation to the antibody trough, is very much influenced by antigen concentration, which is why IEP is an adjunctive procedure and not a substitute for SPEP. Immunoelectrophoresis is also useful in screening for the *absence* of a protein (e.g., IgA, α_1-antitrypsin), though the limit of its sensitivity (0.1 mg/ml) does not make it suitable for exact quantitation.

α-Globulins and Acute-Phase Reactants

Several major serum proteins that are acute-phase reactants (APRs) comprise the α-globulins. These include α_1-antitrypsin, α_1-acid glycoprotein, ceruloplasmin, α_2-macroglobulin (α_2-M), and haptoglobin. Striking elevations of this region of the SPEP may be seen as a nonspecific concomitant of a variety of acute and chronic inflammatory states and may provide clues as to the presence of such underlying conditions, but are rarely of diagnostic consequence.

About three quarters of the α_1 band is α_1-antitrypsin (α_1-AT), with a second major component being α_1-acid glycoprotein (see Fig 4–1). α_1-fetoprotein, other glycoproteins, α_1-lipoprotein, antichymotrypsin, group-specific component (GC) globulin, inter-α trypsin inhibitor, and the transport proteins transcortin and transcobalamin I also have α_1 mobility. Depressed or seemingly flat α_1 may be seen in α_1-AT deficiency, severe hypoproteinemia of various causes, or aged sera. α_1-fetoprotein is usually not a component of adult sera but may be seen in newborn blood or in liver cancer, where it can often be detected by double diffusion. α_1-lipoprotein is an important component of high-density lipoprotein (HDL), is generally present in higher levels in women than in men, and may be elevated in hyperlipoproteinemia.

About half of the α_2 band is constituted by α_2-M and haptoglobin in approximately equal amounts (see Fig 4–1). Striking α_2 elevations may be seen in acute-phase states such as occur with neoplasms, following thermal burns, and in chronic infections. α_2-M is a major protease inhibitor specific for chymotrypsin, trypsin, kallikrein, and various esterases. α_2-M levels are higher in women than men, and elevated values are often seen in patients treated with various estrogens. Particularly striking elevations of α_2-M and the α_2 band are seen in patients with nephrotic syndrome and are due to concomitant inflammation, hypoalbuminemia, and exclusion of these proteins from urine because of their large size. α_2-M is a polymorphic protein that can be directly quantitated by radial immunodiffusion (RID).

The function of haptoglobin is largely understood in terms of its acute-phase biology and its ability to form complexes with free hemoglobin that are rapidly cleared by the reticuloendothelial system (RES). Elevated levels are seen in infections and nephrotic syndrome, where the complexes may also be excluded from urine because of size. Decreased levels are seen with intravascular hemolysis of any etiology.

Other minor constituents of the α_2 band are Zn-α_2 and HS-glycoproteins, antithrombin III, ceruloplasmin, and cholinesterase. These may be quantitated by specific enzyme assays.

The β-Globulins

The major components of the β band are transferrin, β-lipoprotein, and C3 (see Fig 4–1). Transferrin is a major iron transport protein, a determinant of the iron-binding capacity, and thus may be elevated in iron-deficiency states. Elevated β-lipoprotein levels are largely responsible for occasionally striking β spikes in biliary obstruction, pregnancy, and certain nonfasting hyperlipidemias; decreased levels are seen in nutritional disorders such as kwashiorkor. C3 can be quantitated by RID or nephelometry, though more sensitive assays of specific hemolytic activity, or of proteolytic cleavage products generated during complement activation, may also be available in specialty laboratories. C3 may be elevated as an APR or depressed in disease states accompanied by classical or alternative pathway complement activation. Fibrinogen, also a β-globulin, is an APR and a major determinant of the erythrocyte sedimentation rate (ESR). Other β-globulins are C4, hemopexin, plasminogen, factor XIII, C1 inhibitor, and transcobalamin II, all of which require specific assays for quantitation. Because of the heterogeneity of immunoglobulins, many, especially those belonging to the IgM and IgA class, may have β mobility on the SPEP. IgA elevations often account for the so-called β-γ bridging characteristic of certain hepatopathies, notably Laennec's cirrhosis.

Evaluation of the γ Region

Excepting small contributions from fibrinogen and C-reactive protein (CRP) in the β-γ region, the γ portion of the SPEP is entirely Ig. As such, it is an excellent screen for the status of humoral, B cell–mediated immunity. In contradistinction to albumin, which has a relatively restricted electrophoretic mobility, the γ-globulins appear diffuse on the normal SPEP, reflecting in turn synthesis by diverse clones of B cells. Whereas albumin abnormalities are largely restricted to decreased levels in association with deficiency or protein-losing states, both qualitative and quantitative abnormalities may become apparent on careful inspection of the γ region.

It should be recalled that about 85% of the total serum Ig is IgG, so that quantitative abnormalities in the γ region largely reflect this class (Fig 4–3). IgA contributes 10%–15% and IgM 5%–10%. The relative level of each

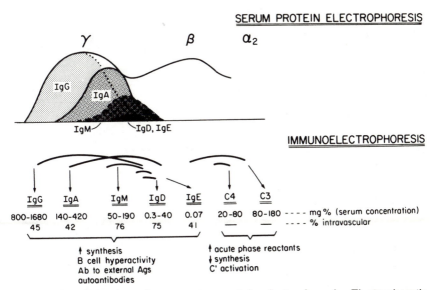

Fig 4–3.—Gamma region on serum protein electrophoresis. Electrophoretic mobility and relative contributions of the five immunoglobulin classes and of complement components, C3 and C4. Increased or decreased levels of these proteins may result from changes in synthetic rate or catabolism/consumption.

Ig class is determined to a considerable extent by the age of the patient and the type of immune response being monitored, and to a lesser extent by sex. IgM is the major Ig in the serum of a neonate, as the maternal placentally transferred IgG decays over the first 21 days post partum and a child's IgG does not reach adult levels until the early teens; IgA may be the predominant antibody class if immunization via the gastrointestinal or upper respiratory tract is monitored. IgM levels are slightly higher in women than in age-matched men, apparently due to X-linked determinants of baseline levels.

Serum γ-globulin levels show wide fluctuations, depending on the state of immunization of the individual. Decreased levels reflect either depressed synthesis or increased catabolism. The former may be due to lack of, or abnormal, B cells, or the presence of suppressive factors (e.g., as are generated in multiple myeloma); the latter may be due to losses via the gastrointestinal or genitourinary tract.[11]

Increases in the γ region on the SPEP are defined as polyclonal, oligoclonal, or monoclonal, depending on the type of clonal expansion characteristic of the particular underlying disorder (Fig 4–4). Polyclonal hyperglobulinemia is characteristic of hyperimmunized states or chronic infections. Oligoclonal banding is occasionally seen in acute infections or

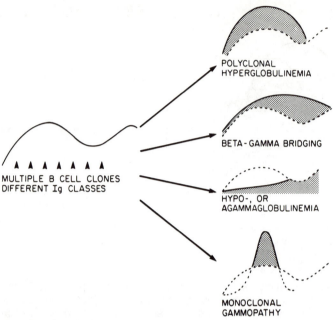

Fig 4–4.—Common abnormalities of the γ region. Polyclonal and monoclonal gammopathy, hypoglobulinemia, and β-γ bridging.

accompanying certain immunologic disorders such as multiple sclerosis (MS), reflecting the predominance of this pattern in the CNS. Monoclonal hyperglobulinemia is an indication of dysproteinemia and requires evaluation to define the specific gammopathy. Autoimmune disorders, such as systemic lupus erythematosus (SLE), are both polyclonal and oligoclonal in that there is both a marked increase in B cell synthetic rate as a manifestation of disease activity, as well as specific antibody activities (e.g., various antinuclear antibodies) of restricted heterogeneity. In Sjögren's syndrome, high levels of circulating immune complex (CIC) material and hyperglobulinemia may be accompanied in some cases by the development of frank B cell dyscrasia, usually of the IgM class. In both diseases high titers of CIC accumulate in serum, partly owing to defective immune specific clearance by RES Fc receptors, considerably influencing the SPEP, as well as potentially causing artifacts on the IEP.

Relevance of the ESR[12]

The ESR provides a screen for SPEP, much as the latter complements the more detailed evaluation of gammopathy by IEP and the direct quantitation of Ig. The value of the ESR is its speed and simplicity; its major utility is in the serial monitoring of patients with inflammatory disorders. Its major disadvantages are lack of specificity and relative insensitivity. The standard method for determination of ESR is that of Westergren, in which 2 ml of venous blood is mixed with 0.5 ml of sodium citrate and allowed to sediment from a 200-mm level in a graduated tube over an hour. Normal values vary somewhat but are usually less than 20–25 mm/hr with higher norms in women and older individuals.

The ESR is directly determined by the viscometric properties of plasma. Highly asymmetric proteins or high molecular weight aggregates may cause profound elevations, accounting for the primary role of fibrinogen in causing acute-phase elevations, as well as often striking elevations in certain macroglobulinemias in which the IgM may be complexed to other serum proteins because of specific antibody activity. Elevated ESRs seen in acute or chronic infections are due to (1) increased fibrinogen, with lesser contributions by ceruloplasmin, haptoglobin, and other APRs, and to (2) polyclonal hyperimmunoglobulinemia.

The contribution of each of these determinants may be evaluated on the routine SPEP.

A relatively normal or inappropriately low ESR in the context of inflammatory disease may be due to viral infection without tissue necrosis or rouleaux formation and red blood cell (RBC) aggregation, as is seen, for example, in polycythemia. The ESR may be moderately increased in anemia, particularly if it is accompanied by shape abnormalities of RBCs such as macrocytosis, spherocytosis, or anisocytosis. Consequently, the complete evaluation of an abnormal ESR includes a blood cell count, peripheral smear morphology, SPEP, and direct determination of Ig and possibly fibrinogen levels.

INTERPRETATION OF THE URINE PROTEIN ELECTROPHORESIS[13–15]

Methodology

Normal urine protein excretion is 40–80 mg/day (average, 50 mg/day), though this may increase significantly as a normal variant following exercise. Urinary protein is a composite of the ultrafiltration of serum and molecular species either originating from the urinary tract or protein fragments proteolytically cleaved or spontaneously developing in urine. Serum ultrafiltrate is predominantly serum albumin (MW 67,000), which normally accounts for over 25% urinary protein excretion, and a group of low molecular weight serum proteins broadly distributed throughout the SPEP (α_1

mobility: acid glycoprotein, α_1-AT, α_1-lipoprotein; α_2 mobility: HS glyco-protein, Zn α_2-glycoprotein, GC globulin, transferrin, hemopexin; β mo-bility: C4, β_2-microglobulin). The low molecular weight proteins are a diverse group of proteins, many of which, such as the Tamm-Horsfall (uromucoid) protein and IgG/IgA and Ig fragments, are of tubular or interstitial origin.

Standard methods will not detect normal proteinuria, and a 100- to 200-fold concentration of a 24-hour collection is required. This may be achieved by vacuum dialysis, dialysis against a high osmotic gradient (e.g., polyvinylpyrrolidone), or by direct precipitation with ammonium sulfate. In most clinical laboratories, ultrafiltration through a filter with a low molecular weight cutoff to remove salts is employed. Concentrated normal urine examined by cellulose acetate electrophoresis has a prominent albumin peak, low α_1, α_2, and β bands, and a low, diffuse γ region (Fig 4–5). The latter is composed primarily of Ig light chains, which characteristically have a faster mobility than the serum γ band.

Significant proteinuria is screened for in the routine dipstick, which develops a colorimetric reaction specific for albumin and will not detect low molecular weight proteinuria of tubular origin or the presence of monoclonal Ig light chains. Suspicion of these proteins should be raised first on the clinical evaluation of the patient and requires determining the 24-hour urine protein excretion. Screening tests of limited utility are precipitation

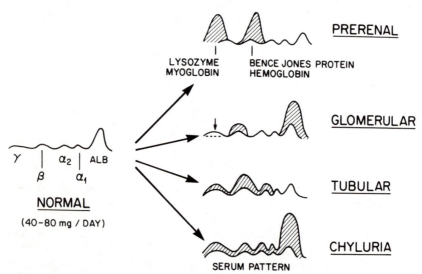

Fig 4–5.—Four major patterns of proteinuria. Abnormalities on the urinary protein electrophoretogram due to prerenal, glomerular, and tubular proteinuria, as well as the pattern seen in chyluria.

with 5% sulfosalicylic acid or other reagents, or colorimetric methods such as the biuret reaction. Significant proteinuria is usually defined as an excretion rate of more than 500 mg/day, with the nephrotic syndrome defined as an excretion rate of more than 4 gm/day. At an excretion rate of more than 1 gm/day, little concentration (10–50×) of urine is required.

Decisions as to more detailed testing should be determined by the clinical status of the patient, and correlated with a complete urinalysis for sediment, pH and osmotic gradient, concomitant abnormalities of the SPEP, and, in selected instances, recognition of systemic complement activation or the presence of specific serologies.

IEP Analysis

Further evaluation of proteinuria by zone electrophoresis or IEP, or both, is indicated if a lymphoproliferative disorder or plasma cell dyscrasia is suspected, and definitely if a monoclonal protein is detected in serum. It should be also a part of the evaluation of all cases of suspected or definite amyloidosis. Urinary electrophoresis of concentrated urine specimens should be correlated with simultaneously collected serum samples; the methodology and reagents are essentially those described previously for serum.

Urinary IEP is used to assess the relative contribution of albumin and globulin fractions and to search for monoclonal proteins. Tubular diseases are characterized by a decreased contribution of albumin and a diffuse increase in α- and β-globulin fractions. This may be confirmed by noting the presence of predominantly low molecular weight proteins (<30,000 daltons) when concentrated urine is examined by modalities such as SDS-polyacrylamide gel electrophoresis. Specific proteins such as β_2-microglobulin, lysozyme, or retinol-binding protein are increased in urine and may be assessed directly by immunodiffusion or specific assays (Table 4–2).

Urinary IEP is used to search for Ig light chains, and as such, its sensitivity is a direct function of the specificity and avidity of the anti-κ and

TABLE 4–2.—LOW MOLECULAR WEIGHT PROTEINS CHARACTERISTIC OF TUBULAR PROTEINURIA

PROTEIN	ELECTROPHORETIC MOBILITY	MOLECULAR WEIGHT	SERUM CONCENTRATION (mg/dl)
α_1-Microglobulin	α_1	25,000	3–6
Retinol-binding protein	α_2	21,000	4.5
β_2-Microglobulin	β_2	11,800	0.15
Ig light chain	β	22,500	. . .
β Trace protein	β	31,000	0.4
γ Trace protein	Post-γ	11,500	. . .
Lysozyme	Post-γ	14,600	. . .

anti-λ antisera employed. Many reference laboratories employ antisera raised against free light chains (e.g., Bence Jones proteins), as well as antibodies against light chain determinants of isolated Igs absorbed of heavy chain reactivity. Urinary IEP should be done with serum as a control. In the presence of large amounts of monoclonal or polyclonal light chains, it may be necessary to test the urine at two dilutions to compensate for concentration artifacts.

Following the diagnosis of a glomerulopathy, tubular disorder, or monoclonal light chain, these diagnostic modalities may be used serially to follow the status of the patient. Spontaneous or induced remissions of urinary polyclonal or monoclonal light chain disease may be monitored by 24-hour protein excretion, direct quantitation, and IEP analysis. Light chain excretion has been used as an index of transplant rejection in patients with kidney homografts. It should be noted, however, that quantitation of urinary light chains by RID may be inaccurate because of the presence of polymers and cross-reacting fragments.

Ultrafiltration from Serum and Glomerular Pathology

Prerenal proteinuria is due to marked increase in specific serum proteins which may occur in pathologic states, overwhelming in turn the normal resorptive capacity of the proximal tubular epithelium. Examples are severe hyperimmunoglobulinemia (polyclonal or monoclonal), myoglobinuria and hemoglobinuria, and the spillage of glycoproteins in association with certain neoplasms. This mechanism is also operative in lysozymuria, due to increased monocyte turnover seen in myelomonocytic leukemia and, to a lesser extent, chronic myelocytic leukemia. Similarly, large loads of monoclonal light chains are responsible for the appearance of Bence Jones protein in urine. The electrophoretic pattern of prerenal proteinuria is thus variable, depending on the protein involved (see Fig 4–5), and may be accompanied by elevated levels of APRs on the SPEP.

Glomerular proteinuria reflects to a varying degree the loss of the sieve function of the glomerular basement membrane. In minimal change disease, as well as in proteinuria due to increased hydrostatic pressure (e.g., renal vein thrombosis, constrictive pericarditis), albumin continues to be selectively ultrafiltered, accompanied by small contributions from low molecular weight α_1 (AT, acid glycoprotein) and β (transferrin) mobility proteins. In orthostatic proteinuria, the glomerular pattern is obtained when the individual is upright and lost when the individual is recumbent.

Serial urinary protein electrophoresis has been used as a screen for determining the selectivity of glomerular proteinuria.[16] This is more accurately assessed by the so-called Selectivity Index, in which the urinary clearance (UV/P) of a series of proteins is plotted against their molecular weights to obtain a ratio. Generally, the relative clearances of IgG (MW 160,000) and transferrin (MW 80,000) will suffice for routine measurements. In conditions such as minimal change disease, the former is essentially excluded from urine. Exercise and prerenal proteinuria tend to be moderately selective, whereas in glomerular infiltrative diseases, such as amyloidosis, the urinary electrophoretogram may resemble closely the SPEP due to complete loss of selective filtration. The clinical value of these coefficients has been questioned, however, and their major use seems to be in monitoring therapeutic trials.

Urinary Proteins

Tubular proteinuria is due to the loss of normal protein resorptive function of the proximal tubular epithelium. It was first described in cadmium poisoning and may be recognized in a number of conditions characterized by proximal tubule dysfunction. These include Fanconi syndrome, lysozymuria, and light chain disease. In these conditions the urinary electrophoretogram characteristically shows a marked decrease in the albumin/globulin ratio compared to glomerular proteinuria (see Fig 4–5). There may be striking increases in α_2 and occasionally in β-globulins, and a relative increase of low molecular weight proteins such as β_2-microglobulin and retinol-binding protein in urine. Lysozyme, if present, is seen as a band with post-γ mobility. The evaluation of tubular proteinuria should include other tests of proximal tubule function, including a search for renal glycosuria, amino aciduria, and hyperphosphaturia, this triad comprising the renal Fanconi syndrome. Proximal bicarbonate tubular defects are apparent as a lowering of the bicarbonate threshold, determined during the induction of metabolic alkalosis.

A fourth form of proteinuria is that accompanying postrenal obstruction, most commonly involving the lymphatics and due to neoplastic infiltration. Chyluria is characterized grossly by a high lipid content and can be seen by Sudan black staining of urine. Albumin levels in urine approximate those of serum. Clotting of samples is due to the presence of fibrinogen which is usually excluded from urine because of its size, even in the most poorly selective glomerular proteinuria.

Proteinuria accompanying renal failure may thus have multiple etiologies, depending on the nature and severity of the pathology. Albuminuria is common, and the extent and contribution of tubular proteinuria and endogenous proteins of renal origin (Tamm-Horsfall, IgA) depend on the degree of tubular and interstitial disease, as well as on the complicating factors of prerenal and postrenal disease and concomitant anemia, hyperviscosity, coagulopathy, and metabolic derangements.

Immunoglobulins and Light Chains[17]

Under normal conditions, plasma cells synthesize approximately equal amounts of heavy and light chains; consequently, only traces of free light chains may be found in the serum. When light chains are produced in excess or exclusively, in so-called light chain disease, they appear transiently in the blood and are rapidly cleared by glomerular filtration, after which they are catabolized by the tubules.[18] The half-life of free light chains is thus only several hours, compared to that of intact Ig, which may be measured in days. Whereas the catabolism of free light chains occurs primarily in the kidney, that of Ig occurs at various sites, prominently in the liver. The serum half-life of Ig light chains is profoundly lengthened after nephrectomy, whereas that of intact IgG is unaffected.[11]

Increased levels of polyclonal light chains in serum may be found in association with inflammatory states, diseases such as systemic lupus erythematosus (SLE) and rheumatoid arthritis (RA), in lymphoproliferative disorders, and in renal failure.[19] Normal polyclonal light chain excretion in the urine is 1.2–7.2 mg/day (mean, 3.4 mg/day), and most of this has β-γ mobility. Diffuse elevations in the β-γ region may be seen in tubular disorders and have been used as a parameter for monitoring acute renal transplant rejection (Fig 4–6). Free light chain in the serum has the same electrophoretic mobility as in the urine but is usually not seen because of rapid clearance. In rare instances, monoclonal light chains may exist in serum as dimers or larger polymers, or both; they may accumulate and may be apparent as moderate-sized β spikes on the SPEP.

Normal urine contains small amounts of IgG (1.2–6.5 mg/day; mean, 3.2 mg/day) and IgA (0.7–2.7 mg; mean, 1.4 mg/day), presumed to originate by local synthesis in the genitourinary tract. Increased levels may accompany renal autoimmune disease, occasional interstitial involvement in plasma cell dyscrasias, or severe glomerular proteinuria. IgM and IgD are not seen in normal urine.

Both normal and pathologic urine may occasionally contain fragments of Ig[20] as well as intact Ig and light chains. Fc fragments may be found normally using sensitive techniques (mean, 0.2 mg/day) and may increase in postexercise urine samples. Other Ig fragments (light chain half-molecules corresponding to VL and CL) may occur in association with plasma cell dyscrasias and are believed to arise either by aberrant secretion or proteolysis occurring in the acid environment of the genitourinary tract. These fragments have provided important information regarding Ig structure, but are not clinically significant. Occasionally they are responsible for a biclonal light chain peak or double arc on IEP. Their more rapid diffusion in agar may complicate the evaluation of urine by RID to quantitate Ig.[21]

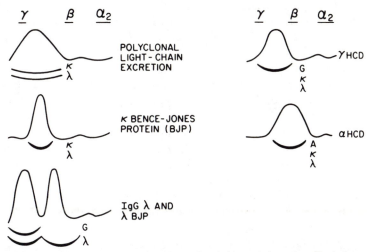

Fig 4–6.—Urinary immunoelectrophoresis of dysproteinemias. Protein and immunoelectrophoretic patterns of concentrated urine seen in polyclonal light chain excretion are compared with patterns seen in various dysproteinemias.

Bence Jones Proteins

Whereas polyclonal urinary light chains may cause diffuse elevation of the β-γ region and react both with anti-κ and anti-λ antisera, monoclonal light chains give a dense band on electrophoresis and react with only one type of light chain constant region determinant. The term "light chain disease" refers to the presence of a monoclonal light chain in the urine; diagnosis of a light chain disease necessitates a search for underlying plasma cell dyscrasia.[22] The term is used synonymously with Bence Jones protein, although the heat test originally used to detect this protein did not require concentrating the urine and would miss 20%–30% of monoclonal urinary light chains by current criteria. The heat test is particularly insensitive if the monoclonal light chain is present in concentrations below 145 mg/dl.

The heat test for Bence Jones protein involves development of a precipitate at 40–60 C on adding acid (usually acetate) to urine to give a pH of 5.0. This precipitate redissolves on boiling. Occasional false positive results are obtained if there are large quantities of polyclonal light chains present, as in inflammatory states and chronic renal insufficiency. Certain other proteins, such as transferrin or hemoglobin, may occasionally give false positive results and the test may be difficult to interpret in the context of considerable albuminuria (e.g., amyloid kidney).

A combination of cellulose acetate electrophoresis and IEP performed on a concentrated specimen of urine is considerably more reliable and sensitive. By these methods, the incidence of monoclonal light chain excretion in myeloma rises from 45% (heat test) to 75% or higher. Bence Jones proteins may exhibit variable electrophoretic mobility; most are β-γ, though some may be found in the γ or α_2 regions. Heterogeneity among Bence Jones proteins reflects differences in primary amino acid sequence (variable region), carbohydrate content, and the presence of dimers and tetramers in urine. Kappa Bence Jones protein polymers are either disulfide or noncovalently linked, whereas λ polymers are primarily disulfide bonded. Thirty percent of patients with Bence Jones proteinuria also have low molecular weight Bence Jones protein fragments, some of which are cleaved at the VC joining region, presumably in urine. These fragments may give extra spikes with faster mobility or double arcs on IEP. Double arcs on IEP may also be due to the concomitant presence of the intact monoclonal Ig and the Bence Jones proteins (see Fig 4–6). A monoclonal arc with anti-Fc antiserum without Bence Jones proteins should suggest γ heavy chain disease (γ-HCD). Bence Jones protein in both serum and urine without a monoclonal arc with anti- μ, -γ or -α heavy chain antisera should prompt a search for IgD or IgE myeloma with appropriate antisera (see Fig 4–6).

The amount of Bence Jones protein in urine is a function of the rate of synthesis and renal catabolism. The former is often followed to assess response to therapy; the latter is considerably influenced by glomerular and tubular pathology. In many cases of primary amyloidosis as well as in myeloma complicated by amyloid, fragments of Ig light chain, consisting of variable region and differing amounts of the constant region, may deposit in glomeruli (as well as elsewhere) in a fibrillar form to produce a nephrotic syndrome. This form of amyloid is designated AL, or "light-chain related" amyloid. Certain light chains appear to have structural amyloidogenicity, manifested generally by inversion of the usual 2:1 kappa-lambda ratio (Table 4–3) and by an increased incidence of certain Vλ subgroups most notably I and VI. Consequently, a careful study of the urine for light chain and λ determinants is always indicated in a proteinuric patient found to have amyloid on renal biopsy.[23, 24]

A direct toxic role of Bence Jones proteins in the induction of proximal renal tubular acidosis and the adult Fanconi syndrome is indicated by the fact that all cases of myeloma and Fanconi syndrome described to date have had Bence Jones proteinuria and, conversely, by the fact that renal disease with tubular atrophy and interstitial fibrosis occurs with increased frequency in light chain myeloma, as well as in IgD myeloma, which is almost always accompanied by Bence Jones proteinuria.[25, 26] That many patients with Bence Jones proteins never develop renal disease suggests that toxicity may relate more to the quantity of Bence Jones protein produced, certain structural features, or local factors that influence precipitation, polymerization, and crystallization. Thus Bence Jones proteins may be associated with spillage of other low molecular weight proteins characteristic of tubular proteinuria.

The differential diagnosis of Bence Jones proteinuria (see Table 4–3) includes multiple myeloma, Waldenström's macroglobulinemia (approximately ⅓ cases), amyloidosis (up to 100% "primary," depending on the series), lymphomas, and μ-HCD. The presence of idiopathic Bence Jones proteins for long periods without progression to clear-cut neoplasm has been described but is uncommon.[27]

ACUTE-PHASE REACTANTS

Definition

APRs are a functionally diverse, electrophoretically heterogeneous group of plasma proteins whose levels increase significantly, and sometimes dramatically, in response to a variety of states that have in common the production of inflammation and tissue damage (Fig 4–7). The acute-phase response is seen in acute bacterial infections, following surgery, in burns, tissue infarction, and acute and chronic inflammatory states. It may be a prominent feature of certain neoplasms, and it is a concomitant of pregnancy. Although fever and leukocytosis are found in some of these states, it is not clear that they are requisite for the sequential changes of APRs, and they may in fact be dissynchronous. Other subtle changes that accompany some acute-phase responses include depressed immune responses and RES function; these effects may be consequences rather than causes of the release of some of these proteins.[12]

Many APRs are glycoproteins and were originally identified by increased hexose content of sera following acute inflammation. They have a rapid

TABLE 4–3.—DIFFERENTIAL DIAGNOSIS OF
BENCE JONES PROTEINURIA*

Multiple myeloma
    IgG—2.3/1
    IgA—2.3/1
    IgD—1/9
    IgE—2/1
Light chain myeloma—1/1.2
Waldenström's macroglobulinemia (2.3/1)
Amyloidosis (AL) (1/1.3)
Lymphoproliferative diseases
With "benign" monoclonal gammopathy
Idiopathic

*Ratios in table are κ/λ.

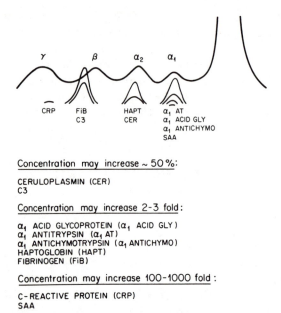

Concentration may increase ~ 50 %:

CERULOPLASMIN (CER)
C3

Concentration may increase 2-3 fold:

α_1 ACID GLYCOPROTEIN (α_1 ACID GLY)
α_1 ANTITRYPSIN (α_1 AT)
α_1 ANTICHYMOTRYPSIN (α_1 ANTICHYMO)
HAPTOGLOBIN (HAPT)
FIBRINOGEN (FiB)

Concentration may increase 100-1000 fold:

C-REACTIVE PROTEIN (CRP)
SAA

Fig 4–7.—Electrophoretic mobilities and relative increases of major serum acute-phase reactants.

serum turnover and appear to be synthesized de novo in response to me-diators released from the site of tissue injury, thus explaining in part lag periods prior to their appearance in blood. The inflammatory potential of injected leukocyte extracts initially suggested a central role for the poly-morphonuclear leukocyte in the pathogenesis of the acute-phase response; more recent studies have more clearly implicated mononuclear cells, pri-marily macrophages.

Different APRs vary considerably in the time course and magnitude of response to tissue injury.[28] All increase after a lag period, which may vary considerably, depending on the particular model under study. Serum col-lected during the lag period has been shown to be capable of transferring the induction of APR between animals or in organ culture systems, which constitutes indirect evidence of the presence of inducing factors. The acute-phase response is characteristically transient, except in chronic in-flammation. Virtually no information is available regarding the factors re-sponsible for turning off the acute-phase response.

In recent years the central role of the liver has become apparent. He-patic weight increases during the acute-phase period and multiple struc-tural and functional changes have been documented. These were shown initially in liver slices or via liver perfusion experiments, and more recently in hepatocyte culture systems. Many, if not all, the APRs are synthesized by the liver, as has been shown by in vitro organ culture, immunohistology, hepatocyte culture, and, most recently, by translation of hepatocyte-derived DNA and specific probes into cell-free systems.

Pathogenesis (Fig 4–8)

Current concepts regarding pathogenesis are largely based on detailed studies of two APRs, the serum amyloid A protein (SAA) and CRP. The serum level of both of these proteins may increase dramatically (up to a thousandfold) following acute inflammation. Both have provided model systems for analysis of the kinetics and biologic significance of the acute-phase response.[29, 30]

Tissue injury initiates a series of events, including activation of the complement and coagulation cascades, which lead in turn to the accumulation of mononuclear cells and polymorphonuclear leukocytes at the site. Release of lysosomal hydrolases from polymorphonuclear leukocytes perpetuates this process and leads to generation of chemotactic factors. Macrophages discharge mediators specifically affecting target cell populations, including bone marrow cells, lymphocytes, and hepatocytes. Release of mediators such as endogenous pyrogen may be triggered by various stimuli (e.g., endotoxin, lymphokines), apparently via distinct receptors on the macrophage. The term interleukin-1 has been used to designate a group of these mediators, notably including endogenous pyrogen (EP), lymphocyte-activating factor (LAF), and SAA stimulating factor (SAA-SF), which have similar molecular weights and chemical properties.[31] Whether this term refers to a single species or a closely related group of molecules is not yet clear. Some of these factors stimulate the synthesis of APR, definitely in the liver

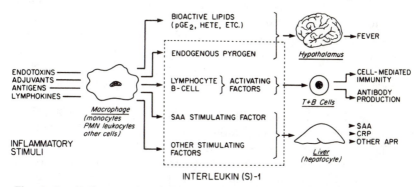

Fig 4–8.—Pathogenesis of the acute-phase response. Stimuli producing acute-phase responses are listed. Note the central roles of the macrophage, interleukin-1, and hepatic production of acute-phase proteins.

and perhaps elsewhere, possibly via membrane receptors on target cells like the hepatocyte, by direct incorporation into the cell and derepression of genome.

APRs are rapidly exported to the blood, appear in some instances (e.g., CRP) to accumulate at the site of tissue injury, and may serve to maintain homeostasis. Some (e.g., fibrinogen) are involved in clotting, many are protease inhibitors (α_1-AT, α_1-antichymotrypsin), and others are known transport proteins (ceruloplasmin, haptoglobin) (see Table 4–1); the relevance of these diverse functions to their physiologic function in tissue injury is unknown. Depressed synthesis of other serum proteins (e.g., albumin, thyroxine-binding prealbumin) also occurs during acute-phase reactions and may be reflected on the SPEP. Many of these proteins are also normally synthesized primarily in the liver, and it may be that low levels are due in some part to the diversion of biosynthetic machinery to the elaboration of APR. Rapid clearance of many APRs from the circulation may be due to localization extravascularly at sites of tissue injury or specific clearance via glycoprotein receptors on hepatocytes.

Methods of Quantitation: Turnover and Synthetic Rates

Modest elevations of C3 during the acute-phase response may be masked if there is significant concomitant systemic complement activation, as occurs, for example, in SLE. Ceruloplasmin is responsible for over 95% of copper transport, binds 6–8 atoms of copper per molecule, and may be determined by its blue color or by oxidase activity; depressed levels may occur in Wilson's disease, other liver diseases, nephrotic syndrome, sprue, kwashiorkor, and in neonates. Biologic properties in vitro that may be significant for the acute-phase response include inhibition of the auto-oxidation of some lipids and a role as scavenger of oxygen-derived free radicals.

Elevations two to three times normal may be seen with α_1-acid glycoprotein, α_1-AT, α_1-antichymotrypsin, haptoglobin, and fibrinogen (see Fig 4–7). These proteins may be measured by antigenic assay (RID or electroimmunoassay) or by their functional properties (protease inhibitory activity, peroxidase activity, or by direct measurement of hemoglobin-haptoglobin complexes).

The half-life (t ½) of most APRs have been determined by following the disappearance of iodine-labeled proteins in normal volunteers; only limited information is available regarding turnover during the acute-phase response. The t ½ of most of these proteins in normals is on the order of 3–5 days, considerably shorter than that of albumin (14.8 days) or IgG (21 days).[32] Some (e.g., SAA) appear to turn over even more rapidly.

The total body pool of several APRs appears to be significantly extravascular, a feature which may be an important variable in acute inflammatory states. Equilibration kinetics between body compartments has not been extensively studied. For these reasons, increased levels of individual APRs may not be fully reflected in the serum concentration. Synthetic rates have been measured in organ cultures by injecting labeled amino acids into the animal before sacrifice and isolation of the liver. The earliest studies of this sort were done with fibrinogen and demonstrated that the rate of synthesis may increase more than 400%, even though increases of only 270% were documented by direct quantitation in serum.[32]

CRP and SAA Protein

C-reactive protein is a serum protein normally present in a concentration of less than 1 µg/ml. Levels may rise several hundredfold during an acute-phase response, peaking at 2–3 days and falling rapidly. The appearance of this protein was initially monitored by its ability to form a complex with the C-polysaccharide of pneumococcus cell wall. More recent screening methods employ a capillary precipitin reaction or RID; detailed serial studies have utilized radioimmunoassay (RIA).

CRP is one of a group of molecules designated pentraxins because of their tendency to form pentamers that have a typical doughnut shape on cross section by electron microscopy. The molecule is phylogenetically old and appears to have served the functional role of antibody in some primitive fish. It resembles certain immunoglobulins in its phosphoryl choline binding properties; complexing with polycations has been shown to activate the classical pathway of complement in vitro. Among other in vitro properties that may be relevant to its physiologic role are binding to damaged cell membranes, platelets, and to a subset of T lymphocyte and other mononuclear cells. CRP may also subserve a primitive immune response as an opsonin for bacteria. Immunohistologic studies have shown it to localize at sites of tissue injury and vasculitis.[30, 33]

SAA protein is an α_1-globulin that is present in concentrations of less than 50 µg/ml in normal serum. Its name derives from the fact that it shares amino terminal homology with the major tissue protein (AA) in secondary amyloid deposits incurred as a consequence of a variety of chronic infectious or inflammatory conditions. The nature of the assumed precursor-product relation of these two proteins (SAA → AA), however, is still unclear.

SAA is a polymorphic apolipoprotein that circulates as a complex with HDL3. Levels rise acutely following an inflammatory stimulus, peaking within 24 hours to levels as high as 1 mg/ml. Rapid decline is seen in man with successful antibiotic treatment of bacterial infection. SAA has been shown to be synthesized by hepatocytes by immunohistologic study of liver, by assay of organ homogenates, by serial measurements in the supernatants of short-term hepatocyte cultures, and, most recently, by isolation of the mRNA for SAA from the liver. Studies on the mouse have shown that SAA mRNA goes up 500-fold following endotoxin injection, peaking at about 9 hours and accounting for as much as 2.5% of total hepatic protein synthesis.[29, 30]

SAA is a sensitive marker of the acute-phase response and is synthesized in response to SAA-SF, a macrophage-derived inducer that appears to be identical to interleukin-1. Whether other triggers exist for hepatocyte SAA synthesis or whether SAA may also be synthesized elsewhere remains to be defined. Some evidence suggests that SAA may subserve an important immunoregulatory function; much remains to be learned regarding its physiologic function, however.

Interpretation in Specific Disease States

Although an understanding of APRs is useful for the interpretation of the ESR and SPEP, specific measurements of these proteins have little clinical utility. Panels of APR have been measured serially in studies to determine the extent of tissue injury (e.g., in myocardial infarction), as a monitor for the development of septic complications (e.g., abscesses) in acute infection, to follow the postoperative state, and in attempts to define tumor loads and the presence and extent of metastases, all with limited success. Similarly, the distinction between bacterial and viral infections (without associated tissue necrosis), between inflammatory (e.g., RA, ankylosing spondylitis) and noninflammatory (e.g., degenerative joint disease) conditions can usually be made on clinical grounds and rarely require measurement of APRs. Serial measurement of the ESR is equally valuable for monitoring response to therapy in diseases such as polymyalgia rheumatica. Nevertheless, the development of RIAs for CRP and SAA has provided important model systems for the elucidation of the acute-phase response, and RIAs may assume greater diagnostic and therapeutic utility as our understanding of the pathogenesis of these disorders increases.

α_1-ANTITRYPSIN

Current Concepts

α_1-Antitrypsin is a 54,000-dalton molecular weight glycoprotein that is the major constituent of the α_1-globulin band of the SPEP. Under normal circumstances, it accounts for the bulk of antiprotease and 90% of the trypsin inhibitory capacity of serum. Normal blood levels are 100–200 mg/dl and are increased in inflammatory states, carcinoma, after surgery, and in pregnancy. Levels are elevated in patients taking estrogens and oral contraceptives, as well as following exposure to cigarette smoke.

Although defined initially in terms of its trypsin inhibitory function, it is likely that the major antiprotease activity of α_1-AT physiologically is directed against elastase activity of polymorphonuclear leukocytes and, to a lesser extent, macrophages. This is based on the known association of α_1-AT deficiency with chronic obstructive pulmonary disease (COPD), and the fact that elastase instilled intratracheally duplicates the lesions of emphysema in experimental animals.[34]

α_1-AT is similar to other APRs in being synthesized in the liver and having a relatively rapid half-life (4–5 days). It is also similar in being polymorphic when assessed by techniques such as isoelectric focusing. The exact basis and significance of this polymorphism are somewhat unclear but may relate to the composition and length of four carbohydrate side chains on the protein backbone of the molecule.

The association of α_1-AT deficiency with COPD was first described in 1963,[35] and its association with childhood cirrhosis was described in 1968.[36] Homozygous α_1-AT deficiency is associated with early-onset panlobular emphysema with a predilection for the lower lobes, usually manifesting during the third to fourth decades of life. The disease is more prevalent in women, and there is considerable evidence that heterozygotes also have enhanced susceptibility to chronic bronchitis and emphysema. Conversely, most patients with centrilobular COPD seen in general practice do not have α_1-AT deficiency. About 15% of homozygous α_1-AT-deficient children will develop liver disease, which manifests initially as a cholestatic jaundice during the first 3–4 months of life. This usually subsides, to be followed by the development of cirrhosis in late childhood or early adolescence. Liver biopsy specimens show inclusion bodies in the hepatocytes containing material with α_1-AT immunoreactivity but apparently devoid of sialic acid. Similar findings have been noted in biopsy specimens from some adults with α_1-AT and COPD. It is thus apparent that not all α_1-AT-deficient patients develop clinical disease.[37]

Methods of Quantitation

In heterozygous α_1-AT deficiency, serum protein levels are 60% of normal; in homozygous deficiency states, serum protein levels are less than 10% of normal. The latter is usually grossly apparent on the SPEP as a marked diminution, or even absence, of the α_1-globulin band. α_1-AT can be quantitated antigenically by rocket electroimmunoassay[38] or functionally as the ability to inhibit the enzymatic activity of a unit quantity of trypsin added to the serum sample. The latter is termed trypsin inhibitory capacity (TIC) and is expressed in milligrams of trypsin inhibited per milliliter of sample. Electroimmunoassay assumes that each polymorph of α_1-AT is recognized with equal avidity by a given antiserum. As further phenotypes of the protein are recognized and defined, this assumption may prove incorrect. Improperly handled sera may give a falsely low TIC due to loss of inhibitory activity; thus, correlation with antigenic analysis is important in the definition of a true deficiency state.

Phenotype determination is done by acid (pH = 4.95) starch gel electrophoresis of serum, which displays the protein as a series of bands of different electrophoretic mobility that may be compared with known standards. M is the most common phenotype, and Z and S the phenotypes most often associated with deficiency states. Z and S phenotypes are displaced cathodally relative to the more common phenotypes and also have slower electrophoretic mobility. Often they are not well visualized in this system, and further verification by crossed immunoelectrophoresis or immunofixation methods is necessary. The former combines starch gel electrophoresis with IEP in agarose-containing anti-α_1-AT antiserum and displays each phenotype as an eliptical precipitin arc extending into the agarose. Additional resolution of some α_1-AT phenotypes has been achieved by agarose gel electrophoresis.[39] By these means, over 20 alleles have been defined that are inherited codominantly and that comprise the so-called protease inhibitor (PI) locus.[40]

Interpretation in Specific Disease States

Elevated α_1-AT levels occur in acute-phase responses and in patients taking estrogens; this effect may be blunted in the context of a preexisting, undetected heterozygous deficiency state. Aside from screening studies, routine determination of α_1-AT is rarely indicated. Such surveys have shown no increase of α_1-AT deficiency or specific phenotypes in populations of COPD patients, and no definite association with other disease states. The major indications for α_1-AT determinations are atypical emphysema in a young person or nonsmoker or as part of the evaluation of childhood cirrhosis. A normal α_1-AT level, determined either antigenically or by TIC, effectively excludes deficiency states. Depressed levels are compatible with heterozygous or homozygous deficiency; the latter requires quantitation of levels less than 10% of normal. Relevance of depressed α_1-AT to disease state may then be confirmed by phenotype analysis, demonstrating most commonly the Z allele; in childhood cirrhosis, further corroboration is provided by the characteristic liver biopsy and immunohistologic findings.

SERUM IMMUNOGLOBULINS: PATTERNS

Polyclonal Hyperglobulinemia

Diffuse elevation of the γ region on the SPEP (see Figs 4–3, 4–4) is one of the most common and least specific abnormalities seen in large screening studies of pathologic sera. Because of the globular nature and symmetry of the Ig molecule, hyperglobulinemia rarely suffices to account for elevation of the ESR, though it is often a concomitant of inflammatory conditions in which significant increases in fibrinogen may occur. Polyclonal hyperglobulinemia appears to result from multiple mechanisms. In chronic liver diseases and infections, major factors are chronic antigenic stimulation, B cell mitogenicity of endotoxins, and loss of normal hepatic filter function for the gastrointestinal tract via the portal system. In autoimmune diseases, such as SLE, there is considerable evidence for intrinsic B cell hyperactivity, which may be associated with loss of T cell suppressor activity during periods of disease activity. Both in the chronic inflammatory liver disorders (chronic hepatitis, cirrhosis) and in the collagen diseases, specific antibodies may appear (antinuclear antibodies, rheumatoid factors, etc.) and are due to activation of multiple clones of B cells. In the case of antiglobulin-producing B cells, these also appear to be expressed to a highly limited extent in normal subjects. Polyclonal hyperglobulinemia may also be seen in association with chronic inflammatory states (e.g., inflammatory bowel disease, sarcoidosis), neoplasms, and occasionally in an idiopathic form, which may be familial or premalignant.

Generally, polyclonal hyperglobulinemia reflects the IgG class; elevations of IgA and IgM must be several-fold normal to be apparent and are more accurately quantitated by RID. High IgA levels may be a concomitant of clinical or subclinical infection of the upper respiratory or genitourinary tracts or of inflammatory bowel disease. An IgM response is characteristic of primary immunization, and elevated IgM levels may be seen early in certain infections, notably hepatitis A. IgM levels may be elevated in primary biliary cirrhosis. The characteristic antimitochondrial antibody seen in this disorder involves this Ig class.

Occasional patients are found to have hyperglobulinemia of relatively restricted mobility without a clear-cut M spike. This phenomenon is thought to represent activation of a limited number of B cell clones and is termed "oligoclonal gammopathy." It is occasionally seen in early infections or accompanying the CSF oligoclonal gammopathy that is characteristic of MS. Whether IEP is used for further evaluation of polyclonal hyperglobulinemia depends solely on the clinical status of the patient. IEP is especially indicated if cryoglobulinemia or a heavy chain disease is suspected, as these entities may only manifest as a diffuse elevation of the γ region of the SPEP.

Monoclonal Gammopathies[41-43]

Screening surveys have made it clear that the prevalence of monoclonal gammopathy in the general population, as well as the association with various disease states, is greater than had been previously appreciated.[44] It is also apparent that patients with lymphoproliferative disorders and plasma cell dyscrasias may present with just an abnormal antibody activity or M spike due to a monoclonal Ig, long before the development of overt disease. The IEP patterns seen in polyclonal hyperglobulinemia are compared with patterns seen in various dysproteinemias in Figure 4–9.

M proteins are usually apparent as narrow peaks in the γ region of the SPEP. In multiple myeloma, there may be depression of the remainder of the γ region due to suppressive factors elaborated, or induced by, the ma-

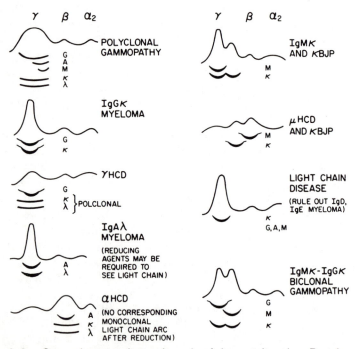

Fig 4–9.—Serum immunoelectrophoresis of dysproteinemias. Protein and immunoelectrophoretic patterns seen in polyclonal hyperglobulinemia are compared with patterns seen in various dysproteinemias.

lignant plasma cells (see Fig 4–4). IgA M spikes tend to be more cathodal and may be found in the β or even α_2 regions. This is rarely of diagnostic utility, however, as the electrophoretic range of IgG is considerably greater than, and overlaps that of, IgA and IgM. Generally, monoclonal gammopathies are clearly seen on the densitometry tracing of the routine cellulose acetate electrophoresis of serum. Therefore, IEP is seldom indicated if no M spike is seen on the SPEP. Exceptions to this rule are the heavy chain diseases, in which the SPEP is often normal, and certain cases of light chain disease or IgD myeloma. In these instances, the decision to proceed to IEP should be guided by the clinical assessment of the patient.

The further workup of a monoclonal gammopathy includes an initial screen quantitation of IgG, IgM, and IgA by RID or nephelometry, and IEP of serum and urine. Quantitation of Ig is not done primarily to assess the level of the abnormal Ig, but rather to determine the level of normal Ig. Profound hypoglobulinemia of normal Igs is a major predisposing factor to infection in the plasma cell dyscrasias. Quantitation of abnormal Igs by RID is often erroneous because (1) polyclonal antisera to normal heterogeneous Ig determinants may not recognize the monoclonal protein with equal avidity, so that the M protein may diffuse further into the agar than equal amounts of normal Ig; (2) IgM macroglobulins may be present in both 7S monomers and 19S polymers[45] and IgA gammopathies as multiple polymers, creating several rings of different diameters on the RID plates; (3) the M protein may have antibody activity and may circulate bound to antigens as high molecular weight immune complexes (e.g., mixed cryoglobulins, rheumatoid factors) that precipitate near the well and don't diffuse out; (4) Fc fragments of Ig, as seen in heavy chain diseases, are recognized by standard anti-heavy chain antisera, but diffuse more rapidly and give falsely elevated levels.[21]

IEP should be performed in all instances of monoclonal gammopathy with monospecific antisera to γ, α, and μ heavy chain, as well as κ and λ light chain determinants. Polyvalent antisera to pooled Ig or normal human serum are often run for comparison. High-titer, rigorously absorbed antisera are essential, with known controls run in parallel. Because of their rarity, IgD and IgE myeloma proteins are not usually included in the IEP but can be screened by double diffusion of serum against anti-D and anti-E antisera. One third of IgD myelomas[46] and all cases of IgE myeloma reported to date have been found to have sizable M spikes on the SPEP.

The location and configuration of the precipitin arc are functions of the concentration and electrophoretic homogeneity of the protein. Sera containing large amounts of M protein may need to be run at more than one dilution, as excess antigen will cause precipitate to form at the edge of the trough; rarely, it is necessary to concentrate a sample to visualize low levels of a monoclonal Ig or light chain (see Fig 4–2). IgM and IgA arcs are narrower and occur closer to the point of application than IgG, making it somewhat harder to appreciate subtle areas of restricted mobility. Electrophoresing the sample for longer periods of time may clarify monoclonality. Normal levels of IgM approach the level of sensitivity of the IEP (1 mg/ml), so that the IgM precipitin arc may not be seen at all in cases of slight hypoglobulinemia. Cryoproteins may precipitate at room temperature to give an oval ring around the well due to high molecular weight complexes and a faint linear anodal precipitin due to antibody excess, as only a small amount of IgG electrophoreses into the agar (see Fig 4–2). Aberrant arcs may result from complexing of IgA to other serum proteins via free disulfide groups, a phenomenon not unusual in IgA myeloma.

Intact M proteins should exhibit homologous restricted mobility with either κ or λ light chain. An occasional sample containing a polymeric Bence Jones protein may exhibit two bands on the SPEP and a double light chain arc, indicating the simultaneous presence in serum (or urine) of the intact Ig and light chain; the electrophoretic mobility of the latter is usually closer to the β region than the former. The heavy chain diseases are a group of gammopathies in which an abnormal heavy chain fragment is produced, characterized by a deletion of all or part of the variable region of the molecule or hinge, or both. Bence Jones proteins may occur also in μ-HCD, but are not seen in α- or γ-HCDs.[47, 48] Heavy chain fragments, being structurally similar to Fc fragments, may exhibit γ-β (γ-HCD), α_2-β (α-HCD), or even α_1 (μ-HCD) mobility, but no homologous light chain arc is detectable on serum IEP. The heavy chain of IgA and occasionally of IgM may mask light chain determinants, making them inaccessible to standard anti-light chain antisera and giving the appearance of a heavy chain disease on IEP. Often, a "phantom" lucency is seen along κ or λ light chain arcs corresponding to the monoclonal α or μ arc. In these cases, prior reduction of serum with 2-mercaptoethanol or dithiothreitol will reveal the light chain arc. Conversely, finding a monoclonal light chain arc without heavy chain arc of similar configuration or mobility, especially if λ, should suggest the possibility of IgD myeloma or primary or myeloma-associated amyloidosis. Over 90% of IgD myelomas are λ, and 90% are associated with Bence Jones proteinuria.[46] Even when a clearly myelomatous marrow aspirate is lacking,[23] most cases of AL amyloid in some series have λ Bence Jones proteins. Occasional serum samples are found to have biclonal and, rarely, triclonal gammopathies. Most commonly, these are of undetermined significance, although they may be associated with myeloma or lymphoproliferative disease.[49]

Urine electrophoresis on a concentrated specimen will confirm the presence of Bence Jones proteinuria in many instances. Once the condition is identified, further workup for secondary renal involvement by multiple myeloma or macroglobulinemia should be pursued.[25] Bence Jones proteins are found in up to 80% of cases of myeloma and in 30%–50% of cases of Waldenström's macroglobulinemia; κ-λ ratios generally reflect normal serum ratios (2:1); idiopathic Bence Jones proteinuria that may be an abortive variant of myeloma has also been described. Heavy chain fragments typically occur in the urine in α- and γ-HCD[50, 51]; in μ-HCD the μ chain fragment is restricted to the serum, and Bence Jones proteins may be detected in urine.[52]

The differential diagnosis of IgG and IgA monoclonal gammopathy in-

TABLE 4–4.—Gammopathies

MALIGNANT
  Multiple myeloma
    Balanced heavy and light chain → G, A, D, E
      paraproteins
    Light only → light chain disease
    Excess light chain production → paraprotein +
      Bence Jones proteinuria
  Plasmacytoma
  Plasma cell leukemia
  Monoclonal IgM
    Waldenström's macroglobulinemia
    Chronic lymphocytic leukemia (CLL)
    Lymphosarcoma
    Hodgkin's and non-Hodgkin's lymphomas
  Amyloidosis (AL)
    With myeloma (↑ incidence in light chain
      disease)
    "Primary"
  Heavy chain diseases (deleted H chain fragment)
    γ-HCD (atypical lymphoma)
    μ-HCD (CLL variant)
    α-HCD (intestinal lymphoma)
  Associated with nonreticular neoplasms
    Colorectal > prostate > breast

SECONDARY
  Rheumatic diseases
    Sjögren's syndrome, other
  Hepatobiliary diseases
    Chronic hepatitis, cholecystitis, other
  Chronic infection or inflammation
  Cold agglutinin disease (IgMκ)
  Papular mucinosis (IgG subclass 1λ)
  Immunodeficiency diseases

UNDETERMINED SIGNIFICANCE
  Transient
  Persistent

---

cludes multiple myeloma and heavy chain disease, while that of IgM gammopathy includes Waldenström's as well as secondary cases of macroglobulinemia (Table 4–4). Both may be associated with a variety of chronic inflammatory and neoplastic states[53–55] or can occur as what Kyle has termed "gammopathy of undetermined significance,"[56] i.e., gammopathy without apparent underlying disease. The significance of this entity(ies) is still somewhat unclear, but some long-term follow-up studies have suggested that a significant percentage of these patients eventually develop multiple myeloma or amyloidosis.[56, 57] Since M proteins are increasingly common after age 50,[44] detection in a young person is of more consequence clinically and requires even more careful follow-up.

Further evaluation of a defined monoclonal gammopathy should include a complete blood cell count and bone marrow aspiration and biopsy. If the suspicion of myeloma is high, repeated aspirations, as well as a bone survey and scan, may be indicated if the initial examination is negative. About 1% of cases of multiple myeloma are associated with plasma cell leukemia, and equal percentages with skeletal or extramedullary plasmacytomas. Features suggestive of malignancy are depressed serum albumin levels or hypoglobulinemia, anemia, and the concurrent presence of Bence Jones proteins or osteolytic bone lesions.[58–60]

The diagnosis of heavy chain disease is suggested by the characteristic clinical picture. γ-HCD often presents as a macroglobulinemia or atypical lymphoma, with prominent adenopathy[50]; α-HCD presents as intestinal lymphoma,[51] and μ-HCD occurs in the setting of chronic lymphocytic leukemia (CLL).[52]

If an IgM monoclonal protein is identified, the patient should be evaluated for Waldenström's macroglobulinemia. The diagnosis of this disease is often difficult, and it is increasingly apparent that the spectrum of its presentations may be quite broad.[61] Often these patients present with symptoms due to antibody activity or abnormal physical properties of the macroglobulin (Table 4–5). The differential diagnosis should include CLL, diffuse lymphocytic lymphosarcoma, and histiocytic lymphoma. A serum viscosity test may be indicated if symptoms suggestive of hyperviscosity syndrome are present or if the IgM level is greater than 2.0 gm/dl.[62] A significant percent of IgA myelomas also are associated with the development of hyperviscosity, by virtue of polymer formation and binding to other serum proteins. Additional evaluation should include a search for rheumatoid factor activity and cryoglobulinemia.

Lastly, in the evaluation of a monoclonal gammopathy it should be recalled that as many as one third of patients will be asymptomatic. Lack of a definitive diagnosis on initial evaluation should not dissuade the clinician from careful follow-up and serial evaluations to observe for the development of overt malignancy.

TABLE 4–5.—SYMPTOMS RELATED TO
GAMMOPATHIES

Hyperviscosity syndromes (IgM > IgA > IgG)
Cryoglobulinemia
Bence Jones proteins
   Myeloma kidney
   Fanconi syndrome ($\kappa > \lambda$)
Clotting and bleeding disorders
   Anti-factor VIII, IX (IgM + IgG)
   Antifibrin monomer (IgG)
Infections (hypogammaglobulinemia)
Hemolytic anemia—cold agglutinin disease
   (IgMκ)
Amyloidosis (VL $\pm$ CL; $\lambda > \kappa$)
Xanthoderma, xanthotrichia (IgG antiriboflavin)
Hypercholesterolemia, xanthomatosis
   (IgA; IgG anti-β-lipoprotein)

Hypoglobulinemia

Hypoglobulinemia has been variously defined in different published series. It is generally accepted, however, that IgG values below 0.3 mg/dl on the standard SPEP or below 250 mg/dl on RID correlate with symptomatology, most notably an increased incidence of infections.

The evaluation of hypoglobulinemia depends on the age of the patient and differs significantly in children and adults. Childhood hypoglobulinemia is frequently congenital and should be interpreted in light of the normal ontogeny of the humoral immune system in young children. Thus IgG deficiency may manifest only after age 1–2 months, when placentally transferred maternal IgG is catabolized and the infant IgG level fails to rise. At age 1 year, the IgM level should be 75% of the adult level, whereas the IgA level is only 20%.

The evaluation of hypoglobulinemia in infancy is essentially the evaluation of immune deficiency and is discussed at length elsewhere in this volume (see Chap. 13). Most common is selective IgA deficiency, a heterogeneous group of disorders representing intrinsic B cell and abnormal suppressor activities, which are often asymptomatic.[63] IgA deficiency is rarely apparent on the SPEP, but may be seen as the absence of an α arc on IEP of serum. RID will confirm the diagnosis. Less common causes of hypoglobulinemia in infancy are X-linked, or Bruton's agammaglobulinemia, which usually manifests very early and is characterized by an absolute lack of B cells, and common variable hypogammaglobulinemia, in which B cells are present and the abnormality is one of terminal B cell differentiation or T cell regulatory function.

In children, the diagnosis may be suggested by recurrent infections, severe dermatologic allergies, or early development of autoimmune disease.

Further evaluation includes the study of lymphocyte subsets, lymph node or tonsilar morphology, and functional assays of cell-mediated immunity.

Hypoglobulinemia in adults is almost always acquired. Defective synthesis may be seen in malignancies such as multiple myeloma or CLL. Ten percent of patients with myeloma will have significant hypogammaglobulinemia, usually with concomitant Bence Jones proteins. Hypoglobulinemia is not unusual in amyloidosis, and a drop in serum Igs has been stated in older literature to herald the development of tissue amyloid in myeloma patients. IgA deficiency may be seen as an isolated finding in collagen diseases such as SLE and RA.

Protein-losing states may result in clinically significant hypoglobulinemia due to losses via the gut, kidney, or skin (Table 4–6). These diagnoses are suggested by the clinical symptoms (e.g., malabsorption, nephrotic syndrome, severe burns). Synthetic rates are normal and turnover studies usually unnecessary. Further evaluation of hypoglobulinemia in the adult should thus include quantitation of Ig levels, urinary and serum IEP, and a careful search for etiologies of protein-losing enteropathy or nephropathy.

CRYOGLOBULINS

Cryoglobulins are serum Igs that possess the property of reversible precipitation in the cold. They are laboratory concomitants of a variety of infectious, neoplastic, and autoimmune diseases, are often of diagnostic importance, can be used to follow the course of specific therapies, and appear to play a role in the immunopathogenesis of some disease states characterized by clinical vasculitis and immune complex glomerulonephritis.

Current Concepts

Cryoglobulins may be simple (type I) or mixed (types II and III) (Table 4–7).[64] The former consist of only one Ig class and are invariably monoclonal proteins, almost always IgG or IgM. Well documented cases of IgA myeloma and Bence Jones proteins that are cold-precipitable have been

TABLE 4–6.—HYPOGAMMAGLOBULINEMIA

Decreased synthesis
  Primary immunodeficiency
  B cell dyscrasia
    Myeloma, chronic lymphocytic leukemia, other
Increased loss
  Renal (nephrosis)
  Gastrointestinal (protein-losing enteropathy)
  Skin (burns)

TABLE 4–7.—CLASSIFICATION OF CRYOGLOBULINEMIA*

	TYPE I	TYPE II	TYPE III
Definition	Mono	Mono–poly	Mixed poly
SPEP	IgM ~ IgG >> IgA M spike	IgMκ Variable	IgM-IgG Broad Ig peak
RF activity	No	Yes	Yes
Serum concentration	May be high	Usually high	Usually Low
Precipitate	Flocculent	Gelatinous	Gelatinous
Time appears	< 24 hr	Variable	Up to 7 days
Cryotemperature	Variable (may be low)	Variable	Variable
CF	Rare	Frequent	Frequent
Cryoprecipitability	Intact Molecule BJP cryoprecipitate rare	Complex IgM-IgG	Complex IgM-IgG
Symptomatic	Few	⟷	Most
Purpura	±		+ + + +
Arthralgias	±		+ + + +
Raynaud's phenomenon	+ + + +		+ +
Gangrene	+ + + +		+
Renal disease	Endomembranous deposits (immune complex nephritis rare)	Immune complex nephritis; endomembranous deposits	Immune complex nephritis
Course	Often rapid	May be rapid if nephropathy or neuropathy	
Associated conditions	B cell neoplasms	B cell neoplasms, idiopathic	Connective tissue diseases, infections, liver diseases, idiopathic

*SPEP, serum protein electrophoresis; RF, rheumatoid factor; CF, complement fixation; BJP, Bence Jones proteins; mono, monoclonal; poly, polyclonal.

described but are relatively rare. Simple cryoglobulins are often present in copious amounts and are readily apparent on refrigeration of more than 5 cc of serum. They are almost always associated with overt multiple myeloma or macroglobulinemia, comprising 5%–15% of the M proteins seen in these states. Cryoprecipitability is very dependent on pH, ionic strength of the medium, and solute concentration, requires an intact molecule, and can be abolished by minor chemical modifications of side groups. Three theories have been suggested to explain cryoinsolubility among these proteins: (1) Specific structural abnormalities might result in conformational changes which favor polymerization as large aggregates in the cold. This might result from specific V region, or idiotypic, sequences, possibly reflecting a common antibody activity (i.e., cross idiotype). It might also be due to abnormal or variant constant region determinants. (2) All Igs are to some minor extent cryoinsoluble, and these proteins are an exaggeration of a normal but general solubility phenomenon. (3) Simple cryoglobulins may in fact not be simple at all, but may have weak antibody activity, directed either against their own Fc determinants or perhaps against other serum proteins, the avidity of which is increased in the cold. Some evidence for the first and last possibilities has accumulated from the observation of a greater incidence of certain subclass (IgG2) and light chain (IgMκ) determinants among these proteins than would be expected from chance, as well as antiglobulin activity when sensitive RIAs are employed. In some instances cryoprecipitability has been related to the presence of sialic acid residues on the Ig, or to binding to lipoproteins. In other well studied cases, however, no detailed physical, chemical, or sequence anomaly has been identified; these findings, as well as the observation of small amounts of cryoglobulins in normal individuals, have suggested the second possibility.[65]

Mixed cryoglobulins (MCs) consist of more than one class of Ig. These proteins have been shown in most instances to be in fact reversibly cold-insoluble rheumatoid factor, with antiglobulin activity invariably being in the IgM fraction. The IgM may be monoclonal (type II), in which case it is IgMκ in over 95% of cases, or polyclonal (type III). Mixed cryoglobulins are cryoprecipitable by virtue of the complexing of IgM with IgG. Kinetic analyses have shown that the binding constant of the complex at room temperature is considerably lower than that of most rheumatoid factors and relatively low for antigen-antibody reactions in general. Thus, it is easy to dissociate these complexes by adding concentrated salt solutions or dilute acetic acid. The individual components may then be separated on the basis of size (19S IgM and 7S IgG), and will only cryoprecipitate when added together again in the cold. Rheumatoid factor is detectable in the IgM fraction of all MCs, either by agglutinating activity or by more sensitive

RIA. Heterologous IgG may be substituted, but preferential cryoprecipit-ability with autologous IgG, and perhaps with certain subclasses (IgG3) of IgG, seems to be the rule.[65]

Many MCs are able to activate complement in vitro and are associated with evidence of systemic hypocomplementemia in vivo. In most cases, both in vitro and in vivo, selective activation of the classical pathway is found, though occasionally only involving early components (C1, C2, C4). This limited activation may be due to the normal limiting influence of the regulatory proteins, factor 1-H and C4-binding protein.[66] This phenome-non may explain why occasional patients are found to have cryoproteins, striking depression of C4, and yet little in the way of symptoms. Mixed cryoglobulins composed only of IgA and IgG have been shown to selectively activate the alternative pathway of complement. The role of complement in the phenomenon of cryoprecipitability is unclear, with some suggestion that the two properties are separable by physicochemical characteristics.

In recent years it has become clear that antibody activities other than classic rheumatoid factor antiglobulin activity directed against IgG Fc may be found in MCs.[67] This was first demonstrated as antigenic and structural cross-idiotypy among IgMκ monoclonal components of MC. It was also suggested by the finding that some IgM reacted best (and occasionally ex-clusively) with an IgG fraction when the latter was complexed to a partic-ular antigen.[68] Specific DNA and anti-DNA antibody activity is enriched in MC occurring in association with SLE, and HBsAg and anti-HBsAb in MC occurring during the prodrome of hepatitis B virus (HBV) infection, in HBsAg carriers, in patients with chronic active hepatitis (CAH), and in patients with vasculitic manifestations of HBV infection resembling clinical polyarteritis nodosa. Specific anti-idiotype activity in the IgM fraction of MCs has been shown, specifically directed against F(ab)$_2$ determinants of autologous and heterologous cryoglobulin IgG. In some cases, these are directed to antibody binding sites specific for HBsAg.[69]

Such observations suggest a direct role for MCs in the immunopathoge-nesis of disorders in which they occur. Corroboration for this concept has come from the observation of systemic complement activation when the serum of patients with known cryoglobulinemia is studied, as well as the finding of specific cryocomplex components and, in some instances, specific antigen and antibody activity in vasculitic or renal lesions when they are examined immunohistologically.

Methods of Collection and Identification

Blood is clotted at 37 C and the serum separated warm. If whole blood is allowed to sit for too long a time at 4 C, a significant amount of cryoprecipitate may come down with the clot. This common error may lead to underestimates of the level of cryoglobulin present and even the false appearance of hypoglobulinemia on the SPEP if the cryoprotein comprises a significant percent of the total Ig. The amount of serum collected should be determined in part by the clinical status of the patient and the index of diagnostic suspicion. Generally, 10–20 ml of blood will suffice.

If a cryoglobulin is present, the serum rapidly becomes opalescent at 4 C and a precipitate should be evident the next day; occasionally 3–7 days of observation may be necessary. Voluminous flocculent precipitates that appear quickly and often above 4 C are likely to be simple myeloma proteins or macroglobulins; occasionally cryocrystalglobulinemia may be seen, usually with IgG monoclonal proteins. Gelatinous precipitates are more likely to be MCs and may vary considerably in amount. Rarely, serum will gel rather than precipitate at low temperatures.

The cryoprecipitate is then spun down and washed with cold phosphate-buffered saline until the yellow color of contaminating plasma is no longer apparent. A whitish opalescent suspension of precipitate mixed in PBS should clarify completely when run under warm running tapwater. Erythrocytes and residual fibrin can be removed by spinning the solution at 37 C, and then reprecipitating the cryoglobulin from the supernatant. The level of the cryoprecipitate can be determined by assessing the cryocrit in a hematocrit tube spun at 4 C, or by directly quantitating the total protein in the washed precipitate.

Isolated cryoprecipitate is tested by double diffusion against antisera to γ, μ, and α heavy chain determinants and albumin, and the plate is developed at 37 C. A precipitin line with antihuman albumin indicates that further washing of the cryoprecipitate is necessary. IEP of the whole serum and the purified cryoprecipitate may show the presence of M proteins and establish the light chain type of the IgM component of an MC. Monoclonality may be somewhat difficult to establish in a purified cryoprotein by IEP because of the tendency of IgM to precipitate near the application well at room temperature. In these cases, fractionation in 0.1M acetic acid may be necessary. Over 95% of monoclonal IgM in MC has κ light chains, more specifically belonging to the VκIIIb subgroup.

The serum evaluation of a patient with cryoglobulinemia should include IEP, quantitative Igs, a test for rheumatoid factor activity (often found in strikingly high titers), and a complement screen consisting of at least C3 and C4 determinations (Fig 4–10). Antinuclear serologic studies should be performed if the patient has suspected SLE, and HBsAg and HBsAb should be assayed if there is clinical or laboratory evidence of liver disease or other reason to suspect HBV infection. If particularly high levels of IgM

MIXED CRYOGLOBULINEMIA

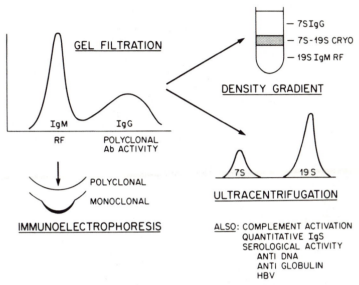

Fig 4–10.—Further workup of a patient with mixed cryoglobulinemia, following the identification of a cryoprotein in blood.

are found, serum viscosity should be measured. As MCs are in fact circulating immune complexes, more sensitive measures of immune complex levels (C1q binding, Raji cell, etc.) are rarely necessary.

Clinical Correlations (Table 4–8)

A search for cryoglobulins is indicated in any patient with clinical or pathologic vasculitis and/or glomerulonephritis of undetermined etiology. They may be found in the evaluation of collagen diseases, particularly when associated with vasculitis. Associations with lupus nephritis, rheumatoid vasculitis, Sjögren's syndrome, and polyarteritis nodosa have been noted in well studied case reports and small series.[63, 66] Cryoglobulins should also be sought as part of the workup of occult infection, as they may be seen in patients with subacute bacterial endocarditis, chronic HBV infection, and diseases such as leprosy, malaria, and syphilis. Any monoclonal cryoglobulin, whether simple or mixed, should suggest the possibility of underlying lymphoproliferative disease or plasma cell dyscrasia. This may require a bone marrow examination or, in the case of IgM monoclonals, considera-

TABLE 4–8.—CRYOGLOBULINEMIA: CLINICAL
ASSOCIATIONS

Infections
  Viral
    Infectious mononucleosis (29%–95%)
    Cytomegalovirus postperfusion syndrome (34%)
    Acute hepatitis B (± non-A, non-B) prodrome
      (77%)
    Chronic HBV infection (46%)
    Adenovirus infection
  Bacterial
    Subacute bacterial endocarditis (up to 90%)
    Lepromatous leprosy (± erythema nodosum) (up
      to 95%)
    Acute poststreptococcal nephritis (50%–75%)
    Lymphogranuloma venereum
    Postintestinal bypass with arthritis
    Syphilis (15%–38%)
    ?Lyme arthritis; extra-articular disease (up to
      45%)
  Fungal
    Coccidioidomycosis
  Parasitic
    Kala-Azar
    Toxoplasmosis
    Tropical splenomegaly syndrome
    Echinococcosis
    Malaria
    Schistosomiasis
Autoimmune diseases
  Systemic lupus erythematosus (16%–89%)
    Nephritis, hypocomplementemia
  Rheumatoid arthritis (20%–25%)
    Vasculitis, Felty's syndrome
  Polyarteritis nodosa (HbsAg positive and negative)
  Sjögren's syndrome (± macroglobulinemia)
  Scleroderma (Raynaud's phenomenon)
  Sarcoidosis
  Thyroiditis
  Henoch-Schönlein purpura (47%–64%)
  Endomyocardial fibrosis (41%)
Lymphoproliferative diseases
  Macroglobulinemia (primary and secondary)
  (Atypical) lymphoma
  Chronic lymphocytic leukemia
  Immunoblastic lymphadenopathy
Renal disease
  Proliferative glomerulonephritis
Liver diseases
  Cirrhosis (Laennec's, postnecrotic)
  Biliary cirrhosis (up to 90%)
  Chronic hepatitis
Familial
Essential—syndrome of purpura, arthralgias, nephritis

tion of CLL, lymphoma, and angioblastic lymphadenopathy in the differential diagnosis.

Careful studies have shown low levels of cryoglobulins in most normal individuals. Levels of 10–80 μg/ml (mean, 30 μg/ml) have been found when 50-ml aliquots of blood were studied, and a significant number of these found to be MCs.[64] These cryoproteins are universally polyclonal and provide some substantiation for the concept that they may be part of the spectrum of a normal solubility phenomenon. Pathologic cryoproteins occur at cryocrits of 1% or higher, corresponding to protein concentrations above 0.2 mg/ml. Therefore, methods described for screening for cryoproteins in pathologic sera would not be sufficiently sensitive to pick up normal levels of cryoglobulins.

Clinical symptoms that should suggest checking for cryoglobulins are palpable purpura, severe cold intolerance, and peripheral gangrene or ulcers without clear-cut vascular or other etiology. Cold urticaria has been described in three cases of IgA-IgG MC, but cryoglobulinemia is quite uncommon in most cases of cold-induced urticaria. Familial cryoglobulinemia (in one study, associated with serum complement abnormalities of selective early classical pathway activation) has been described in a few kindreds, but is quite rare.

A particular clinical syndrome that has been associated with the presence of MCs is that of purpura-arthralgias-weakness and renal disease. The syndrome occurs predominantly in middle-aged women and is characterized by the development of immune-complex glomerulonephritis in about one half of the cases, and often the development of generalized vasculitis.[70] A significant percentage of these patients have clinical and laboratory evidence of subclinical liver disease and serologic findings suggestive of a role for HBV in the pathogenesis of disease. This association has been corroborated by the finding of HBsAg and HBsAb enriched in cryoprecipitates, anti-idiotypic specificity related to anti-HBsAb activity, and the demonstration of HBsAg in some cases of vasculitic, nephritic, and hepatic lesions by immunofluorescence and immunoperoxidase techniques.[67, 69]

Once established, the presence of a cryoglobulin may be of some utility clinically. Although the absolute level or cryocrit correlates only poorly with symptomatology in large series, in individual patients serial determinations may closely reflect the clinical response to therapy. This has proved to be the case in small series of patients with progressive renal disease, neuropathy, or major vessel involvement of other organs who were treated with cytotoxic agents and aggressive plasmapheresis regimens. Interestingly, although a drop in cryocrit correlated well with proteinuria or decreasing azotemia, parallel changes were not seen in the complement abnormalities or rheumatoid factor titer.[71]

PYROGLOBULINS[72]

Pyroglobulins are Igs that form a gel at 56 C. They differ from Bence Jones proteins in that the precipitate does not dissolve on further heating but is irreversible. Usually, they are found incidentally in the course of heating sera to 56 C to inactivate complement for serologic testing.

All pyroglobulins identified to date have been M proteins and have accounted for about 3% of paraproteins in large series screened for this entity. About half of all cases are associated with multiple myeloma; macroglobulinemia is less common, as are other lymphoproliferative disorders (lymphosarcoma) and neoplastic states. Two cases of IgA pyroglobulins have been reported, as well as isolated instances of coexistent cryoglobulinemia and pyroglobulinemia.

Pyroglobulins are not associated with distinctive symptomatology. The molecular basis of the phenomenon is obscure, though it appears to be dependent on the intact molecule and cannot be reliably localized to heavy or light chains or to variable or constant region determinants. Its major importance is as a laboratory artifact associated with certain plasma cell dyscrasias, and as a convenient way of isolating some monoclonal proteins.

COLD-PRECIPITABLE FIBRINOGENS

Identification

Cryofibrinogenemia has traditionally been defined as the occurrence of reversibly cold-precipitable protein in anticoagulated blood that can be shown antigenically or functionally to be fibrinogen. An important exclusion is that of cryoglobulinemia, which should not be present in a control sample of serum. The initial description of cryofibrinogenemia in 1955 defined it as a protein that could be made to clot with thrombin, to distinguish the phenomenon from the so-called cold-insoluble globulin of plasma, a β-globulin that was not thrombin coagulable. The latter is now recognized to be plasma fibronectin.

Recent studies have made it clear that the phenomenon of cold insolubility of fibrinogen in plasma may in fact result from at least two different mechanisms (Fig 4–11), one of which does not require the actual presence of fibrinogen. In true cryofibrinogenemia, soluble complexes of fibrinogen-fibrin precipitate in the presence of fibronectin. Since only small amounts of the latter are required, it has been suggested that the fibronectin serves as a "nucleus" for cryoprecipitation by noncovalent and covalent linkages to fibrin. All three components contribute to the phenomenon, and it can be induced in normal plasma by addition of thrombin or thrombin-like en-

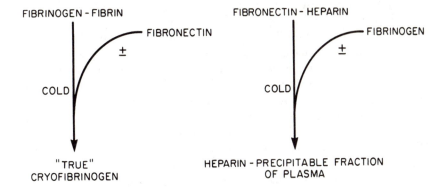

Fig 4–11.—Cold-precipitable proteins of plasma.

zymes. This entity has been best studied as a concomitant of chronic intravascular coagulation.

A second form of plasma cold insolubility occurs after the addition of a sulfated mucopolysaccharide such as heparin. This entity was first described as a concomitant of endotoxemia but has since been shown in human plasma in a variety of other clinical states. Here, heparin-fibronectin complexes form, apparently at a site on the molecule distinct from the locus of interaction with fibrin. These complexes are cryoprecipitable, but with reduced threshold in the presence of fibrinogen. The latter is incorporated into the complex secondarily during cryoprecipitation, which accounts for its variable and occasionally minor contribution to some of these cryoprecipitates. This interaction may be relevant to the function of fibronectin as a cell adhesive and opsonic protein.[73]

Cryoprecipitation in both systems presumably reflects conformational changes of fibrin-fibrinogen or fibronectin occurring in these complexes. Like cryoglobulinemia, cold insolubility is sensitive to conditions of solute concentration and pH, but the molecular basis for the effect is unknown.

Clinical Correlations

Older reports noted the presence of "cryofibrinogen" in about 3% of random blood samples.[74] Prominent clinical associations are neoplastic states, including both hematologic (myeloma, leukemias) and solid malignancies, and thromboembolic disease. It has frequently been found in the evaluation of the hypercoagulable state that is seen as a concomitant or presenting feature of certain malignancies (e.g., Trousseau's syndrome).[75] In such patients, serial measurements might provide some guide as to response to therapy or in following the course of disease. Other associations noted in large series have included pregnancy, the use of oral contraceptives, diabetes mellitus, cold-sensitivity states, and an essential form.

Recent awareness that cold insolubility in plasma may be due to fibrin or fibronectin with secondary cryoprecipitation of fibrinogen, and that true cryofibrinogenemia is a relatively rare phenomenon, have cast considerable doubt on the significance of older studies and the clinical utility of this test. Whether there are significant amounts of "cryofibrinogen" in normal plasma is unknown.

In screening plasma for cold insoluble precipitates, it is also important to examine serum for the simultaneous presence of cryoglobulins. Five to ten cubic centimeters of citrated plasma is collected and allowed to stand overnight at 4 C. Important considerations are (1) adequate amounts of citrate (9:1 vol/vol blood:citrate) in the syringe or tube to prevent calcium induction of fibrin formation; (2) rapid collection to avoid fibrin formation in the syringe; (3) no heparinization and no heparin in a line from which the blood may be taken. If these precautions are observed, the presence of any precipitate in plasma on at least two separate occasions is probably abnormal. Further characterization of the precipitate as primarily fibrin, fibronectin, or a truly abnormal fibrinogen requires detailed biochemical analysis in a specialty coagulation laboratory.

CEREBROSPINAL FLUID IGS

Methods of Identification

On standard lumbar puncture, the normal CSF protein level is less than 45 mg/dl. Since normal serum has a total protein content of 8 gm (8,000 mg/dl), it is apparent that CSF protein concentration is less the 0.6% that of blood.[76] The composition of CSF protein reflects several physiologic processes, as follows. (1) *Filtration*—presumed to occur at the level of the cerebrovascular endothelium. Proteins filtered into the CSF from the blood are of low molecular weight. For example, albumin is represented proportionately to its level in serum, but larger molecules such as IgM are excluded. (2) *Equilibration*—labeling studies involving the injection of tagged Ig in normal volunteers have shown equilibration to the CSF to take 4 days for IgG, 3 days for albumin. Thus, a rapid rise in the serum protein concentration may not be reflected immediately in the CSF if the blood-brain barrier is intact. (3) *Local synthesis*, responsible for selective rises in Igs in immune reactions involving the CNS, also appears to be responsible for the higher concentrations of some CSF proteins, such as prealbumin (5% in CSF vs. 0.004% in serum) and transferrin than would be expected from their molecular size. In addition, proteins that appear to be unique to CSF—the so-called τ (tau) fraction (with β-γ mobility), as well as β trace and γ trace proteins—are also assumed to originate by local synthesis. (4) *Degradation and clearance*—little is known of the processes involved here, although the absorptive capacity of the arachnoid villi and the ability of glial cells, pericytes, or Fc receptor–bearing cells in the brain to degrade proteins or remove immune complexes are presumably involved. Protein levels in the subarachnoid space are often higher than in cisternal or ventricular fluid, reflecting flow of CSF and possibly differences in synthetic rates between various parts of the brain.[77]

Because of the small amount of protein present, CSF must be concentrated about 200-fold before it can be displayed by cellulose acetate electrophoresis. In practice, this method is rarely of any clinical utility, and more sensitive techniques such as agarose, SDS-polyacrylamide, and two-dimensional gel electrophoresis have been utilized for detailed studies. Normal CSF is composed of approximately 5% prealbumin, 60% albumin, 5% α_1-, 7% α_2-, 14% β- (mostly transferrin), and 9% γ-globulin (Fig 4–12).

A rise in CSF protein concentration may thus reflect one or more of the following phenomena. (1) Increased serum levels. The selectivity pattern would remain unchanged (e.g., increased prealbumin and decreased γ-globulin) but might reflect increased levels of specific proteins in the serum. This would account for the appearance of a paraprotein in the CSF. (2) Increased admixture due to breakdown of the blood-brain barrier. Here the CSF protein concentration would approach that of serum. This pattern is seen normally in neonates due to immaturity of the blood-brain barrier and occurs in meningitis and other such inflammatory conditions involving the CNS. (3) Local synthesis. (4) Impaired resorption. Interruption of CSF flow by spinal tumors, tuberculous meningitis, etc. can cause striking rises in CSF protein. The integrity of the blood-brain barrier can be screened by noting the serum-CSF albumin ratio, which should be about 230 normally. Since albumin is not known to be produced in the CNS, a drop in this ratio may be due to leakage from the serum.

IEP and RID of concentrated CSF fluid are generally of limited clinical utility. Ig precipitin arcs may show a more restricted mobility compared to serum due to oligoclonal local synthesis of specific antibodies (Fig 4–13), and transferrin and prealbumin have been noted to have somewhat different mobilities than found in serum. Quantitation of specific proteins, especially Igs, requires more sensitive methods such as electroimmunoassay,[78] RIA, or enzyme-linked (ELISA) assays.

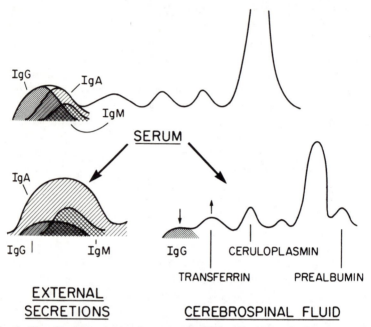

Fig 4–12.—Protein electrophoresis of CSF and external secretions. Figure shows normal variations from the pattern obtained in serum.

CSF Ig Synthesis

A selective increase in CSF γ-globulin concentration was first reported in 1942[79] in patients with multiple sclerosis (MS), but may also be seen in conditions such as meningoencephalitis, tuberculous meningitis, and syphilis. The increase may be recorded as the ratio of CSF γ-globulin or IgG to total CSF protein or albumin. Measurements of albumin, total globulin, or IgG in serum collected at the same time will establish the relevance of abnormal ratios. Normal CSF IgG content is less than 5.5 mg/dl; IgA, less

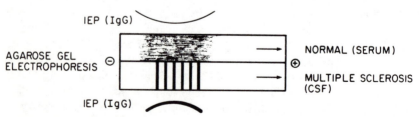

Fig 4–13.—Oligoclonal pattern. Restricted electrophoretic mobility and banding on agarose gel electrophoresis.

than 0.6 mg/dl; and IgM, less than 1.3 mg/dl. The IgG serum-CSF ratio has been established as 369 in studies on normal volunteers. Tourtellotte and Ma[80] have developed a formula for calculating CSF Ig synthetic rate that allows for admixture that might reflect breakdown of the blood-brain barrier, by including a correction factor for leakage of albumin from the serum:

$$\left(\text{IgG CSF} - \frac{\text{IgG serum}}{369} \right) - \left(\text{Alb CSF} - \frac{\text{Alb serum}}{230} \right) \left(\frac{\text{IgG serum}}{\text{Alb serum}} \right) 0.43$$

When these measurements are used, normal Ig synthesis in the CSF is less than 4.5 mg/day. The MS patient, on the other hand, may make up to 100 mg (average 16 mg) IgG per day in the CNS, figures that have been directly verified in some labeling studies.

Screens for CSF Ig synthesis include CSF Ig-CSF total protein (usually ~ 8%) and $\frac{\text{IgG CSF/serum}}{\text{albumin CSF/serum}}$ (usually <12%). Some 75%–85% of MS patients have increased CSF Ig synthesis, as do all patients with subacute sclerosing panencephalitis, 50% of patients with neurosyphilis, 40%–50% of patients with meningitis, and occasional patients with Guillain-Barré syndrome or other disorders. It is thus apparent that an increased CSF Ig synthetic rate is characteristic but not diagnostic of a variety of diseases affecting the CNS.

Abnormal Patterns—Oligoclonal Banding

Additional qualitative Ig abnormalities can be demonstrated in CSF of more than 90% of MS patients and add specificity to the diagnosis of the disorder. These abnormalities include (1) selective increases of IgG compared to other Ig classes,[78] (2) increased levels of the IgG1 subclass, a feature recently shown to be linked to G1m (1) allotype,[81] (3) increase in κ/λ ratio compared to normal, and (4) oligoclonal banding.[82] All these abnormalities are thought to reflect Ig production by a limited number of B cell clones in the CNS, possibly adjacent to plaques. Oligoclonal Ig synthesis has been corroborated directly by measurement of in vitro synthetic patterns by CSF lymphocytes isolated from MS patients.

Oligoclonal banding is apparent as multiple areas of restricted mobility (usually 6–10) in the normally diffuse γ region (see Fig 4–13). Early studies utilized agarose gel electrophoresis[83] and required concentration of 5–10 ml of CSF several hundredfold for direct visualization by protein staining of gels. Electrophoresis may be combined with immunofixation, in which anti-Ig is applied to and diffuses into the gel. Extraneous proteins are then washed out, and the Ig-anti-Ig precipitates, as is visualized with a protein stain. More recently, SDS-polyacrylamide gel electrophoresis, isoelectric focusing, and isotachophoresis methods have been done on unconcentrated CSF for direct demonstration of banding.

Oligoclonal banding occurs in about 80% of patients with MS, but may also be seen in 40% of patients with other inflammatory diseases of the CSF.

Clinical Correlations

The main value of measuring CSF Ig is to confirm the clinical diagnosis of MS. Oligoclonal banding is presumably one measure of an abnormal immune system and may even be reflected systemically in a minority of patients (serum hyperglobulinemia, oligoclonal banding in serum). Recent work using techniques described in Chapters 3 and 6 has shown CICs and depressed suppressor cell number and function in many MS patients. The pathogenic significance of these abnormalities is unclear, and it is possible that their quantitation may be of diagnostic importance in the near future. At present, the main value of establishing an increased CSF Ig synthetic rate or oligoclonal banding is to exclude a variety of degenerative diseases of the CNS. Similarly, the clinical utility of these parameters in early diagnosis is uncertain, and fluctuations only generally follow clinical exacerbations and remissions.

OTHER BODY FLUIDS

The representation of various Ig classes in extravascular compartments is partly a function of their physical properties; for example, IgM is almost exclusively vascular because of its large size. The major Ig class of external secretions (upper respiratory, saliva, intestinal, lacrimal, urinary) is IgA, owing to the presence of lymphoid tissue (gut associated and bronchus associated) in the submucosa of the gut and respiratory tract committed to producing predominantly this class of Ig. Whereas IgA constitutes only 15%–20% of the total Ig of serum, it constitutes more than 80% of the total Ig of saliva (see Fig 4–12).[84]

The Ig composition of internal secretions (CSF, synovial fluid, pleural fluid, peritoneal fluid), on the other hand, generally reflects that of serum, with the exclusion of IgM because of its size. Local synthesis of Ig may also influence the composition of internal secretions. The effect of these factors on the CSF has been noted above. The total Ig content of the synovial fluid of a patient with active rheumatoid synovitis is higher than would be expected from serum transudation because of loss of the semipermeability of the synovial membrane due to inflammation. Additionally, the IgG and IgM contents are higher than expected because of local synthesis of IgG and IgM rheumatoid factor by subsynovial germinal centers. Lastly, IgG in synovial fluid may have a more restricted electrophoretic mobility than serum due to the major contribution of clones of plasma cells synthesizing antibodies with antiglobulin or antinuclear antibody activity.

IgA in external secretions is predominantly (90%) dimeric, in contradistinction to serum IgA, which is 85% monomeric. The IgA2 subclass is a minor component of serum but is increased in external secretions. Dimeric IgA in external secretions is bonded to two glycoproteins—the J chain (MW 15,000) and secretory component (SC) (MW 60,000). The former is synthesized by plasma cells, the latter by epithelial cells. J chain is associated with polymeric Igs of IgA and IgM classes; a small amount of IgM also has SC attached. The function of SC is to protect IgA in external secretions from proteolytic digestion. Patients with selective IgA deficiency are often found to have free SC in external secretions and a compensatory increase in IgM.[84]

It has been estimated that the gut mucosa synthesizes 3 gm of IgA per day, most of which is excreted. Animal studies have indicated that 80%–85% of the IgA in saliva is made locally.[85] This is also true of nasal mucosa and is evidenced by striking rises in specific IgA antibody after infection by viruses that localize in the mucosa of the upper respiratory tract (e.g., rhinoviruses, respiratory syncytial virus, myxoviruses).[86] In atopics, there is considerable evidence for IgE secretion by lymphoid tissue of the nasopharynx, correlating only poorly with serum IgE. Recent work has shown that as much as 20% of the B cells of the gut mucosa may bear surface IgE, and most of this is apparently exported to the blood. The mucosal immune response is tightly and finely regulated by T cell circuits.

Quantitation of Ig in external secretions may be inaccurate due to the presence of polymers and complexed Ig, interference by proteolytic digestion products of Ig, and admixture with serum. There is a steady decrease in the IgA contribution (83% → 19%) and an increase in the IgG contribution (6% → 75%) as samples are obtained serially downward through the trachea into the bronchial tree. Lavage fluid from the lower respiratory tract is a mixture between that found in nasopharyngeal secretions and serum.[87] Comparison of specific Ig or antibody activity with simultaneous measurements in serum considerably enhances the specificity of formulas for calculating secretory function.[88]

CONCLUSIONS

The proper evaluation of Igs in serum and other body fluids requires a knowledge of Ig structure, function, and turnover rates. Considerable basic information has accumulated that may be used in the interpretation of commonly available immunologic tests. The assessment of Igs and other serum proteins is a search for indications of inflammatory processes, deficiency states, and an overall evaluation of humoral immunity. Restricted heterogeneity and frank dysproteinemia reflect the clonality of the B cell line, as well as neoplastic transformation of lymphocytes and plasma cells. These considerations provide a basis for the further interpretation of specific antibody activities, cell surface markers, and cell-mediated immunity.

ACKNOWLEDGMENTS

Research was supported by NIH grants Nos. AG01973 and AM26588, and by the Arthritis Foundation, Inc.

Karen Randall prepared the manuscript.

REFERENCES

1. Allison A.C.: *Structure and Function of Plasma Proteins*. New York, Plenum Press, 1974, vol. 1; 1976, vol. 2.
2. Ritzmann S.E., Daniels J.C. (eds.): *Serum Protein Abnormalities: Diagnostic and Clinical Aspects*. Boston, Little, Brown & Co., 1975.
3. Putnam F.W. (ed.): *The Plasma Proteins*. New York, Academic Press, 1977, vol. 1–3.
4. Tiselius A.: A new apparatus for electrophoretic analysis of colloidal mixtures. *Trans. Faraday Soc.* 33:524, 1937.
5. Kohn J.: A cellulose acetate supporting medium for zone electrophoresis. *Clin. Chim. Acta* 2:297, 1957.
6. Smithies O.: Zone electrophoresis in starch gels and its application to studies of serum proteins. *Adv. Protein Chem.* 14:65, 1959.
7. Grabar P., Burtin P.: *Immunoelectrophoretic Analysis*. New York, American Elsevier, 1964.
8. Ouchterlony O.: Diffusion-in-gel methods for immunological analysis. *Prog. Allergy* 6:30, 1962.
9. Kochwa S.: Immunoelectrophoresis (including zone electrophoresis), in Rose N.R., Friedman H. (eds.): *Manual of Clinical Immunology*. Washington, D.C., American Society for Microbiology, 1976, pp. 17–35.
10. Grabar P., Williams L.A. Jr.: Methode permettant l'étude conjugée des propriétés electrophorétiques et immunochemiques d'un mélange de protéines: Application à serum sanguin. *Biochim. Biophys. Acta* 10:193, 1953.
11. Waldmann T.A., Strober W.: Metabolism of immunoglobulins. *Prog. Allergy* 13:1, 1969.
12. Kushner I.: The acute-phase reactants and the erythrocyte sedimentation rate, in Kelley W.N., Harris E.D. Jr., Ruddy S., et al. (eds.): *Textbook of Rheumatology*. Philadelphia, W.B. Saunders Co., 1981, pp. 669–676.
13. Berggard I.: In Manuel Y., Revillard J.P., Betuel H. (eds.): *Proteins in Normal and Pathological Urine*. Basel, S. Karger, 1970.
14. Pruzanski W., Ogryzlo M.A.: Abnormal proteinuria in malignant diseases. *Adv. Clin. Chem.* 13:335, 1970.
15. Kyle R.A.: Analysis of immunoglobulins in urine, in Duarte C.G. (ed.): *Renal Function Tests*. Boston, Little, Brown & Co., 1980, pp. 291–326.

16. Hardwicke J., Cameron J.S., Harrison J.F., et al.: Proteinuria studied by clearance of individual macromolecules, in Manuel Y., Revillard J.P., Betuel H. (eds.): *Proteins in Normal and Pathological Urine*. Basel, S. Karger, 1970, pp. 111–152.

17. Solomon A.: Bence Jones proteins and light chains of immunoglobulins. *N. Engl. J. Med.* 294:17, 91, 1976.

18. Wochner R.D., Strober W., Waldman T.A.: The role of the kidney in the catabolism of Bence Jones proteins and immunoglobulin fragments. *J. Exp. Med.* 126:207, 1967.

19. Damacco F., Waldenström J.: Serum and urine light chain levels in benign monoclonal gammopathies, multiple myeloma and Waldenström's macroglobulinemia. *Clin. Exp. Immunol.* 3:91, 1968.

20. Vaughan J.H., Jacox R.F., Gray B.A.: Light and heavy chain components of gamma globulins in urines of normal persons and patients with agammaglobulinemia. *J. Clin. Invest.* 46:266, 1967.

21. Gilliland B.C., Mannik M.: Immunologic quantitation of proteins in serum, urine, and other body fluids, in Vyas G.N., Stites D.P., Brocher G. (eds.): *Laboratory Diagnosis of Immunologic Disorders*. New York, Grune & Stratton, 1975, pp. 13–30.

22. Stone M.J., Frenkel E.P.: The clinical spectrum of light chain myeloma: A study of 35 patients with special reference to the occurrence of amyloidosis. *Am. J. Med.* 58:601, 1975.

23. Isobe T., Osserman E.F.: Patterns of amyloidosis and their association with plasma cell dyscrasia, monoclonal immunoglobulins and Bence Jones proteins. *N. Engl. J. Med.* 290:473, 1974.

24. Glenner G.G.: Amyloid deposits and amyloidosis. *N. Engl. J. Med.* 302:1283–1292, 1333–1343, 1980.

25. De Fronzo R.A., Cooke R., Wright J.R., et al.: Renal function in multiple myeloma. *Medicine* 57:151, 1978.

26. Gorevic P.D., Franklin E.C.: Multiple myeloma and related diseases: Amyloidosis and cryoglobulinemia, in Zabriskie J.B., Becker L., Villareal H., et al. (eds.): *Clinical Immunological Diseases of the Kidney*. New York, John Wiley & Sons, 1982.

27. Kyle R.A., Maldonado J.E., Bayrd E.D.: Idopathic Bence Jones proteinuria: A distinct entity. *Am. J. Med.* 55:222–226, 1973.

28. Gordon A.H.: The acute phase plasma proteins, in Bianchi R., Mariani G., McFarlane A.S. (eds.): *Plasma Protein Turnover*. Baltimore, University Park Press, 1976, pp. 381–394.

29. Sipe J.D., Rosenstreich D.L.: Serum factors associated with inflammation, in Oppenheim J.J., Rosensteich D.L., Potter M. (eds.): *Cellular Functions in Immunity and Inflammation*. New York, Elsevier-North Holland, 1981, pp. 411–429.

30. C-reactive protein and the plasma protein response to tissue injury. Conference, *Ann. NY Acad. Sci.* 389:1–482.

31. Dinarello C.A., Wolff S.M.: Molecular basis of fever in humans. *Am. J. Med.* 72:799, 1982.

32. Koj A.: Acute phase reactants, in Allison A.C. (ed.): *Structure and Function of Plasma Proteins*. New York, Plenum Press, 1974, vol. 1, pp. 73–131.

33. Pepsy M.B.: C-reactive protein fifty years on. *Lancet* 1:653, 1981.

34. Guenter C.A., Welch M.H., Hammersten J.F.: Alpha-1-antitrypsin deficiency and pulmonary emphysema. *Annu. Rev. Med.* 22:283, 1971.

35. Laurell C.B., Eriksson S.: The electrophoretic α1-globulin pattern of serum in α1-antitrypsin deficiency in patients with pulmonary emphysema. *Scand. J. Clin. Invest.* 15:132, 1963.
36. Sharp H.L., Bridges R.A., Kruit W., et al.: Cirrhosis associated with alpha-1-antitrypsin deficiency: A previously unrecognized inherited disorder. *J. Lab. Clin. Med.* 73:934, 1969.
37. Morse J.O.: Alpha-1-antitrypsin deficiency. *N. Engl. J. Med.* 299:1045–1048, 1099–1105, 1978.
38. Laurell C.B. (ed.): Electrophoretic and electroimmunochemical analyses of proteins. *Scand. J. Clin. Lab. Invest.* 29, suppl. 124, 1972.
39. Laurell C.B.: Quantitative estimation of proteins by electrophoresis in agarose containing antibodies. *Anal. Biochem.* 15:45, 1966.
40. Talamo R.C., Bruce R.M., Langley C.E., et al.: *Alpha-1-Antitrypsin Laboratory Manual.* Washington, D.C., U.S. Dept. of Health, Education, and Welfare, publication No. (NIH) 78-1420, 1978.
41. Franklin E.C.: Electrophoresis and immunoelectrophoresis in the evaluation of homogeneous immunoglobulin components, in Bach F.H., Good R.A. (eds.): *Clinical Immunobiology.*, New York, Academic Press, 1976, vol. 3, pp. 21–36.
42. Spiegelberg H.L.: Detection and subtyping of monoclonal immunoglobulins, in Nakamura R.M., Dito W.R., Tucker E.S. III (eds.): *Immunoassays in the Clinical Laboratory*, ed. 2. New York, Allen R. Liss, 1979, pp. 243–271.
43. Kyle R.A.: Classification and diagnosis of monoclonal gammopathies, in Rose N.R., Friedman H. (eds.): *Manual of Clinical Immunology*, ed. 2. New York, American Society for Microbiology, 1980, pp. 135–150.
44. Axelsson U., Hallen J.: A population study on monoclonal gammopathy. *Acta Med. Scand.* 191:111, 1972.
45. Solomon A.S., Kunkel, H.G.: "Monoclonal" type, low molecular weight protein related to γ M macroglobulins. *Am. J. Med.* 42:958, 1967.
46. Jancelewicz Z., Takatsuki Sugai S.: IgD myeloma: Review of 133 cases. *Arch. Intern. Med.* 135:87, 1975.
47. Frangione B., Franklin E.C.: Heavy chain diseases: Clinical features and molecular significance of the disordered immunoglobulin structure. *Semin. Hematol.* 10:53, 1973.
48. Franklin E.C., Frangione B.: Structural variants of human and murine immunoglobulins. *Contemp. Top. Mol. Immunol.* 4:89, 1975.
49. Kyle R.A., Robinson R.A., Katzmann J.A.: The clinical aspects of biclonal gammopathies: Review of 57 cases. *Am. J. Med.* 71:999, 1981.
50. Franklin E.C., Lowenstein J., Bigelow B., et al.: Heavy chain disease: A new disorder of serum γ globulins. Report of a first case. *Am. J. Med.* 37:332, 1964.
51. Seligmann M., Danon F., Hurez D., et al.: Alpha chain disease: A new immunoglobulin abnormality. *Science* 162:1396, 1968.
52. Forte F.A., Prelli F., Yount W.J., et al.: Heavy chain disease of the μ (γm) type: Report of the first case. *Blood* 36:437, 1970.
53. Michaux J.L., Heremans J.F.: 30 Cases of monoclonal immunoglobulin disorders other than myeloma or macroglobulinemia. *Am. J. Med.* 46:562, 1969.
54. Isobe T., Osserman E.F.: Pathologic conditions associated with plasma cell dyscrasias: A study of 806 cases. *Ann. NY Acad. Sci.* 190:507, 1971.
55. Zawadki Z.A., Edwards G.A.: Nonmyelomatous monoclonal immunoglobulinemia. *Prog. Clin. Immunol.* 1:105–156, 1972.
56. Kyle R.A.: Monoclonal gammopathy of undetermined significance: Natural history of 24 cases. *Am. J. Med.* 64:814, 1978.

57. Axelsson V.: An 11-year follow-up of 64 subjects with M components. *Acta Med. Scand.* 201:173, 1977.
58. Waldenström J.: *Diagnosis and Treatment of Multiple Myeloma.* New York, Grune & Stratton, 1970.
59. Snapper I., Kahn A.: *Myelomatosis.* Baltimore, University Park Press, 1971.
60. Kyle R.A.: Multiple myeloma: Review of 869 cases. *Mayo Clin. Proc.* 50:29, 1975.
61. Mackensie M.R., Fudenberg H.H.: Macroglobulinemia: An analysis of 40 patients. *Blood* 39:874, 1972.
62. Block K.J., Maki D.G.: Hyperviscosity syndromes associated with immunoglobulin abnormalities. *Semin. Hematol.* 10:113–121, 1973.
63. Ammann A.J., Hong R.: Selective IgA deficiency: Presentation of 30 cases and a review of the literature. *Medicine* 50:223, 1971.
64. Brouet J.C., Clauvel J.P., Danon F., et al.: Biological and clinical significance of cryoglobulins. *Am. J. Med.* 57:775, 1974.
65. Grey H.M., Kohler P.F.: Cryoimmunoglobulins. *Semin. Hematol.* 10:87, 1973.
66. Haydey R.P., DeRojas M.P., Gigli I.: A newly described control mechanism of complement activation in patients with mixed cryoglobulinemia (cryoglobulins and complement). *J. Invest. Dermatol.* 74:328–332, 1980.
67. Gorevic P.D., Kassab H.J., Levo Y., et al.: Mixed cryoglobulinemia: Clinical aspects and long-term follow-up of 40 patients. *Am. J. Med.* 69:287, 1980.
68. Wager O., Rasanen J.A.: Mixed cryoglobulinemia in relation to autoimmune aberrations, in Bonomo L., Turk J.L. (eds.): *Proceedings of the International Symposium on Immune Complex Diseases.* Milan, Carlo Erba Foundation, 1970, p. 140.
69. Geltner D., Franklin E.C., Frangione B.: Anti-idiotypic activity in the IgM fractions of mixed cryoglobulins. *J. Immunol.* 125:1530, 1980.
70. Meltzer M., Franklin E.C., Elias K., et al.: Cryoglobulinemia: A clinical and laboratory study—II. Cryoglobulins with rheumatoid factor activity. *Am. J. Med.* 40:837, 1966.
71. Geltner D., Kohn R.W., Gorevic P.D., et al.: The effect of combination therapy (steroids, immunosuppressives, and plasmapheresis) on 5 mixed cryoglobulinemia patients with renal, neurologic and vascular involvement. *Arthritis Rheum.* 24:1121, 1981.
72. Zinneman H.H.: Cryoglobulins and pyroglobulins, in Good R.A., Litman G.W. (eds.): *Comprehensive Immunology.* New York, Plenum Press, 1978, vol 5, pp. 323–343.
73. Mosseson M.W., Anrani D.L.: The structure and biologic activities of plasma fibronectin. *Blood* 56:145, 1980.
74. Smith S.B., Arkin C.: Cryofibrinogenemia. *Am. J. Clin. Pathol.* 58:524, 1972.
75. Sack G.H. Jr., Levin J., Bell W.R.: Trousseau's syndrome and other manifestations of chronic disseminated coagulopathy in patients with neoplasm: Clinical, pathophysiologic and therapeutic features. *Medicine* 56:1, 1977.
76. Brackenridge C.J.: Cerebrospinal fluid protein fractions in health and disease. *J. Clin. Pathol.* 15:206, 1962.
77. Rapaport S.I.: *Blood-Brain Barrier in Physiology and Medicine.* New York, Raven Press, 1976.
78. Schneck S.A., Claman H.N.: CSF immunoglobulins in multiple sclerosis and other neurological diseases: Measurement by electroimmunodiffusion. *Arch. Neurol.* 20:132, 1969.
79. Kabat E.A., Moore D.H., Landow H.: An electrophoretic study of the protein

components in cerebrospinal fluid and their relationship to the serum proteins. *J. Clin. Invest.* 21:571, 1942.

80. Tourtellotte W.W., Ma B.I.: Multiple sclerosis: The blood-brain barrier and the measurement of de novo central nervous system IgG synthesis. *Neurology* 28:71, 1978.

81. Salier J.P., Goust J.M., Pandey J.P., et al.: Preferential synthesis of the G1m[1] allotype of IgG1 in the central nervous system of multiple sclerosis patients. *Science* 213:1400, 1981.

82. Lisak R.P., Eshgegian K.: Oligoclonal immunoglobulins in cerebrospinal fluid in multiple sclerosis. *Clin. Chem.* 26:1340, 1980.

83. Johnson K.P., Arrigo S.C., Nelson B.J.: Agarose electrophoresis of cerebrospinal fluid in multiple sclerosis. *Neurology* 27:217, 1977.

84. Tomasi T.B. Jr.: Secretory immunoglobulins. *N. Engl. J. Med.* 287:500, 1972.

85. Clancy R., Bienenstock J.: Secretion immunoglobulins. *Clin. Gastroenterol.* 5:231–247, 1976.

86. Rossen R.D., Butler W.T.: Immunologic responses to infection at mucosal surfaces, in Knight V. (ed.): *Viral and Mycoplasma Infections of the Respiratory Tract.* Philadelphia, Lea & Febiger, 1973, pp. 23–52.

87. Kaltreider H.B.: Expression of immune mechanisms in the lung. *Am. Rev. Respir. Dis.* 113:347, 1976.

88. Matthews K.P.: Calculation of secretory antibodies and immunoglobulins. *J. Allergy Clin. Immunol.* 68:46, 1981.

5

Autoimmune Diseases

John J. Condemi, M.D.

INTRODUCTION

SINCE THE EARLIEST descriptions of the immune system, the ability of an individual to react to a wide variety of foreign insults, such as microorganisms and parasites, and internal changes, such as cancer cells, while not responding to one's own self, has intrigued researchers and is now attracting the attention of the clinician. Clinicians are interested because they encounter an increasing number of diseases and a wide range of clinical situations in which autoimmune phenomena apparently contribute to the symptoms. Clinical interest has been stimulated further by the therapeutic interventions that are now available or will be available in the near future to restore the function of the immune system to its major role in the prevention rather than production of disease.

As early investigators began to appreciate the importance of the immune system for host defense, the first descriptions of autoimmune phenomena in the early 1900s aroused sufficient anxiety to cause Ehrlich to coin the term "horror autotoxicus" to describe the horrible situation in which an individual would attempt to destroy himself.[1] This horror at physiologic self-destructive mechanisms was certainly justified with the delineation of the many autoimmune disease states. What has changed since that time, however, is the recognition that the production of autoimmunity is a common phenomenon, often under normal immune regulation, and that in some situations, such as the response to cancer cells, it may benefit the individual. The clinician is often called on to decide if the autoimmune phenomenon described in a certain disease is truly responsible for tissue injury, if it is an autoimmune phenomenon of no clinical significance, or if it is an autoimmune response that may have clinical significance, such as in diagnosis or following the clinical course, but no pathogenic significance. Although the autoimmune response may be in either limb of the immune system, it is the response secondary to circulating antibodies that

113

is most easily detectable and best understood. The technology to measure delayed hypersensitivity has not been developed to the point that tests are commonly available, nor is the role of delayed hypersensitivity in autoimmunity clearly understood. Autoimmunity can therefore be defined as the failure of an individual's immune system to recognize self. Consequently, an immune response develops to antigens normally present in tissue. Table 5–1 lists diseases for which there is good evidence of autoimmunity in the production of disease. Table 5–2 lists diseases in which autoimmune responses are thought to contribute to pathogenesis. Table 5–3 lists autoimmune responses considered to be of diagnostic or pathogenic significance. Table 5–4 lists autoimmune manifestations that are not considered to contribute to disease or to be of diagnostic value.

Grouping of Autoimmune Diseases

Human autoimmune diseases can be divided into three main groups: organ-specific diseases, non-organ-specific diseases, and non-organ-specific diseases that produce lesions in one or a few organs. Organ-specific diseases are characterized by chronic inflammatory changes in a specific organ. The autoantibodies that are demonstrated exhibit specificity for the antigens of the diseased organ. Examples of this group are autoimmune

TABLE 5–1.—Autoimmune Diseases Fulfilling
Witebsky's Criteria[2]

Systemic lupus erythematosus
Hashimoto's thyroiditis
Graves' disease
Myasthenia gravis
Insulin-resistant diabetes with anti-insulin receptor antibodies
Anti-glomerular basement membrane nephritis
Goodpasture's syndrome
Pemphigus

TABLE 5–2.—Suspected
Autoimmune Diseases Not
Fulfilling Witebsky's Criteria[2]

Rheumatoid arthritis
Insulin-dependent diabetes
Autoimmune insulin syndrome
Gastritis
Pernicious anemia
Addison's disease
Pemphigoid
Chronic active hepatitis
Primary biliary cirrhosis

TABLE 5–3.—ANTIBODIES OF DIAGNOSTIC
SIGNIFICANCE

LE cell in systemic lupus erythematosus (SLE)
Anti-double-stranded DNA in SLE
Anti-SM in SLE
Anti-histone in drug-induced lupus erythematosus
Anti-SS-A and SS-B in Sjögren's syndrome
Antinucleolar in scleroderma
Anticentromere in CREST syndrome
Anti-insulin receptor in diabetes mellitus
Anti-glomerular basement membrane in nephritis and
    Goodpasture's syndrome
Anti-acetylcholine receptor in myasthenia gravis
Anti-intercellular antigen of stratified epithelium in pemphigus
Anti-lamina lucida in pemphigoid
Antireticulin in dermatitis herpetiformis

TABLE 5–4.—ANTIBODIES OF LOW DIAGNOSTIC
SIGNIFICANCE

Anti-single-stranded DNA in systemic lupus erythematosus
Rheumatoid factor in rheumatoid arthritis
Antithyroglobulin for thyroiditis
Antimicrosomal antibody for thyroiditis
Anti-skeletal muscle antibody in myasthenia gravis
Anti-islet cell antibody in insulin-dependent diabetes
Anti-B_{12} nonblocking antibodies in pernicious anemia
Antisperm antibody in infertility (by indirect immunofluorescence)

---

hemolytic anemia, idiopathic thrombocytopenic purpura, idiopathic leuko-
penia, Goodpasture's syndrome, myasthenia gravis, Graves' disease, pemphigus, juvenile diabetes, and Addison's disease. The non-organ-specific
diseases include systemic lupus erythematosus (SLE) and rheumatoid arthritis (RA). Non-organ-specific diseases that produce lesions in one or few
organs include primary biliary cirrhosis and chronic active hepatitis. Organ-
specific autoantibodies for which there is no associated pathogenic or diagnostic role are not considered here.

In the evaluation of any given patient, it should be recognized that there
is a tendency for more than one autoimmune disorder to occur in the same
individual. For example, patients with autoimmune thyroiditis have a
much higher incidence of pernicious anemia than would be found in a random population sample. Similarly, patients with pernicious anemia have a
higher frequency of thyroiditis and thyrotoxicosis than the general population. In addition, symptoms may be due to more than one mechanism, as
happens in SLE, where it is not uncommon to find organ-specific manifestations such as hemolytic anemia, idiopathic thrombocytopenia, and leu-

kopenia, as well as non-organ-specific manifestations. There can also be combinations of important and unimportant autoimmune responses, as happens in myasthenia gravis, where the antibody to acetylcholine receptor produces disease but the antibody to myosin is of little clinical importance.

Autoimmune diseases are generally defined by the presence of an antibody or sensitized lymphoid cell to an autoantigen. In 1959 Witebsky suggested certain criteria that should be fulfilled before a disease is included among the autoimmune diseases[2]: (1) The autoimmune response must be regularly associated with the disease. (2) The antigen responsible for the disease in man, when administered to animals, must be capable of inducing a similar disease in animals. (3) The immunopathologic changes induced in animals and observed in man should be similar. (4) The disease should be transferable by either serum or cells from a diseased animal to a normal animal. The diseases or manifestations listed in Table 5–1 fulfill these criteria, while those listed in Table 5–2 have considerable evidence supporting a role for autoimmunity but, in general, are lacking animal models.

Sensitivity and Specificity

Whereas Witebsky's criteria are helpful in determining conclusively whether a disease is of autoimmune etiology, they do not help the clinician in deciding the usefulness of the tests available in diagnosis or management. The value of a test depends on its sensitivity and specificity. The sensitivity of a test is the probability that patients with that disease will have a positive test result. A very sensitive test would yield positive results in 95%–100% of patients with a given disease. In very sensitive tests, one can exclude the diagnosis if the test result is negative. The specificity of a test is the probability that those who have a negative test result do not have the disease (normals) and the frequency with which a positive test occurs in other diseases. The specificity may therefore vary, depending on whether one is comparing the frequency of a positive test result in a diseased population with its frequency in healthy normal subjects or in patients with other diseases. We can take as an example the creatine phosphokinase (CPK) level in a patient with a myocardial infaction (MI). This is a sensitive test which is positive in most patients with MI, and it effectively separates patients with chest pain due to MI from patients with chest pain and no MI and from normal subjects without chest pain. In this setting, it is a highly sensitive and highly specific test for MI. The specificity of an elevated CPK level for the diagnosis of MI decreases significantly, however, if it is used as a screening test for MI in an outpatient office setting. In this situation, most patients with an elevated CPK level most likely have a disease or a clinical state other than MI. The test remains sensitive for

MI, but its specificity decreases significantly because the CPK level is more likely to be elevated as a result of tissue injury, activity, hypothyroidism, or muscle disease than as a result of MI. The clinician must use a combination of history, physical examination findings, and clinical status to interpret the laboratory test results and arrive at a proper diagnosis. The same is true of laboratory tests to detect autoimmune diseases.

Most commonly available tests for autoimmune diseases are serologic tests that detect autoantibody. The autoantibody is usually present in varying amounts and may be reported as the dilution or as the reciprocal of the dilution which gave the last positive result. For example, the immunofluorescence test for the detection of antinuclear antibody (ANA) is performed first with undiluted serum, designated as neat, and then with serum sequentially diluted to 1/40, 1/80, 1/160, 1/320 of its initial strength. (If the ... 1/320, one part of the serum is added to 319 parts of a diluent.) ...0 dilution gave the last positive result, the laboratory may report ...g positive at 1/80 or at the reciprocal, 80. Figure 5–1 shows the ...y and specificity of autoantibody tests when the autoantibody is ... in varying amounts. In an ideal situation, where the autoantibody ...t in both normal subjects and diseased patients, one would like to ...dilution that is diagnostic for a specific disease. This means that ...h the test may be positive in patients without the disease, once a ...titer is achieved (cutoff), there is a high probability that the individual has the disease. A test with a definite cutoff titer would have high sensitivity and high specificity. This precision is rarely achieved in tests

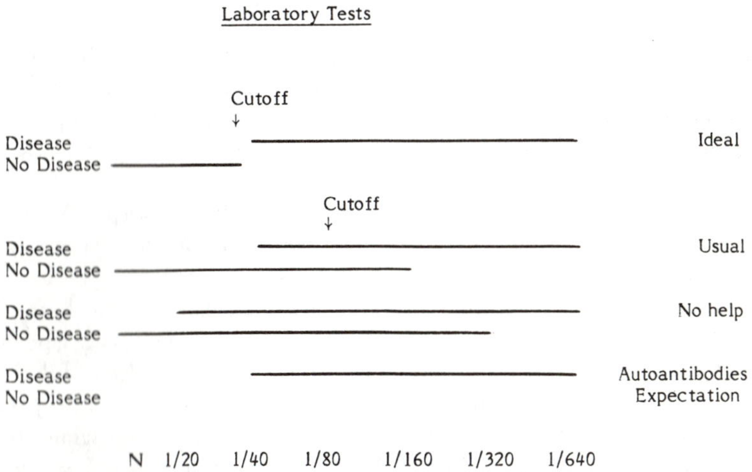

Laboratory Tests

Fig 5–1.—Schematic depiction of sensitivity and specificity of autoantibody tests in which autoantibody is present in varying amounts.

used for the detection of autoantibodies, but such a diagnostic titer does exist for the antibody for the acetylcholine receptor site in myasthenia gravis.

More usually, however, there is some overlap between normal subjects and diseased patients at titers in the diagnostic range. At those titers the test is not specific (overlap zone), and one must use additional information to decide whether a patient has a given disease. Nevertheless, when the autoantibody is present in high titers, it is very likely that the individual has the disease. Tests that give these results are very sensitive and specific only at high titers. This situation describes the ANA test.

A third possibility is considerable overlap between diseased and disease-free individuals. A test of this sort has very little clinical value except when it is negative, in which case it can be used to rule out the disease in question. The test would be very sensitive but not specific. This describes the antibody for single-stranded DNA (ssDNA). In addition, this describes the ANA and rheumatoid factor (RF) tests, if patients with other rheumatic diseases are substituted for nondiseased individuals.

A fourth possibility, which most clinicians might expect of tests for autoimmune diseases: patients with an abnormal laboratory test result have the disease, but not all patients with the disease have abnormal tests. Such a test would be very specific and moderately sensitive. I wish to emphasize, however, that this is an unusual occurrence in patients with autoimmune diseases, but it does describe the antibody for native double-stranded DNA (nDNA).

Proposed Mechanisms

In anticipation that in the future we will be able to treat the immune-mediated diseases more specifically by decreasing autoantibody production or the cellular immune response, a brief understanding of how autoimmune phenomena can occur is appropriate. Five mechanisms are possible, as described below.

SEQUESTRATION ANTIGEN THEORY.—According to the sequestration antigen theory, antigens that do not normally circulate or have access to the immune system will stimulate the immune system once they gain intravascular entry or once the immune system has been exposed to them. This mechanism was believed to explain immune responses to sperm (aspermia), thyroglobulin (thyroiditis), and eye lens protein (sympathetic ophthalmia). In essence, the immune system never recognized certain materials present in the body as self because it was not exposed to these antigens during early development. There is presently little enthusiasm for the sequestration antigen theory as a general explanation for autoimmune diseases because, as assays for the presence of antigens in the circulation became more sensitive, it also became apparent that sperm and thyroglobulin may be present normally in the circulation in small amounts without the development of autoantibodies. Sympathetic ophthalmia, which is considered a T cell–mediated disease, may be explained by this mechanism.

ALTERED ANTIGEN OR NEOANTIGEN THEORY.—According to this theory, antigens recognized as self are altered so that the immune system no longer recognizes them as self. This alteration can come about by chemical means, as occurs in contact dermatitis, or by biologic changes, as occur in the development of new antigens on malignant cells, or through alteration of host protein by infectious agents. Although viruses have been suggested in this explanation for autoimmune phenomena, few data support this concept in autoimmune diseases. However, the neoantigen theory does explain the development of RF and contact dermatitis.

SHARED OR CROSS-REACTIVE ANTIGEN THEORY.—According to this theory, there are exogenous antigens that are similar to self antigens. The immune system, in responding to the exogenous agent, in some manner subsequently loses the ability to distinguish self as self and produces antibodies or T cells that react with self. This theory explains the presence of autoantibodies in paroxysmal cold hemoglobinuria caused by *Treponema pallidum*, the hemolytic anemia noted in mycoplasma infections, and postvaccinal and postinfectious encephalomyelitis, and is thought to explain rheumatic fever due to streptococcal infections.

NONIMMUNOLOGIC STIMULATION OF EITHER T OR B CELLS.—This mechanism has been demonstrated in Epstein-Barr virus (EBV) infection in which B cells are infected by EBV and stimulate antibody production in the B cells. If the B cell is capable of producing autoantibody, it will do so under the stimulation of the EBV infection. This explains the autoantibody production noted in infectious mononucleosis.[3]

ALTERATION OF NORMAL HOMEOSTATIC MECHANISMS.—At present, alterations of the normal immune response are considered to be the most likely explanation for most autoimmune phenomena. The immune response is now recognized to be a complex, integrated network of interactions among macrophages, T cells serving specialized memory, helper, suppressor, or effector functions, and B cells which require a continuous exchange of information in order to be stimulated or suppressed.[4] There is evidence that decreased suppressor T cell function occurs in patients with aldomet-induced hemolytic anemia[5] and SLE[6] and in the normal process of aging. This decrease in suppressor T cell function may allow B cell autoantibodies or self-reactive T cells to be produced that result in autoimmune phenomena. Increased activity of helper T function may be the mechanism by which some drug-induced autoimmune phenomena occur.[7] Other factors that may contribute to altering the normal inhibition of autoimmunity are genetics and hormones.[8] There is considerable evidence, both from experimental studies on animals and from correlative studies on humans, that genes associated with the major histocompatibility locus antigen (HLA) are important in immune regulation and in the pathogenesis of autoimmunity. Indirect evidence of the importance of genetic factors is supplied by the observation that autoimmune phenomena occur with increased frequency in certain families. The importance of hormones in the immune response is suggested by the observation that most of the human autoimmune diseases are much commoner in women than in men. Autoantibodies also increase with age, but in most situations this does not increase the incidence of disease.

The production of autoimmunity is a complex situation characterized by a breakdown of normal homeostatic mechanisms at several points due to several factors. As we learn about the normal response to antigens, we will also learn about the autoimmune response; as we learn to manipulate the normal, so shall we be able to manipulate the ability of the immune system to react to self.

I will first discuss the autoantibodies in the non-organ-specific diseases, SLE, RA, and scleroderma, because they are the diseases for which tests are commonly available and most widely ordered.

NON-ORGAN-SPECIFIC DISEASES AND ANTIBODIES

Antinuclear Antibodies and the LE Cell Phenomenon

Historically, the first test for the demonstration of ANA was the demonstration of the LE cell phenomenon. The LE cell, which was first described by Hargraves et al. in 1948,[9] results from the phagocytosis of altered nuclear material by polymorphonuclear leukocytes. Alteration of the nuclear material results from the reaction of ANA with nuclear DNA histone. This reaction results in the influx of water, altering the free nuclear material, and acts as an opsonin, thereby enhancing phagocytosis by the polymorphonuclear leukocytes. The hematoxylin body found in the tissue of patients with SLE, and the LE cell inclusion of the LE cell, are thought to be of similar origin.

In the last 2 decades, other tests have largely replaced the LE cell test to demonstrate ANAs. However, more than one surprised physician has made a diagnosis of SLE based on the unexpected appearance of the LE cell in pericardial, pleural, or spinal fluid. Although the LE cell test is less sensitive than the routinely available immunofluorescence test for ANA, it is more specific. Harvey et al. believe that up to 80% of SLE patients will have a positive LE test at some time in the course of their disease.[10] The apparent sensitivity of the LE cell test decreases significantly, however, when one considers that only 20% of SLE patients may be positive at a given time. In general, because of sensitivity, the ANA tests are routinely ordered when SLE is considered, and the LE cell preparation is ordered when other ANA-specific tests are negative to help confirm a diagnosis of SLE. The LE cell preparation is less likely than ANA-specific tests to be positive in normal subjects and in patients with other collagen vascular diseases, such as RA, polymyositis, or chronic active hepatitis. I regard it as a valuable test for distinguishing SLE from other rheumatic diseases (the LE cell preparation is therefore moderately sensitive and moderately specific for SLE).

Antinuclear Antibodies (Figs 5–2 through 5–5)

Although several assays are available, the indirect immunofluorescent (IIF) technique (see Chap. 2) is the one most commonly used to detect ANA. The ANA consists of a number of antibodies specific for nuclear antigens. In the IIF technique, organ sections from animal or man have been used, as well as tissue culture, as substrates for the detection of ANA. To understand the results reported by a given laboratory, one must know the significance of a given titer, the frequency of positive reactions, and the fluorescence patterns seen in normal subjects and in patients with other diseases. These may all vary according to the substrate used.

Much has been made of the patterns of immunofluorescence (nuclear rim, speckled, homogeneous, and nucleolar staining) that are observed in

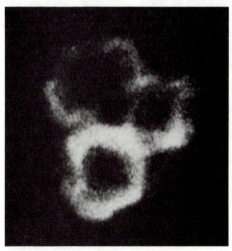

Fig 5–2.—Indirect immunofluorescence antinuclear antibody test on peripheral blood leukocytes: rim pattern.

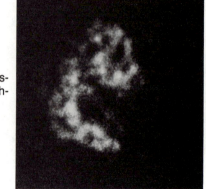

Fig 5–3.—Indirect immunofluorescence antinuclear antibody test on peripheral blood leukocytes: speckled pattern.

different patients, but their usefulness in clinical diagnosis is limited by two factors. First, most SLE sera have a mixture of ANA, as demonstrated by changes in the fluorescence pattern at different dilutions of the serum. The explanation for this observation is that the antibody responsible for the solid pattern may be in lower titer, so that as the serum is diluted, the pattern disappears; if the antibody responsible for the rim or speckled pattern is present in higher titer, these patterns will be evident at the higher dilutions. Second, no specific pattern is specific for any one disease except the nucleolar staining pattern. A pure nucleolar pattern, when present at high antibody titer (>1,000), is almost diagnostic for scleroderma.[11] Al-

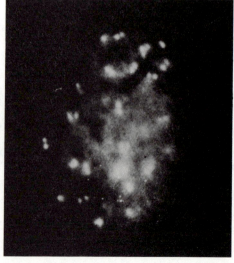

Fig 5–4.—Indirect immunofluorescence antinuclear antibody test on tissue culture preparation: positive speckled pattern associated with antibodies to centromeres. This cell is in metaphase. (Reproduced courtesy of Eric Schenk, M.D.)

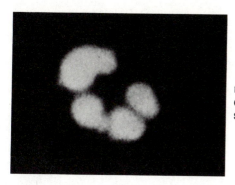

Fig 5–5.—Indirect immunofluorescence antinuclear antibody test on peripheral blood leukocytes: solid pattern.

though specific, this test is not very sensitive; it may be positive in only 20% of patients with scleroderma, and usually these patients can be diagnosed clinically because of the extensive skin involvement.

The patterns of fluorescence do, however, appear to be related to specific antibodies directed against specific nuclear antigens. The homogeneous staining pattern is due to antibody to insoluble DNA histone and can be seen in all the connective tissue diseases. It may also be the antibody responsible for the LE cell preparation. The reason one can observe a positive homogeneous pattern and a negative LE cell preparation is that the antibody is not present in a high enough titer to produce a positive LE cell preparation. A rim pattern of fluorescence is seen mainly in sera from patients with SLE and is associated primarily with antibodies to DNA. This pattern, however, can be seen in sera from patients who do not have SLE and in sera that do not contain a demonstrable antibody to DNA. The speckled pattern of fluorescence is due to antibodies of many specificities and is seen in all connective tissue diseases. Antibodies that produce this pattern are demonstrated less frequently in substrates of human origin and more frequently when tissue culture substrates are used. Further studies on the antigens causing the speckled pattern have revealed clinically relevant information that is discussed in the section on extractable nuclear antigens.

IIF for the demonstration of ANA has an established place in the workup of patients with SLE and should be used as a screening test, to be followed by more specific diagnostic tests. It is positive in 95%–98% of patients with SLE and has a high degree of sensitivity, but it is frequently positive as well in patients with other connective tissue diseases, in family members of individuals with SLE, and, in low titer, in normal individuals.[12] For these reasons, it is not specific—it cannot be used to distinguish patients with SLE from those with similar diseases. In addition, if one considers the prevalence of SLE in a population to be 1 in 2,000, which is a generous prevalence, and that the test may yield positive results in up to 7% of normals, it is understandable why IIF is not used as a screening test in asymptomatic individuals. One is more likely to obtain a false positive test result in a normal person than a true positive result in a patient with SLE. As stated, the ANA test is positive in various connective tissue diseases, including 30% of patients with RA[13] and 50% of patients with scleroderma.[14] Although the ANA titers in patients with RA and scleroderma tend to be lower than in patients with SLE, high titers do occur with sufficient frequency in these diseases that high titer alone does not support a diagnosis of SLE.

DNA Antibodies

Of the specific ANA, anti-DNA antibodies are most readily obtainable. Among these antibodies are those with the highest specificity for the diagnosis of SLE. As stated previously, the LE cell preparation demonstrates antibody to a DNA histone complex, and although it is more specific than the ANA assay, a positive response does occur in other diseases. Antibodies to nDNA are highly specific for the clinical diagnosis of SLE, although there are rare reports of such antibodies being found in RA and chronic active hepatitis.[15] Anti-nDNA antibodies occur maximally in 70%–75% of active, untreated cases of SLE. Their levels fluctuate with disease activity and tend to be low in patients who are in remission, whether the remission is spontaneously or treatment induced, high in patients with active disease, and low in patients with few signs and symptoms. Patients with minimal signs and symptoms are usually examined in an outpatient setting, and in this type of patient and in this setting, the test has a high specificity but a low sensitivity. Unfortunately, there is no single sensitive and specific test available for evaluating a patient with minimal signs or symptoms. In addition to being of diagnostic help, the test can be used to identify patients at risk for renal disease. Most patients with active nephritis have appreciable titers of antibody to nDNA.[16] Until recently, the most commonly used assay for antibody to nDNA was the Farr test. In this test, nDNA is obtained from human cell lines or microorganisms. The nDNA is radioactively labeled and incubated with the serum to be tested. A reaction is allowed to occur, and the immunoglobulin fraction is precipitated with 50% ammonium sulfate. If the radioactive nDNA has attached itself to antibody, some radioactivity will appear in the pellet and the percentage bound can be determined by knowing how much radioactive nDNA was added to the serum and how much remained in solution. The sensitivity and specificity of the Farr test depend on good preparations of nDNA that are free of single-stranded determinants.

The difficulty of preparing pure nDNA led to the development of another test that is gaining increasing popularity for the detection of antibody to nDNA. This is an IIF method that uses *Crithidia luciliae* as a substrate.[17] *Crithidia luciliae* is a trypanosome which grows easily in culture at room temperature and contains within its kinetoplast circular double-stranded DNA that is immunochemically nDNA. The test has the advantage of a purified antigen and is easy to perform. A disadvantage is that titers of antibody can only be crudely determined by sequential dilutions of the patient's serum. Since it is a very specific test, most laboratories report results as positive or negative only. Therefore, IIF with *C. luciliae* is not being used to measure activity of disease, as one can use the antibody to nDNA as determined by the Farr technique.

Antibodies to ssDNA occur in almost all patients with SLE but are also found in patients with a number of inflammatory diseases, including all the collagen vascular diseases. A test for anti-ssDNA antibody is therefore much less specific than the ANA test, and most laboratories no longer offer it routinely. The antibody does appear to have some pathogenic significance because it can be eluted from the kidneys of patients with SLE and renal disease.

Antibodies to Extractable Nuclear Antigens

Antigens of the nonhistone (acidic) nuclear proteins are commonly known as the extractable nuclear antigens (ENA). They became the object of intense interest after it was demonstrated that some ENAs may be of diagnostic significance in distinguishing one rheumatic disease from another. Antibodies to ENA all have a speckled pattern of immunofluorescence, but different substrates have varying amounts of the antigens, so the frequency of positive results will vary with different substrates. To determine the specificity of the antibody producing the speckled pattern, other techniques must be used, such as Ouchterlony double diffusion or passive hemagglutination. These tests use specific antigens extracted from tissues such as calf thymus or tissue culture cells. The antigens responsible for the speckled pattern are designated SM (the first two letters of the patient's name in whose serum such antibodies were first demonstrated), nuclear ribonucleoprotein (NRNP), and SS-B. These antigens can be detected on mouse kidney or rat liver substrates. The antigen called HA by other investigators is the same as SS-B.[18] Antibody to SS-A does not give positive fluorescence on these substrates. The designations SS-A and SS-B stand for soluble substance A and B, which are obtained by extraction from Wil-2 cells, a human lymphoblastoid cell line.[19] When the immunofluorescent technique with Wil-2 cells is used, antibodies to SS-A result in a speckled pattern of fluorescence, whereas antibodies to SS-B result in a homogeneous pattern.

The antibody to the SM antigen, when present, is highly specific for SLE.[14] Unfortunately, it is detected only in about 25% of SLE patients; but it has not been detected in other rheumatic diseases. Therefore, the test is very specific but not sensitive for SLE.

Antibody to NRNP occurs in about 40% of SLE patients and is of great clinical interest because patients with such antibodies rarely make antibody to nDNA, have a low incidence of nephritis, and generally have a favorable prognosis.[20] These antibodies, however, are not specific for SLE and can be found in patients with RA and scleroderma. In addition, they are found in high titers in patients who have overlap features of SLE, scleroderma, and polymyositis, a condition commonly referred to as the mixed connective tissue disease (MCTD) syndrome.[21] While it is true that such patients may have high titers of NRNP, to the exclusion of other antinuclear antibodies, some patients who have high titers of antibodies to NRNP do not have clinical features of MCTD and can be diagnosed as having SLE[22] or scleroderma.[14] In addition, some patients with typical features of MCTD may have both SM and anti-DNA antibodies with no antibodies to NRNP and are therefore at risk for development of renal disease. The typical MCTD patient is either in the early stages of scleroderma or has SLE, and the antibody profile is of help in determining the eventual clinical course. These types of observations have suggested that the clinical course is more tightly linked with serology rather than with the presenting clinical features.

By the Ouchterlony double diffusion technique, precipitins can be demonstrated to SS-A in 70% of patients and to SS-B in 48% of patients with Sjögren's syndrome, in 9% and 3%, respectively, of patients with RA with Sjögren's syndrome, and in 0% of patients with SLE.[19] In another study, the antibody to the SS-B antigen by Ouchterlony double diffusion was detected in 13% of sera from patients with SLE, but in 68% of sera from patients with Sjögren's syndrome, either primary or associated with other rheumatic diseases.[23] These antibodies are therefore of moderate sensitivity and specificity for Sjögren's syndrome.

Histone Antibodies

Antibodies to histones produce a rim or homogeneous pattern of nuclear staining when tissue is used as a substrate. The technique confirming that antibody to histones is present utilizes .1N hydrochloric acid as a histone-extracting solvent in a tissue substrate (usually mouse kidney slices) and IIF. IIF is performed on two tissue slices, one that has not been extracted with .1N HCl and one that has been extracted with HCl. If strong nuclear staining is noted on a slide bearing unextracted tissue and disappears or significantly decreases on a slide bearing HCl-extracted tissue, the antibody is reacting with histones. Since these antibodies are present in only 35% of patients with SLE, it is not a sensitive or specific test for SLE, but it is of value in evaluating patients who have SLE-like syndromes induced by procainamide and hydralazine. In this population of patients, the histone antibody is the predominant antibody and is present in 96% of patients with active disease.[24] The test is therefore useful in a negative sense: if one suspects that a patient has hydralazine- or procainamide-induced LE syndrome and the test is negative, as indicated by appropriate staining of both the extracted and unextracted tissue, then it is unlikely that the patient has drug-induced SLE.

Other Antibodies in SLE

Although this chapter deals with ANA, patients with SLE have a multitude of antibodies to other antigens. These are listed in Table 5–5. This fact is important in evaluating patients who are ANA-positive and are suspected of having SLE but who do not have sufficient clinical symptoms to establish a diagnosis of SLE.[25] In these ANA-positive, SM- and DNA-antibody-negative patients, clinical or serologic tests should be performed to determine if other antibodies are present. Clinical or serologic confirmation

TABLE 5–5.—Other Autoantibodies
in SLE

Membranes
Red blood cells
Platelets
Granulocytes
Lymphocytes
Circulating proteins
Rheumatoid factor
Circulating anticoagulant
Cytoplasmic antigens
Ribosomal ribonuclear protein
Mitochondrial
Microsomal
Organ-specific
Thyroid epithelial cells
Gastric parietal cells
Adrenal cortical cells
Neuronal cells
Heart
Other
Cardiolipin
Collagen

of the presence of other antibodies would help establish the diagnosis of SLE in a patient who is SM- or DNA-antibody-negative.

Others antibodies of importance are antibodies to cytoplasmic antigens, which have been designated RO and LA by Provost[26] and which are not detectable by IIF. By the Ouchterlony double diffusion technique, these antibodies occur in 30% and 10% of SLE patients, respectively. They also occur in about 5% of patients with RA, scleroderma, and polymyositis. RO and LA antibodies are of interest because there is a small number of patients who are ANA-negative on conventional substrates but who have clinical features of SLE and only cytoplasmic antibodies. These ANA-negative SLE patients are characterized by extensive dermatitis, especially of the photosensitive type, and are also RF-positive. RO and LA antibodies have also been demonstrated in the serum of both the mother and her newborn when the newborn has a lupus-like dermatitis at birth, suggesting that these antibodies may contribute to the dermatitis noted in patients with SLE.

Scleroderma

The ANAs detected by IIF are often found in low titers in the sera of patients with scleroderma. The frequency varies from 40%–90%, depending on the substrates used, but in general ANA tests are of very little clinical value in evaluating patients with scleroderma. There are, however, two antibodies that are important in the diagnosis of scleroderma—the antinucleolar antibody and the antibody that detects chromosome centromeres. Antinucleolar antibodies react with a low molecular weight nuclear RNA and are found in about 20% of patients.[11] This test is therefore very specific but not sensitive.

The anticentromere antibody is sensitive and moderately specific in patients with the CREST syndrome, a subset of patients with scleroderma. The CREST syndrome has minimal skin involvement but entails calcinosis (c), Raynaud's phenomenon (r), esophageal dysfunction (e), sclerodactyly (s), and telangiectasia (t). Although this syndrome is thought to be a mild form of scleroderma, the mildness refers only to the skin involvement. Patients with the CREST syndrome can also develop pulmonary fibrosis, hypertension, and hepatic involvement of scleroderma. IIF detection of the anticentromere antibody is performed on tissue culture cell lines with a high mitotic index to obtain cells that are in metaphase. The commercially available Hep-2 human epithelial cell line is commonly used. A positive test result has been found in 98% of patients with CREST syndrome, 29% of patients with Raynaud's disease, 7% of patients with MCTD, 2% of patients with SLE, and 12% of patients with systemic sclerosis.[27] The test is of value in determining which patients with the CREST syndrome will remain free of extensive skin involvement and in evaluating patients who present with Raynaud's phenomenon. In general, a positive test indicates that the patient should be examined extensively and followed closely for the development of systemic disease.

Rheumatoid Factors

The term "rheumatoid factor" evolved from the observation of Waaler[28] and Rose[29] that serum from a high proportion of patients with RA agglutinated sheep RBCs sensitized with rabbit antibodies to sheep RBCs. Although these factors have been demonstrated to be anti-antibodies or anti-immunoglobulins, the term rheumatoid factor has persisted because of their association with RA, even though it is now recognized that RF auto-antibodies are associated with a wide variety of disease states, and also occur with increased frequency in the elderly. RF antibodies are directed against specific antigenic determinants on the Fc fragments of human or animal IgG. They exist in the three major classes of immunoglobulins (IgA, IgG, IgM; also in IgD), although they usually exist in serum in the IgM fraction. They are now thought to comprise a broad spectrum of antibodies with a wide range of specificities for the Fc fragment of IgG.

Other anti-immunoglobulins have been identified that have specificities for the antibody-combining sites, called anti-idiotypes, and for other portions of the immunoglobulin molecule. These are not RF antibodies because their specificities are for sites other than the Fc fragment of IgG.

Methods of Measurement

Several different methods have been developed for measuring RF. The most commonly used test is the latex agglutination test.[28-30] Latex particles are coated with aggregated human 7S IgG and are then incubated with human serum, either on a slide or in a test tube. Agglutination of the particles indicates the presence of RF. An estimation of titer is obtained by performing serial dilutions of the serum. Other particles such as bentonite have been used; the agglutination principles are the same.

In some laboratories, the sensitized sheep RBC agglutination test (Waaler-Rose test) is still employed. In this test sheep RBCs are coated with rabbit 7S antibody to sheep RBCs. The ability of serum to agglutinate these rabbit 7S antibody-coated sheep RBCs indicates the presence of antibody to IgG. A variation of this test involves the use of formalized or tannic acid–treated RBCs to allow a more stable bond between the IgG and the RBC.

Diagnostic Significance of Tests for RF

RF is not specific for any disease entity. The RF titer increases with age and may be found in very high titers in a few healthy young adults. RF tests are moderately sensitive for RA, yielding positive results in 60%–90% of patients with RA, and the positivity increases with duration of disease. In addition, almost 100% of patients with rheumatoid nodules are RF-positive. Thus, although the test is sensitive for RA, its specificity is significantly decreased by its high prevalence in patients with many infections, such as subacute bacterial endocarditis, syphilis, schistosomiasis, tuberculosis, leprosy, and, transiently, in patients who have been immunized.[31] The wide range of infectious states associated with positive RF tests suggest that extensive or persistent exposure to antigens induces RF production. It may be that after antibody has reacted with antigen it acquires a new configuration that is recognized as foreign and therefore is capable of eliciting an immune response. By this theory, RF production is a normal immune response under the control of the usual modulating factors.

Other diseases in which the RF titer is known to be increased include idiopathic fibrosis, silicosis, asbestosis, sarcoidosis, chronic active hepatitis, mixed cryoglobulinemia, hypergammaglobulinemia-purpura, and the collagen vascular diseases.[32] Because of this high frequency of positive RF results in normals and in patients with other diseases, the RF is of no help as a screening test for RA, nor is it of any help in establishing the diagnosis of RA. If one suspects that a patient has RA clinically, a positive test would confirm the diagnosis. However, since 10%–40% of patients with RA have a negative test result, one can still make the diagnosis of RA using clinical criteria. The RF is therefore a test that is moderately sensitive but poorly specific for RA.

ORGAN-SPECIFIC DISEASES AND ANTIBODIES

Autoimmune Thyroid Disease—Thyroiditis

Autoimmune diseases of the thyroid fulfill Witebsky's criteria and have served as the model for organ-specific autoimmune diseases. Thyroiditis is one of the most common of the endocrine diseases. Depending on the clinical course, pathology, and serology, it may present in a variety of forms, including Hashimoto's thyroiditis, nonspecific chronic thyroiditis, lymphocytic thyroiditis of adolescence and childhood, and chronic atrophic thyroiditis. These disorders have in common the presence of antibodies to thyroid gland, a lymphocytic infiltration of the gland, a higher incidence in women, and coexistence with pernicious anemia, idiopathic adrenal failure,

Sjögren's syndrome, RA, chronic active hepatitis, and SLE. These are all diseases considered to be of autoimmune etiology and with familial clustering. The autoimmune etiology has been established in an animal model.[33] In addition, Graves' disease, or primary hyperplasia, is due to a diffuse stimulation of the gland by thyroid-stimulating immunoglobulin, originally described as long-acting thyroid stimulator (LATS). This stimulator seems to act in the same manner as thyroid-stimulating hormone (TSH).[34] The serologic diagnosis of autoimmune thyroiditis is based primarily on the detection of antibodies to thyroglobulin, to microsomes, to thyroid cell surface antigens, and to colloid component antigens. In practice, because of availability, the tests performed are for antibodies to thyroglobulin and microsomes.

Antibodies to Thyroglobulins

Although antibodies to thyroglobulins can be detected by several techniques, they are usually detected by the passive hemagglutination assay (see Chap. 2).[35] In this procedure, thyroglobulin is isolated and RBCs are sensitized to it. The thyroglobulin-sensitized RBCs are then incubated with the serum to be tested. If the patient has antibodies to thyroglobulin, agglutination occurs. A titer is obtained by diluting the serum and determining the final dilution capable of producing agglutination. A more sensitive technique is radioimmunoassay,[36] and a less sensitive technique is IIF. By using IIF, one may detect all four antibodies on sections of human thyroid tissue. The more sensitive assay gives both a higher titer and a higher frequency of positive tests in a given disease. As one might expect, the more sensitive the assay, the less specific it becomes for autoimmune thyroiditis. By radioimmunoassay, 100% of patients with thyroiditis, 98% of patients with Graves' disease, and 20% of controls are positive.[36]

The highest titers of antibody to thyroglobulin are associated with Hashimoto's thyroiditis. By the hemagglutination technique, 85% of patients have titers greater than 1:32. On occasion, similar high titers can also be seen in patients with nonimmune thyroid diseases, such as toxic diffuse goiter, nontoxic nodular goiter, and thyroid carcinoma, and in 5% of normals. Normal individuals rarely have titers over 1:256, and titers over 1:1,000 are considered diagnostic for Hashimoto's thyroiditis. In addition, about 50% of relatives of patients with Hashimoto's thyroiditis, chronic thyroiditis, or diffuse toxic goiter have measurable titers of thyroid antibodies, and antibody levels increase with age.[34] Normal individuals and relatives of patients with overt thyroid disease who have measurable titers may have subclinical thyroid autoimmune disease rather than an autoantibody of no clinical significance.[37] IIF, being less sensitive than the hemagglutination technique, gives lower titers in patients with Hashimoto's disease but is usually negative in patients with goiters or thyroid carcinoma and in normal subjects. This technique is therefore moderately sensitive and specific. The hemagglutination assay is sensitive and moderately specific. The radioimmunoassay is very sensitive and nonspecific. Very high titers, however, are diagnostic of Hashimoto's thyroiditis.

Antibodies to Thyroid Microsomes

The first recognition of autoantibodies to microsomes was obtained by IIF and using human thyroid tissue. The specificity of the cytoplasmic staining of the thyroid parenchyma-lining follicles for microsomes was determined by absorbing the serum with the microsomal fraction of thyroid tissue homogenates and noting that the serum no longer stained the cytoplasm. Presently, most general laboratories use the passive hemagglutination technique, which is available commercially in a kit. It appears to be as sensitive and specific as IIF.[37] Sera from 95% of patients with Hashimoto's thyroiditis and 87% of patients with Graves' disease have been reported to be positive by both techniques. In addition, 20% of patients with nonimmune thyroid disease, including thyroid cancer, may be positive. High titers, however, strongly suggest thyroiditis or Graves' disease.[38] The presence of antibodies to thyroid microsomes is therefore sensitive but only moderately specific for thyroiditis.

Other Autoimmune Reactions

Patients with autoimmune Hashimoto's thyroiditis also have an increase in the thyroid cell surface antibody and the colloid component antibody other than thyroglobulin. Both of these antibodies can be detected by IIF. In addition, there is a cytotoxic assay to measure the thyroid cell surface antibody.[39] In the cytotoxic assay, viable human or rhesus monkey thyroid cells can be killed by the cell surface antibodies from patients with thyroiditis. Cell-mediated immunity has also been demonstrated in patients and animals with thyroiditis, but less frequently than autoantibodies and with less organ specificity. The role that these antibodies and cell-mediated immunity play in the production of thyroiditis is not clear. Since these tests are essentially research assays, their sensitivities and frequencies have not been established.

Graves' Disease

The hyperthyroidism of Graves' disease is a consequence of stimulation of the thyroid by circulating immunoglobulins, which can be detected in several ways. There is no commercially available test. In a sensitive assay based on the ability of sera from patients with Graves' disease to compete with the ability of radioactive-labeled TSH to bind to its receptor on human thyroid membrane, 60%–100% of patients with Graves' disease are positive and can be distinguished from patients with toxic nodular goiter and from normal controls.[40] In addition to antithyroglobulin antibodies (in 50% of patients) and antimicrosomal antibodies (in 87%), there are now case reports of patients with Graves' disease who also have immune complex–mediated manifestations.[41]

It should be clear that in the evaluation of a patient with thyroid disease the immunologic studies must be combined with chemical tests, radioisotope studies, physical examination, and family history in order to arrive at a specific diagnosis.[42] In addition, one must be aware of the increased frequency of these antibodies in patients with nonimmunologic thyroid diseases, other endocrinopathies, pernicious anemia, and rheumatic diseases and in the aged.

Myasthenia Gravis

Clinical evidence has long suggested a role for autoimmune phenomena in myasthenia gravis. The evidence consisted of pathology of the neuromuscular junction lesion, an abnormal thymus, remission of the disease in some patients with thymectomy, the presence of other autoantibodies, such as ANA, antithyroid antibody, and RF, the transient occurrence of neonatal myasthenia gravis in children born to myasthenic mothers, and the presence of autoantibodies to striated muscle.

With the identification of an antibody to the acetylcholine receptor, and as a result of studies on animals, myasthenia gravis has been shown to fulfill Witebsky's criteria for an autoimmune disease. An acetylcholine receptor antibody is detected in 95% of patients with myasthenia gravis, and rabbits and other animals injected with electric eel acetylcholine receptors develop a myasthenia syndrome. Animals with the clinical manifestations of myasthenia have clinical, pathologic, pharmacologic, and electrophysiologic features similar to those noted in man. Passive transfer of serum from an involved animal to a nonimmunized animal will induce the disease within 24 hours.[43] As tests for the detection of antibody to the acetylcholine receptor become more standardized, one can expect that this will be a routine procedure in the diagnosis of myasthenia gravis. Three such tests are described below.

ANTIBODY TO STRIATED MUSCLE.—The only test commonly available for myasthenia gravis is for striated muscle cell antibodies. IIF is currently used for detecting this antibody. Striated muscle of rat, guinea pig, or man is used as the substrate. Although thymus is not commonly used, it is also possible to demonstrate antibody to muscle antigen in thymus tissue. The antibody reacts to both the I band of the sarcomere and the A band of the myofibril of skeletal muscle. Undiluted serum from normal subjects ordinarily yields a positive result, so the test should be performed at high dilutions. Depending on the laboratory, significant dilutions are above the 1:40 to 1:50 range. Any finding in less diluted serum should not be considered significant. Antibodies to striated muscle occur in only 40% of all patients with myasthenia gravis, and therefore the test is not a sensitive one. However, it is positive in 90%–100% of patients with myasthenia gravis and thymoma, in 25% of patients with thymoma and no myasthenia gravis, and in 30% of patients with myasthenia gravis and no thymoma.[44, 45] These kinds of relationships suggest that the thymus is very important in the production of this autoantibody. At present the test is not considered to be of diagnostic or of pathologic significance.

Antibody to acetylcholine receptors.—While tests for antibodies to acetylcholine receptors are not currently available, it is certain that these antibodies are of major pathologic significance in patients with myasthenia gravis. The demonstration of this antibody utilizes a fraction of cobra venom called α-bungarotoxin, which is capable of binding to the acetylcholine receptors. This material is radiolabeled, and the ability of a patient's serum to inhibit binding of the radiolabeled bungarotoxin to the acetylcholine receptor indicates the presence of an autoantibody to the receptor. The acetylcholine receptor is obtained from the electric organ of eels and is solubilized so that the reaction can occur in an aqueous medium. Positive inhibition occurs if 20% of the radiolabeled α-bungarotoxin is inhibited from reacting with the acetylcholine receptor of the electric eel. In limited series, 30%–70% of patients with myasthenia gravis have had inhibition above the 20% level and 95% have had some inhibition. No control patient has had positive inhibition above the 20% level. Recently, an immunofluorescence technique has been developed to make the detection of this antibody more practical. Evidence exists for a relationship of this antigen to the thymus in that acetylcholine receptor antigen is present on the surface of thymic epithelial cells.

Cellular immunity.—There is also evidence that patients with myasthenia gravis do have delayed sensitivity in vitro to the acetylcholine receptor. This evidence is suggested by blast transformation of peripheral blood lymphocytes isolated from patients with myasthenia gravis and stimulated with acetylcholine receptor preparations obtained from the electric organ of the eel.[43]

Diabetes Mellitus

For many years, there has been circumstantial evidence of an autoimmune component in insulin-dependent diabetes. The evidence consisted of an increased frequency of multiple endocrinopathies in the same patient and an increased frequency of autoantibodies in some patients with insulin-dependent diabetes.[46] Consistent with an autoimmune pathogenesis were the findings of an insulitis[47] and animal models in which diabetes could be produced actively and passively.[48]

This circumstantial evidence has recently been supported by immunologic studies documenting that autoimmunity to insulin is responsible for some of the manifestations in a small group of insulin-dependent diabetic patients. These manifestations can be divided into three groups: (1) autoimmune insulin syndrome, (2) insulin-resistant diabetes with antireceptor antibodies, and (3) insulin allergy. Insulin-resistant diabetes due to antibodies to exogenous insulin is not an autoimmune disease, but it will be discussed because it is an immune response that may bear on the treatment of diabetes mellitus. In the juvenile-onset diabetic, although there is an autoimmune response, there is also evidence that this response is secondary and follows viral injury to the islet cells.

Immunologic Tests

CELL-MEDIATED IMMUNITY.—There is evidence for a cellular immune response to pancreatic islet cells. This evidence was obtained by incubating pancreatic homogenates with peripheral blood lymphocytes from diabetic patients. By this technique, 65% of diabetic patients exhibited inhibition of leukocyte migration.[49] This inhibition was taken as evidence of cellular immunity and was attributed to the production of migration inhibitory factor by lymphocytes obtained from diabetic patients when stimulated by pancreatic tissue. In addition, lymphocytes from patients with insulin-dependent diabetes are cytotoxic to cultured human insulinoma cells.[50] In a recent study, lymphocytes were obtained from peripheral blood samples of patients with insulin-dependent diabetes and transferred to athymic nude mice, so that no cell destruction would occur, and the animals developed diabetes.[51]

INSULIN ANTIBODIES.—The presence of insulin-binding antibodies on radioimmunoassay of sera of diabetic patients was first reported by Berson et al. in 1956.[52] By this technique and by direct skin testing with insulin, antibodies have been detected in all immunoglobulin classes.[53]

ISLET CELL ANTIBODIES.—IIF is used to detect antibodies to islet cells. The substrate is unfixed group O human pancreas obtained from cadaver kidney donors or fresh undigested human pancreas. The staining of importance is the cytoplasm of cells in the islets, but experience is required to determine the cell stained.[54]

Autoimmune Insulin Syndrome

About 20 cases have been reported of patients who have had insulin antibodies in association with hypoglycemia without any prior exposure to exogenous insulin. In these patients, one must rule out the self-administration of insulin that is not reported to the physician.[55]

Insulin-Resistant Diabetes with Antireceptor Antibodies

The clearest association of autoimmunity and diabetes is seen in patients who have autoantibodies to insulin receptors.[56] These patients also have acanthosis nigricans.[56] As one might expect, these patients are typically insulin resistant, and some require astronomical amounts of insulin to stimulate the insulin receptor site. There is an animal model for this form of diabetes, and so the disease fulfills Witebsky's criteria for an autoimmune disease.

The antibody nature of the insulin resistance in these patients has been demonstrated on their circulating monocytes. Monocyte resistance to the effect of insulin could be passively transferred from the serum of these patients to normal cells. The inhibiting factor is IgG. Radioactive insulin is used to demonstrate this antibody. When radioactive insulin is incubated with normal cells from healthy subjects, specific binding occurs at the insulin receptor sites. When these cells are incubated with serum containing anti-insulin receptor antibodies prior to exposure to the radioactive insulins, the binding of the radioactive insulin is decreased significantly compared to cells exposed to normal serum. In acute experiments, this antibody is capable of inducing the full range of insulin actions on monocytes and is similar to LATS in patients with Graves' disease. With chronic exposure of cells in culture to these antibodies, however, the stimulating effect of the antibody is only temporary and is followed by several hours of lack of cell response to insulin. Such tissue culture experiments suggest that these patients are in the refractory stage of cell response to insulin. Some patients have improved spontaneously, while others have required cytoxan and prednisone, or prednisone alone, to induce remission. In one patient, an exchange plasma transfusion was effective in lowering antibody titers and temporarily producing some clinical improvement, as indicated by increased responsiveness to insulin.[57] In addition, these patients may be ANA-positive and may have other autoimmune diseases such as SLE and Sjögren's syndrome or ataxia-telangiectasia.[58]

Insulin Allergy

Some immunologic reactions to insulin take the form of insulin allergy. Patients with insulin allergy demonstrate an IgE response to insulin, and the allergy can be detected by routine skin testing. On skin testing, patients have immediate wheal and flare reactions, and on administration of insulin, they may experience systemic reactions such as urticaria, angioedema, hypotension, and wheezing. All such patients have positive immediate skin tests when insulin from animal sources is used, and some have positive skin tests when human insulin is used.[59] These patients become allergic to human insulin by the shared or cross-reactive antigen model.

Insulin Resistance

Most patients with insulin-resistant diabetes have high titers of antibodies to administered insulin. Insulin resistance is said to exist whenever normal amounts of insulin elicit a less than normal biologic response. Since the average rate of endogenous insulin secretion does not exceed 60 units per day, any patient requiring an excess of 60 units per day has some degree of insulin resistance. A diagnosis of insulin-resistant diabetes due to anti-insulin antibodies requires the demonstration of antibodies to insulin, ordinarily by using radioactively labeled insulin in a competitive binding assay.[60]

Autoimmunity in Insulin-Dependent Diabetics

Although autoimmunity in insulin-dependent diabetics has not been proved, there is some evidence for it. The evidence is by five associations: (1) there appears to be an association of diabetes with other autoimmune endocrinopathies; (2) there is a high prevalence of autoantibodies to nonpancreatic antigens in patients with diabetes; (3) an inflammatory process in the pancreas, similar to that recognized in autoimmune endocrinopathies, is seen in some patients with diabetes mellitus; (4) circulating antibodies to islet cells are noted in 31% of patients with insulin-dependent diabetes; and (5) there is also evidence of a cell-mediated immunity to islet cells, using a leukocyte migration inhibition test.

Serum Antibodies to Islet Cells

By IIF, islet cell antibodies can be demonstrated in 31% of patients with insulin-dependent diabetes in about 6% of non-insulin-dependent diabetics, and in .5%–1.7% of nondiabetic normals with low titers. Nondiabetic patients with other autoimmune endocrinopathies or nondiabetic first-degree relatives of patients with insulin-dependent diabetes mellitus also show a slight increase in islet cell antibodies (8%–9%) above normal. These autoantibodies do not react with insulin but do react with intracellular membranes, which accounts for the cytoplasmic staining noted on human pancreatic tissue. As with all autoantibodies in the organ-specific antibody group, a question remains as to whether these islet cell antibodies play a pathogenic role in the development of insulin-dependent diabetes, or if they are simply markers of β cell destruction.[61] Antibodies detected by this technique are not sensitive and only moderately specific.

Immunologic Aspects of Kidney Disease

The participation of immunologic mechanisms in the pathogenesis of human glomerulonephritis is well established. In most forms of renal disease the injury is a consequence of immune complexes, which account for 70%–80% of the glomerulitidies. The other form of immune system–mediated renal disease occurs by autoantibodies to glomerular basement membrane (GBM) and accounts for 2%–5% of patients with glomerulonephritis.

Immune Complexes

The role of immune complexes is discussed in Chapter 6; in this section I will discuss only the immunologic tests available for establishing the diagnosis of anti-GBM nephritis and Goodpasture's syndrome. Cellular immunity is not thought to play a major role in these diseases.

Autoantibodies to GBM

Autoantibodies to GBM are responsible for some cases of rapidly progressive crescentic glomerulonephritis, as well as for the manifestations of Goodpasture's syndrome. Patients with this form of nephritis have similar serologic findings and renal immunopathology as patients with Goodpasture's syndrome but do not have evidence of pulmonary involvement. The diagnosis of anti-renal basement membrane antibody disease is established by direct immunofluorescence (DIF). In this procedure, a renal biopsy is performed and DIF is used to determine whether antibody or complement is localized to the area of inflammation. Patients with anti-renal basement membrane antibody disease have a bright, linear accumulation of IgG along the GBM.[62] The routine histologic studies should also reveal crescentic glomerulonephritis. The combination of linear deposition of immunoglobulin and crescentic glomerulonephritis is sufficient to establish the diagnosis of renal disease due to anti-basement membrane antibody. The pattern suggests the diagnosis but does not establish it, because it can also be seen in various forms of sclerosing glomerulonephritis, as well as in kidneys of some patients with hypertension or SLE.

More conclusive evidence for anti-GBM disease is obtained by demonstrating the presence of anti-GBM antibodies in the serum of patients. This may be done by IIF, using normal kidney tissue as a substrate and layering the patient's serum on this substrate to determine if antibody to the basement membrane is present. The presence of anti-GBM antibody is indicated by the attachment of the fluorescein-labeled anti-human immunoglobulin antibody to the GBM. By IIF, positive results are obtained in 60%–85% of patients.

A more sensitive radioimmunoassay that uses purified GBM is positive in 80%–95% of patients.[63] The serologic test is specific for anti-GBM nephritis, and the reason why it is not positive in 100% of cases is that the antibody may be present in such low concentrations in the serum that it is undetectable. In this situation, most of the antibody that is produced is attached to the GBM, and only after these antigenic sites are saturated will the excess circulate in the serum. Patients who have had nephrectomies may have a rapid rise in anti-GBM antibody because the GBM is no longer available for combination with antibody and all the antibody produced is present in the serum.

This form of renal disease has been reproduced experimentally in a number of animals, and the disease has also been transferred from human serum to squirrel monkeys.[61] In patients with pulmonary manifestations, such as those that occur in Goodpasture's syndrome, IgG deposition similar to that found in the kidney is also noted along the pulmonary alveolar basement membrane.[62] The tests for anti-GBM antibody are therefore moderately sensitive but very specific by IIF, and both sensitive and specific by radioimmunoassay.

Immunologic Aspects of Skin Disease

Bullous diseases, which include pemphigus, pemphigoid, and dermatitis herpetiformis, are routinely diagnosed by DIF. In addition, DIF is helpful in the diagnosis of lichen planus and skin manifestations due to lupus erythematosus. The only disease of this group that fulfills Witebsky's postulates is pemphigus. The others, except lichen planus, have evidence that autoimmunity is contributing to the pathology; in lichen planus, the immunopathology is of diagnostic importance but not pathogenic significance.

DIF, which is used to establish a diagnosis and is able to detect the presence of immunoglobulin, complement, and fibrinogen in biopsy specimens of skin lesions, has been facilitated by the use of a holding medium. This is a medium that allows tissues to be stored at room temperature for several months while retaining their histologic features.[64, 65] Prior to the development of a holding medium, tissue had to be flash-frozen and kept frozen until use.

Pemphigus

DIF in pemphigus detects IgG in the intercellular substance of the epidermis and stratified epithelium of involved skin (Fig 5–6).[65] IgG is found in all the clinical varieties of the disease, such as vulgaris, vegetans, foliaceous, and erythematosus. The positive stain can be detected in both involved and adjacent uninvolved tissue. In addition to immunoglobulin localization to the skin, patients have a serum antibody to the intercellular substance of stratified epithelium that can be detected with IIF.[67] The best substrate for the demonstration of this antibody is monkey esophagus; when this is not available, rat or guinea pig esophagus is a reasonable alternative. In some cases, however, the antibody can only be demonstrated on monkey esophageal tissue.[68] The titer of the pemphigus antibody often parallels the severity of the illness and can be used to monitor treatment. There are reports of the antibody being detected before the skin and mucosal lesions appeared. The titer will begin to fall before clinical remission

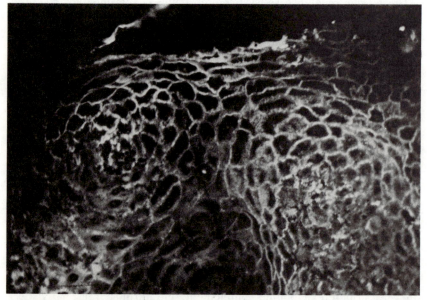

Fig 5–6.—Direct immunofluorescence test performed on skin of a patient with pemphigus: pattern indicates presence of IgG in the intercellular area. (Reproduced courtesy of Eric Schenk, M.D.)

is noted and rise before a relapse of the disease.[69] These observations are taken to imply pathologic significance of the pemphigus antibody. However, the antibody often appears in the serum of burn patients,[70] and a number of drugs evoke pemphigus-like lesions. These drugs include penicillamine, rifampin, phenylbutazone, and captopril.[71] The drug most frequently incriminated is penicillamine. In these patients, both serum antibody tests and direct staining techniques have been positive. Major experimental evidence that these antibodies contribute to the pathogenesis is that they cause the development of acantholytic lesions in culture,[72] and in passive transfer from patients with disease to animals cutaneous blisters developed.[73] Attempts to immunize animals to this antigen have produced antibodies but no pathologic lesions. The DIF and IIF techniques for detection of antibody to stratified epithelium are very sensitive and moderately specific.

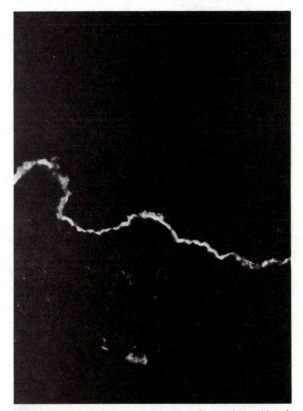

Fig 5–7.—Direct immunofluorescence test performed on skin of a patient with pemphigoid: linear deposition of IgG at the basement membrane between epidermis and dermis. (Reproduced courtesy of Eric Schenk, M.D.)

Pemphigoid

Pemphigoid is a bullous disease in which the separation occurs in the subepidermal area. Bullae may form on normal skin or on an erythematous base. In addition, bullae can occur in the mucous membranes, and in some patients the bullae localize only in the skin or in the mucous membrane. In other patients they are found in both areas. Lesions may also occur in the eyes and genitalia. DIF studies have revealed immunoglobulin localized to the basement membrane zone of the stratified epithelium.[66] The autoantibodies are predominantly of the IgG class but occasionally of the IgM, IgA, IgD, and IgE classes. In addition, complement can frequently be demonstrated in this area. While DIF is positive in almost all cases of bullous pemphigoid, it is positive in only 10% of patients with cicatricial pemphigoid.[74] The pattern may show either a linear deposition or a granular deposition. No clinical significance is attached to these different patterns (Fig 5–7).

IIF detects a circulating antibody in the sera of patients with this disease in 80% of cases.[75] The actual localization of the antibody is in the lamina lucida, which is between the basement membrane and the basal cells.[76] The antibody titer does not appear to show any correlation with the activity or the course of the disease, which suggests that this antibody may not be relevant to the production of the skin lesions. Tissue culture experiments reveal that the antibody does localize to the lamina lucida area, but no changes are noted in the tissue culture. In addition, injection of the antibody into the skin of animals produces localization of the antibody but no pathologic lesions in the skin; however, antibody injection does have a pathogenic effect on rabbit corneal epithelium.[77]

Herpes gestationis, a bullous disease that occurs in late pregnancy and the postpartum period, is positive both by DIF and, in 20% of patients, by IIF of pemphigoid, indicating that this is a form of pemphigoid.[78] Direct staining of the basement membrane zone is also noted in SLE. In this disease, serum antibody is never detected and the pattern is invariably granular. It is thought that localization of immunoglobulin and complement in SLE is due to immune complexes rather than to an anti-basement membrane antibody or lamina lucida antigen. In pemphigoid direct staining is therefore moderately sensitive and specific. The indirect technique for detection of antibody is moderately sensitive but very specific.

Dermatitis Herpetiformis

Dermatitis herpetiformis is a pruritic vesicular eruption that most commonly occurs on the elbows, knees, trunk, and buttocks. Direct staining of the skin adjacent to the vesicular eruption reveals IgA deposits in the fibular material of the dermal papillae.[79] The antigen inducing the autoantibody is reticulin. IIF studies have revealed the presence of antibody in only 25% of patients with untreated disease.[80] The low incidence of this finding may be due to the fact that the antibody is bound to tissues, and only when all the tissue sites have been saturated does the antibody appear in serum. Most patients with dermatitis herpetiformis have asymptomatic gluten enteropathy, and some patients will improve on a gluten-free diet.[80]

The major evidence that dermatitis herpetiformis may be an autoimmune disorder is related to the appearance of other autoantibodies, such as antibodies to gastric mucosa, thyroid, and ANA. Although the role of antireticulin antibody in the production of disease is not clear, it is of tremendous importance clinically in establishing a diagnosis. There is a bullous dermatitis, especially in children, in which linear IgA deposition can be found in the basement membrane zone. These patients appear to have a mixed type of dermatitis clinically that can either be closely related to dermatitis herpetiformis or to bullous pemphigoid.[81, 82] DIF is both sensitive and specific for the detection of reticulin antibody in dermatitis herpetiformis. IIF is not sensitive but is specific for this skin disease.

Discoid Lupus and SLE

Immunologic studies can be extremely important in evaluating rashes in SLE and in distinguishing SLE from discoid lupus erythematosus (DLE). In both SLE and DLE, DIF of involved skin reveals granular deposits of IgG, IgM, and various complement components at the dermoepidermal junction "band of fluorescence" in 90% of cases. In normal appearing skin from sun-exposed areas of the upper extremities, a band test was positive in 54% of patients with SLE but was negative in all patients with DLE (Fig 5–8).[83] If one excludes MCTD, the direct staining of uninvolved skin is therefore a very specific but not sensitive test for distinguishing SLE from DLE. The direct staining of involved skin is sensitive but not specific for distinguishing SLE from DLE, but it is sensitive and specific for distinguishing SLE from other dermatologic disorders. Although patients with pemphigoid have staining in the same area, the linear pattern of pemphigoid and the granular pattern of SLE and DLE are distinctive. However, similar deposits are seen, albeit rarely, in graft-vs.-host reactions, various forms of vasculitis, fixed drug eruptions, and leprosy.[83–87]

A positive band test in uninvolved skin is observed in less than 1% of patients with other ANA-positive or other rheumatic or immunologic dis-

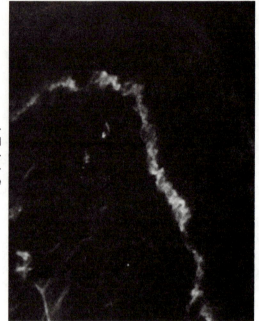

Fig 5–8.—Direct immuno-fluorescence test performed on uninvolved skin of a patient with SLE: pattern indicates presence of IgG at the dermoepidermal junction.

eases.[83, 85] The only rheumatic disease identified with any frequency is MCTD, and many cases are a subset of SLE. In addition, these patients may have nuclear staining by the DIF technique.[87] The sensitivity of a positive band test in uninvolved skin is only moderate for SLE, but the test remains specific if one excludes MCTD.

The clinical significance of a positive band test in uninvolved skin has not been clarified, but most workers agree that there is a correlation between the presence of deposits and clinical activity. There are conflicting reports on its relationship to renal disease. Nevertheless, a sufficient number of patients have a positive band test and no renal disease, so caution should be used in assuming that patients with a positive band test have renal disease. In NZB/NZW mice that develop SLE, the conversion of a positive IgM band test to an IgG band test is associated with a conversion from inactive to active disease. The same association has been suggested for humans.[88] The pathogenesis of the band test is thought to be deposition of immune complexes. Therefore IIF for the presence of a circulating antibody to an antigen in skin basement membrane is negative, which distinguishes SLE from pemphigoid, in which one can frequently detect a circulating antibody.

Lichen Planus

Lichen planus is a violaceous, scaling, papular, pruritic eruption that is usually localized to flexural surfaces, mucous membranes, and genitals. The cause is unknown, but immunologic studies suggest a role for the immune system. In 1973, Waisman reported immunoglobulin and fibrin deposition at the dermoepidermal junction in 95% of patients with lichen planus.[89, 90] These deposits are mainly IgM and may also be detected in uninvolved skin.[91] In the bullous form of lichen planus, a circulating antibody to an antigen in the basement membrane has also been detected by IIF.

The clinical picture of lichen planus is usually adequate to establish a diagnosis except in the bullous forms or when extensive skin lesions are present without mucosal or genital involvement. In these situations, immunofluorescent studies are extremely helpful in arriving at a proper diagnosis.

Gastrointestinal Disease

Autoimmunity based on pathology, immunologic studies, and disease associations has been implicated in a number of disorders of the gastrointestinal tract. The actual contribution of immune responses, however, has been well established in only a few diseases. These include gastritis, pernicious anemia, chronic active hepatitis, and primary biliary cirrhosis. The immune response in gastritis and pernicious anemia is organ-directed and described in this section. The immune response in liver disease is non-organ-directed and is discussed in the next section.

Chronic Gastritis

Recent immunologic studies have led to the suggestion that there may be an immunologic type A and a nonimmunologic type B gastritis.[92] Type A gastritis is associated with a chronic inflammatory response in which lymphocytes and plasma cells predominate in the gastric mucosa. Patients with type A gastritis often have autoimmune endocrinopathies such as Hashimoto's thyroiditis and hyperthyroidism, insulin-dependent diabetes, hypoadrenalism, hypoparathyroidism, and vitiligo.[93] They may also have organ-specific antibodies to these organs without clinical manifestations. The direct evidence for autoimmunity is the demonstration of antibodies to parietal cell and intrinsic factor and the high incidence of pernicious anemia.

Immunologic Tests

Antiparietal cell antibodies.—The techniques used to demonstrate antiparietal cell antibodies include IIF and complement fixation (CF). Eighty percent of patients with gastritis and pernicious anemia are positive by both of these tests.[94] The substrate in the immunofluorescent technique is frozen sections of human fundus mucosa obtained during surgical procedures. The immunofluorescence pattern is localized to the cytoplasm of gastric parietal cells. These antibodies are also seen in patients with Hashimoto's thyroiditis, thyrotoxicosis, adrenal insufficiency, and diabetes mellitus. They may also be found in first-degree relatives of patients with pernicious anemia and occasionally in healthy individuals, especially in women over the age of 60.[95]

Intrinsic factor antibodies.—Intrinsic factor antibodies are found in patients with pernicious anemia with or without gastritis. Two anti-intrinsic antibodies have been described. One is a blocking antibody that combines with intrinsic factor at or near its vitamin B_{12} binding site, thereby inhibiting vitamin B_{12} binding.[96] The second antibody binds to intrinsic factor at a site other than the binding site and is probably of no clinical significance.[97] These antibodies have been demonstrated in both serum and gastric juices. Blocking antibody is detected in roughly 60% of patients with pernicious anemia, and the other antibody in 35%.[97] These antibodies are detected by radioimmunoassays, double diffusion gel assays, or the Farr technique.

Cell-mediated immunity.—The absence of intrinsic factor antibodies in some patients with pernicious anemia and the association of pernicious anemia with hypogammaglobulinemia have led to the speculation that cellular immunity may be the more important immune response.[98] This speculation has prompted studies using human intrinsic factor and lymphocytes from patients with pernicious anemia. In this system, one can detect lymphocyte transformation and the release of an inhibitor of leukocyte migration.[99] Both of these are standard assays for measurement of cellular immunity (see Chap. 3).

Interpretation.—At present, there is no conclusive evidence supporting an etiologic role of circulating gastric autoantibodies or cellular immunity to gastric antigens in the pathogenesis of chronic gastritis and pernicious anemia. It is possible that these immunologic abnormalities are the consequence of an immune response to inflamed gastric mucosa.

The diagnosis of chronic gastritis is established by endoscopy and biopsy. The presence of antibody to parietal cells or to intrinsic factor cannot be used to establish the diagnosis of chronic gastritis or pernicious anemia. The antibody tests are performed to determine if the gastritis is immunologically mediated, as well as to assess the likelihood of pernicious anemia developing in a given patient. The diagnosis of pernicious anemia is based on anemia and the B_{12} absorption test. If a patient has chronic gastritis and antibodies to parietal cells without anemia, follow-up visits should be scheduled and studies for pernicious anemia repeated.

Infertility

The role of autoimmunity (antibody to sperm in males and the isoimmune antibody response to sperm in females) in states of infertility is not well understood. In both males and females, one can detect antisperm antibodies and no other explanation for infertility. This finding suggests that antisperm antibodies may have a pathogenic role in preventing fertilization of the female. The major source of confusion, however, is that these antibodies can be detected as well in normal adult men and women who are able to contribute to the production of a child.

A number of tests are available to demonstrate immune responses to sperm antigens. These include tests that produce agglutination of sperms, immobilization of sperms, tests for spermatotoxicity, IIF, and tests for cellular immunity such as the leukocyte migration inhibition test and blast transformation.[100, 101] Assessment of cellular immunity to sperm antigens is restricted to research laboratories, and the significance of such immunity remains to be determined. The two clinical tests that are available are the agglutination test and the immunofluorescence test. By these assays, antibodies to sperm can be detected in the serum and in the seminal fluid. In females, antibody has also been demonstrated in cervical secretions. Although the role of antibodies in the different fluids has not been correlated with infertility, it appears that antibodies in the secretory fluid are more important in preventing pregnancy than antibodies in serum. In addition, there appears to be a better correlation with infertility with agglutinating antibodies, rather than those antibodies demonstrated by IIF.

Of some pertinence to the agglutination technique is the observation that sperm will agglutinate in specific patterns, such as head-to-head, tail-to-tail, or head-to-tail. Antibodies directed toward sperm head antigens are primarily IgM, whereas those directed toward the tail are primarily IgG.

The basis for the formation of the antibodies is not clear, but most individuals with antisperm antibodies have demonstrable infection or obstruction in the lower urinary tract. A high incidence of sperm antibodies has been found following surgical vasectomy and trauma to the testicles. In one large study of 2,000 serum samples from infertile men, positive agglutination tests with normal sperm of various donors was observed in 3.3% of patients.[102] In a study of 74 women with unexplained infertility, sperm-reactive antibodies producing agglutination were demonstrated in 20%, whereas they were demonstrated in 1% of women with infertility due to known causes.[103] In another study comparing the eventual ability of women to become pregnant who had infertility for no known causes, only 10% of those with agglutinating antibodies for sperm became pregnant, as opposed to 35% in the nonantibody group.[104]

The IIF tests for detection of antibody to sperm uses normal sperm. A number of antibody patterns have been detected, but their correlation with infertility is not established. In addition, there does not appear to be a correlation with antibodies demonstrated by immunofluorescence with the agglutination test, and so this test is not performed in the routine evaluation of fertility. It is difficult to determine when infertility is due to autoimmunity, and determining the sensitivity and specificity of autoimmunity tests is difficult. Since the frequency of positive agglutination is low in patients with infertility, I believe that the test is of low sensitivity. If the incidence of autoimmune infertility were known, it might approach the incidence associated with infertility due to agglutinating antibody, which would make it a more sensitive test. The same problem exists for determining specificity.

Autoimmunity and the Adrenal Gland

Adrenal cortical hypofunction, or Addison's disease, is an uncommon endocrine disease that affects approximately 6 of every 100,000 people. While some cases are due to destruction of the adrenal gland by metastatic tumor, granulomatous disease, or tuberculosis, in most cases the adrenal atrophy occurs in the absence of any apparent cause. In the United States, two thirds of cases of Addison's disease fall into the idiopathic category, and current evidence suggests that it is probably an autoimmune disorder.

The most commonly used test is the IIF test. The substrate is human surgical specimens obtained from patients undergoing adrenalectomy or at autopsy. Adrenal glands from monkeys can also be used. In a positive test, the immunofluorescence is located in the cytoplasm; when the cell is fractionated, the antigen is localized in the microsomal and mitochondrial fractions by the antibodies obtained from patients. The reported incidence of antibodies in patients with idiopathic Addison's disease is 38%–74% and the antibody is present in low titer by IIF. When the titers in patients with Addison's disease are compared with titers in normal subjects, the immunofluorescence test is seen to be specific, since very low titers are found in less than 1% of normal individuals. The specificity decreases, however, when the test is extended to patients with Addison's disease and tuberculosis, because 18% of patients with tuberculosis of the adrenal gland are positive. First-degree relatives of patients with idiopathic Addison's disease have a higher incidence of antiadrenal antibodies, as do patients with idiopathic hypoparathyroidism, autoimmune thyroid disease, and diabetes mellitus. Patients with idiopathic Addison's disease have a higher frequency of other autoimmune disorders, such as thyrotoxicosis, Hashimoto's thyroiditis, and ovarian failure.[105] The association of Hashimoto's thyroiditis or hypothyroidism and idiopathic Addison's disease is termed Schmidt's syndrome.

NON-ORGAN-SPECIFIC DISEASES

The major non-organ-specific diseases are chronic active hepatitis and primary biliary cirrhosis. These are diseases in which autoimmunity is suspected but not supported and in which the diagnostic antibodies are not directed against liver tissue. Although one cannot state at the present time that there is an autoimmune hepatitis, a number of immunologic tests should be ordered in patients with liver disease. These include tests for immunoglobulin levels and detection of autoantibodies against nuclei, smooth muscle, and mitochondria, as well as serologic tests for hepatitis A and B infections.

Chronic Active Hepatitis

Chronic active hepatitis is a syndrome of multiple etiology with a duration of disease of over 6 months and histologic abnormalities that include periportal necrosis of hepatocytes and progressive architectural disorganization. This pathology can now be divided into four subgroups. Type A is the subgroup with significant autoimmune manifestations. In the older literature, this subgroup was often referred to as lupoid hepatitis because of the occurrence of autoantibodies and a positive LE cell test. It is now clear that type A liver disease does not occur in SLE, and the exact role that these autoantibodies play in the production of liver damage has not been established. These patients have hypergammaglobulinemia and antibodies to nuclear and smooth muscle antigens. In addition, they are frequently RF positive. The immunoglobulin elevation is predominantly in the IgG class. The ANA usually demonstrates a homogeneous or ring pattern. The ANA varies with activity of disease, and only rarely are antibodies to nDNA detected.[106] In these situations, the antibody to nDNA is of low titer and occurs only transiently during the most active phase of the disease. The anti-smooth muscle antibody is detected by the immunofluorescent technique using frozen sections of rat stomach as a substrate; however, any tissue containing smooth muscle can be used. The test is positive in 60%–70% of patients, but it is positive in a number of other diseases as well.[107]

These diseases include infectious mononucleosis,[108] infectious hepatitis, viral illnesses, RA, alcoholic liver disease, and a variety of malignancies, depending on the sensitivity of the technique; 3%–14% of normal subjects are also positive. The test is moderately sensitive and moderately specific. On cultured fibroblasts, the smooth muscle antibodies have three specificities. They may be specific for microfilaments (actin and myosin), for microtubules (tubulin), and for intermediate filaments (desmin and vimentin). If one determines the specific antigen determinant of the smooth muscle antibodies, a useful serologic marker is the anti-actin antibody.[109] This test is positive in 70% of patients with chronic active hepatitis. A positive response occurs much less frequently in patients with other liver diseases and not at all in patients with rheumatic diseases. The anti-actin assay, then, is both sensitive and specific.

Type B chronic active hepatitis is associated with the presence of hepatitis surface antigen in the blood. Type C chronic active hepatitis has no distinguishing markers. Type D hepatitis is drug-induced, with oxyphenisatin, a component of some laxatives, acetaminophen, and methyldopa all being suspected. Other potential causative agents are the hepatotoxins, such as carbon tetrachloride.

Primary Biliary Cirrhosis

Primary biliary cirrhosis is a chronic cholestatic disease that is characterized by slow and progressive destruction of the intrahepatic bile ducts. It can occur in association with other symptoms that are usually of rheumatic origin, such as Raynaud's disease, sicca syndrome, or arthralgia.[110] It may also be secondary to scleroderma and to sarcoid.[111] The most common serologic marker detected in 90% of cases is the antibody to mitochondrial antigens. The usual technique for the detection of this antibody is IIF using renal tubular cells that are rich in mitochondria. It is a test of considerable diagnostic value in that it is positive in very low titers in less than 2% of cases of extrahepatic biliary obstruction, which is the major differential diagnostic category. However, it is also positive in 10% of patients with chronic active hepatitis and occasionally in patients with other rheumatic diseases, such as Sjögren's syndrome.[112] It is therefore both a sensitive and specific test for primary biliary cirrhosis.

Other immunologic tests of some assistance in establishing the diagnosis of chronic biliary cirrhosis include determining the presence of hypergammaglobulinemia in the IgM class,[113] immune complexes (positive in 95%),[114] RF (positive in 68%),[115] and ANA (positive in 26%).[107] These latter are not specific for primary biliary cirrhosis and probably indicate that alterations of normal homeostatic mechanisms for the control of autoantibody production have occurred.

APPENDIX

SUMMARY OF AVAILABLE TESTS*

ANTIGEN SPECIFICITY	TECHNIQUE	CLINICAL SIGNIFICANCE FOR SLE		
		Sensitivity	Specificity	Comments
Nuclear	IIF on tissue	High	Low	Routine ANA
Deoxyribonucleoprotein	LE cell test	Moderate	Moderate	LE cell test should only be performed in ANA-positive patients
	IIF: rim or homogeneous nuclear staining, routine substrates			
DNA (double-stranded)	Farr	Moderate	High	Correlated with renal disease in SLE
	IIF on *Crithidia luciliae* substrate; on routine substrates rim pattern			Sensitivity lower in mild or inactive disease
DNA (single-stranded)	Farr	High	Very low	Present in all SLE and many rheumatic and nonrheumatic diseases
Extractable nuclear antigens	IIF, speckled nuclear staining best demonstrated on animal substrate or tissue culture	High	Low	Most patients with SLE will have an antibody capable of producing a speckled ANA pattern
SM	Hemagglutination; agar gel diffusion	Low	High	Detected only in SLE
NRNP	Hemagglutination; agar gel diffusion	Moderate	Low	Present in SLE, other rheumatic diseases, and MCTD

Continued

SUMMARY OF AVAILABLE TESTS*—Continued

ANTIGEN SPECIFICITY	TECHNIQUE	CLINICAL SIGNIFICANCE FOR SLE		
		Sensitivity	Specificity	Comments
SS-B (Ha)	IIF, speckled nuclear staining on mouse kidney, homogeneous pattern on human lymphoblastoid cell line (Wil-2); agar gel diffusion	Low	Low	Moderately sensitive and specific for Sjögren's syndrome
SS-A	IIF, speckled nuclear staining on Wil-2 cells; no staining on routine tests using animal substrates; agar gel diffusion	Low	Low	Moderately sensitive and specific for Sjögren's syndrome
Histones	IIF, rim or homogeneous nuclear staining pattern	Low	Low	Highly sensitive and moderately specific for drug-induced SLE
Cytoplasmic RO	Ouchterlony	Low	High	May be the only positive test in ANA-negative SLE
LA	Ouchterlony	Low	Low	
Nucleolar	IIF	Low	Low	Very specific but low sensitivity for scleroderma with skin involvement
Centromere	IIF, speckled nuclear staining pattern on rapidly dividing cells in tissue culture (Hep-2)	Low	Low	Very sensitive and moderately specific for scleroderma with minimal skin involvement

*IIF, indirect immunofluorescence; SLE, systemic lupus erythematosus; ANA, antinuclear antibody; SS-A and SS-B, soluble substances A and B; NRNP, nuclear ribonucleoprotein.

DISEASE-ORIENTED TESTS*

DISEASE	ANTIGEN	TESTS	CLINICAL SIGNIFICANCE	
			Sensitivity	Specificity
RA	IgG	RF by latex aggregation	Moderate	Low
Thyroiditis	Thyroglobulin	Hemagglutination	High	Moderate
		RIA	High	Low
		IIF	Moderate	Moderate
	Microsomes	Hemagglutination	High	Moderate
		IIF	High	Moderate
Graves' disease	Thyroid receptor	Tests LATS immunoglobulin; not routinely available	High	High
Diabetes mellitus				
Anti-insulin syndrome	Insulin	Radioimmunoassay	High	High
Insulin allergy	Insulin	Direct skin test for detection of IgE	High	High
Insulin-dependent diabetes	Islet cells	IIF	Low	Moderate
	Insulin receptors	Serum of patient inhibits insulin binding to tissue; not available	High	High
Myasthenia gravis	Skeletal muscle	IIF	Low	Low
	Acetylcholine receptor	IIF (not commercially available)	In patients with thymoma: High	Low Low
		RIA (not commercially available)	Moderate High	Low High
Rapidly progressive glomerulonephritis	GBM	DIF	High	Moderate
Goodpasture's syndrome	GBM	IIF	Moderate	High
		RIA	High	High
		DIF	High	High
Pemphigus	Intercellular substance of stratified epithelium	IIF	High	High

Continued

DISEASE-ORIENTED TESTS*—*Continued*

DISEASE	ANTIGEN	TESTS	CLINICAL SIGNIFICANCE	
			Sensitivity	Specificity
Pemphigoid	Dermoepidermal junction	DIF	High	High
	Lamina lucida	IIF	Moderate	High
Dermatitis herpetiformis	Reticulin	DIF	High	High
		IIF	Low	High
Lichen planus	Unknown	DIF	High	High
		IIF	Low	High
Chronic gastritis	Parietal cells	IIF	High	Moderate
	Intrinsic factor	Agar gel diffusion; RIA;		
		Farr; blocking antibody:	High	Moderate
		Nonblocking antibody:	Low	Low
Pernicious anemia	Intrinsic factor	Blocking antibody	Moderate	Moderate
		Nonblocking antibody	Low	Low
Infertility	Sperm	Sperm immobilization	Low	Moderate
		IIF	Moderate	Low
Addison's disease	Adrenal gland	IIF	Moderate	Moderate
Chronic active hepatitis	Smooth muscle	IIF	Moderate	Moderate
	Actin			
Primary biliary cirrhosis	Mitochondria	IIF	High	High
			High	High

*IIF, indirect immunofluorescence; DIF, direct immunofluorescence; RA, rheumatoid arthritis; RF, rheumatoid factor; RIA, radioimmunoassay; LATS, long-acting thyroid stimulator; GBM, glomerular basement membrane.

REFERENCES

1. Ehrlich P., Morgenroth J.: Über Hämolysine, Fünfte Mittheilung, in Himmelweit F. (ed.): *The Collected Papers of Paul Ehrlich*. London, Pergamon Press, 1957, vol. 2, p. 234.
2. Witebsky E.: Historical roots of present concepts of immunopathology, in Graber P., Miescher P.A. (eds.): *Immunopathology: First International Symposium*. Basel, Schwabe, 1959.
3. DeWalle M., Thielemans C., Van Camp B.K.G.: Characterization of immunoregulatory T cells in EBV-induced infectious mononucleosis by monoclonal antibodies. *N. Engl. J. Med.* 304:460, 1981.
4. Reinherz E.L., Schlossman S.F.: Current concepts in immunology. *N. Engl. J. Med.* 303:370, 1980.
5. Kurtland H.H. III, Mohler D.N., Horwitz D.A.: Methyldopa inhibition of suppressor lymphocyte function. *N. Engl. J. Med.* 302:875, 1980.
6. Decker J.L., Steinberg A.D., Reinertsen J.L., et al.: Systemic lupus erythematosus: Evolving concepts. *Ann. Intern. Med.* 91:587, 1979.
7. Miller K.B., and Salen D.: Immune regulatory abnormalities produced by procainamide. *Am. J. Med.* 73:487, 1982.
8. Talal N.: Autoimmunity, in Fudenberg H.H., Stites D.P., Caldwell J.L., et al. (eds.): *Basic and Clinical Immunology*, ed. 3. Los Altos, California, Lang Medical Publishers, 1980, p. 220.
9. Hargraves M.N., Richmond H., Morton R.: Presentation of two bone marrow elements: The "tart" cell and "LE" cell. *Proc. Staff Meet. Mayo Clinic* 23:25, 1948.
10. Harvey A.M., Shulman L.E., Tumulty A., et al.: Systemic lupus erythematosus: Review of the literature and clinical analysis of 138 cases. *Medicine* 33:291, 1954.
11. Miyauaki S., Ritchie R.F.: Nucleolar antigens specific for anti-nucleolar antibody in the sera of patients with systemic rheumatic diseases. *Arthritis Rheum.* 16:726, 1973.
12. Richardson B., Epstein W.V.: Utility of the fluorescent antinuclear antibody test in a single patient. *Ann. Intern. Med.* 95:333, 1981.
13. Barnett E.V., Condemi J.J., Jacox R.F., et al.: Antinuclear factors in systemic lupus erythematosus and rheumatoid arthritis. *Ann. Intern. Med.* 63:100, 1965.
14. Rothfield N.F., Rodnan G.P.: Serum antinuclear antibodies in systemic sclerosis (scleroderma). *Arthritis Rheum.* 11:607, 1968.
15. Notman D.D., Kurata N., Tan E.M.: Profiles of antinuclear antibodies in systemic rheumatic diseases. *Ann. Intern. Med.* 83:464, 1975.
16. Chubick A.: DNA antibodies in SLE and pseudolupus syndrome. *Adv. Intern. Med.* 26:467, 1980.
17. Aarden L.A., DeGroot E.R., Feltkamp T.E.W.: Immunology of DNA *Crithidia luciliae:* A simple substrate for the determination of anti-ds DNA with the immunofluorescent technique. *Ann. NY Acad. Sci.* 254:505, 1975.
18. Akizuki M., Powers R., Holman H.R.: A soluble acidic protein of the cell nucleus which reacts with serum from patients with SLE. *J. Clin. Invest.* 59:264, 1977.
19. Alspaugh M.A., Talal N., Tan E.N.: Differentiation and characterization of autoantibodies and antigens in Sjögren's syndrome. *Arthritis Rheum.* 19:216, 1976.

20. Reichlin M., Mattioli M.: Antigens in antibodies characteristic of systemic lupus erythematosus. *Bull. Rheum. Dis.* 24:756, 1974.

21. Sharp G.C., Irvin W.S., Tan E.M., et al.: Mixed connective tissue disease: An apparently distinct rheumatic disease syndrome associated with a specific antibody to extractable nuclear antigen (ENA). *Am. J. Med.* 42:148, 1972.

22. Maddison P.J., Reichlin M.: Quantitation of precipitating antibodies to certain soluble nuclear antigens in SLE: Their contribution to hypergammaglobulinemia. *Arthritis Rheum.* 20:819, 1977.

23. Kassan S.S., Akizuki M., Steinberg A.D., et al.: Antibody to soluble and nuclear antigen in Sjögren's syndrome. *Am. J. Med.* 63:328, 1977.

24. Tan E.M., Cohen A.S., Fries J.F., et al.: The 1982 revised criteria for the classification of systemic lupus erythematosus. *Arthritis and Rheumatism* 25:1271, 1982.

25. Tan E.M., Portanova J.P.: The role of histones as nuclear autoantigens in drug-related lupus erythematosus. *Arthritis Rheum.* 24:1064, 1981.

26. Provost T.T., Ahmed A.R., Maddison P.J., et al.: Antibodies to cytoplasmic antigens in lupus erythematosus: Serological marker for systemic disease. *Arthritis Rheum.* 20:1457, 1977.

27. Fritzler M.J., Kinsella P.D., Garbutt E.: The CREST syndrome: A distinct serological entity with anticentromere antibodies. *Am. J. Med.* 69:520, 1980.

28. Waaler E.: On the occurrence of a factor in human serum activating the specific agglutination of sheep red blood cells. *Acta Pathol. Microbiol. Scand.* 17:172, 1940.

29. Rose H.M., Rayan C., Pearce E.: Differentiation agglutination of normal and sensitized sheep erythrocytes by sera of patients with rheumatoid arthritis. *Proc. Soc. Exp. Biol. Med.* 68:1, 1948.

30. Singer J.M., Plotz C.N.: The latex fixation test: Application to the serological diagnosis of rheumatoid arthritis. *Am. J. Med.* 21:888, 1956.

31. Bartfeld H., Epstein W.V.: Rheumatoid factors and their biological significance. *Ann. NY Acad. Sci.* 168:1, 1968.

32. Mannik N.: Rheumatoid factors, in *Arthritis and Allied Conditions*, ed. 9. Philadelphia, Lea & Febiger, 1979, p. 504.

33. Rose N.R., Witebsky E.: Studies on organ specificity: V. Changes in the thyroid glands of rabbits following active immunization with rabbit thyroid extracts. *J. Immunol.* 76:417, 1956.

34. Strabosch C.R., Wenzel B.E., Row V.V., et al.: Chromology of autoimmunothyroid disease. *New Engl. J. Med.* 307:1499, 1982.

35. Doniach D.: Humoral and genetic aspects of thyroid autoimmunity. *J. Clin. Endocrinol.* 4:267, 1975.

36. Mori T., Kriss J.P.: Measurements of competitive binding, radioassay of serum, anti-microsomal and anti-thyroglobulin antibodies in Graves' disease and other thyroid disorders. *J. Clin. Endocrinol.* 33:688, 1971.

37. Yoshida H., Amino N., Yagawa K., et al.: Association of serum antithyroid antibodies with lymphocytic infiltration of the thyroid gland: Studies of 70 autopsy cases. *J. Clin. Endocrinol.* 46:859, 1978.

38. Amino N., Hagen S.R., Yamada M., et al.: Measurements of circulating thyroid microsomal antibodies by the tanned red cell hemagglutination technique: Its usefulness in the diagnosis of autoimmune thyroid disease. *J. Clin. Endocrinol.* 5:115, 1976.

39. Pulver-Taft R.J.V., Doniach D., Roitt I.M., et al.: Cytotoxic effects of Hash-

imoto's serum on human thyroid cells in tissue culture. *Lancet* 2:214, 1959.

40. Smith B.R., Hall R.: Thyroid-stimulating immunoglobulins in Graves' disease. *Lancet* 2:427, 1974.

41. Horvath F. Jr., Teague P., Gaffney E.F., et al.: Thyroid antigen-associated immune complex glomerulonephritis in Graves' disease. *Am. J. Med.* 67:901, 1979.

42. Fisher D.A., Oddie T.H., Johnson D.E.: The diagnosis of Hashimoto's thyroiditis. *Clin. Endocrinol. Metab.* 40:795, 1975.

43. Whitaker J.M.: Myasthenia gravis and autoimmunity. *Adv. Intern. Med.* 26:489, 1980.

44. Strauss A.J.L., Van der Geld H.W.R., Kemp P.J., et al.: Immunological concomitants of myasthenia gravis. *Ann. NY Acad. Sci.* 124:744, 1965.

45. Strauss A.J.L., Smith C.W., Cage G.W., et al.: Further studies on the specificity of presumed immune associations of myasthenia gravis in consideration of possible pathogenic implications. *Ann. NY Acad. Sci.* 135:557, 1966.

46. Christy M., Deckert T., Nerup J.: Immunity and autoimmunity in diabetes mellitus. *Clin. Endocrinol. Metab.* 6:305, 1977.

47. Gepts W.: Islet changes suggesting a possible immune etiology of human diabetes mellitus. *Acta Endocrinol.* 83(suppl. 205):95, 1976.

48. Egberg J., Junker K., Kroman H., et al.: Autoimmune insulitis: Pathological findings in experimental animal models and in juvenile diabetes mellitus. *Acta Endocrinol.* 83(suppl. 205):129, 1976.

49. Irvine W.J., MacCuish A.C., Campbell C.J., et al.: Organ-specific cell-mediated autoimmunity in diabetes mellitus. *Acta Endocrinol.* 83(suppl. 205):65, 1976.

50. Maclaren N.K., Huang S.W., Fogh J.: Antibody to cultured human insulinoma cells in insulin-dependent diabetics. *Lancet* 1:997, 1975.

51. Buchard K., Madsbad S., Rygarid J.: Passive transfer of diabetes mellitus from man to mouse. *Lancet* 1:908, 1978.

52. Berson S.A., Yalow R.S., Bauman A., et al.: Insulin I^{131} metabolism in human subjects: Demonstration of insulin binding globulin in circulation of insulin-treated subjects. *J. Clin. Invest.* 35:170, 1956.

53. DeShazo R.D.: Insulin allergy and insulin resistance: Two immunological reactions. *Postgrad. Med.* 63:85, 1978.

54. Orci L., Malaisse-Lagae F., Betens D., et al.: Pancreatic polypeptide-rich regions in human pancreas. *Lancet* 2:1200, 1978.

55. Hirata Y.: Spontaneous insulin antibodies in hypoglycemia. *Diabetes: Proceedings of the Ninth Congress of the International Diabetic Federation.* Amsterdam, Oxford, 1978, pp. 278–284.

56. Flier J.S., Kahn C.R., Roth J., et al.: Antibodies that impair insulin receptor binding in an unusual diabetic syndrome with severe insulin resistance. *Science* 190:63, 1975.

57 Kahn C.R., Flier J.S., Bar R.S., et al.: The syndromes of insulin resistance and acanthosis nigricans. Insulin-receptor disorders in man. *N. Engl. J. Med.* 294:739, 1976.

58. Bar R.S., Levis W.R., Rechler M.M., et al.: Extreme insulin resistance in ataxia telangiectasia: Defect in affinity of insulin receptor. *N. Engl. J. Med.* 298:1164, 1978.

59. Mattson J.R., Patterson R., Roberts M.: Insulin therapy in patients with systemic insulin allergy. *Arch. Intern. Med.* 135:118, 1975.

60. Berson S.A., Yalow R.S.: Insulin (antagónists) and insulin resistance, in Ellenberg M., Rifkin H. (eds.): *Diabetes Mellitus: Theory and Practice.* New York, McGraw-Hill Book Co., 1970, pp. 388–422.

61. Bottazzo G.F., Pujol-Borrell R., Doniach D.: *Humoral and Cellular Immunity in Diabetes Mellitus.* Philadelphia, W.B. Saunders Co., 1981, vol. 1, pp. 139–159.

62. Wilson C.B., Dixon F.J.: The renal response to immunological injury in the kidney, in Brenner B.M., Rector F.C. (eds.): *The Kidney.* Philadelphia, W.B. Saunders Co., 1976, pp. 838–908.

63. Wilson C.B., Dixon F.J.: Antiglomerular basement antibody-induced glomerulonephritis. *Kidney Int.* 3:74, 1973.

64. Michael B., Milner Y., David K.: Preservation of tissue-fixed immunoglobulin in skin biopsies in patients with lupus erythematosus and bullous diseases: Preliminary report. *J. Invest. Dermatol.* 59:440, 1973.

65. Nicengard R.J., Jablonska S., Chorzelski T.P.: Immunofluorescent studies: Comparison of methods of transportation. *Arch. Dermatol.* 114:1329, 1978.

66. Jorden R.E., Triftshauser C.T., Schroeter A.L.: Direct immunofluorescence studies of pemphigus and bullous pemphigoid. *Arch. Dermatol.* 103:486, 1971.

67. Peck S.M., Osserman K.E., Weiner L.B., et al.: Studies in bullous diseases: Immunofluorescent serological tests. *N. Engl. J. Med.* 279:951, 1968.

68. Feiberman C., Stolzner G., Provost T.T.: Pemphigus vulgaris: Superior sensitivity of monkey esophagus in the determination of pemphigus antibody. *Arch. Dermatol.* 117:561, 1981.

69. Fitzpatrick R.E., Newcomber V.D.: The correlation of disease activity in antibody titers in pemphigus. *Arch. Dermatol.* 116:285, 1980.

70. Ablin R.J., Milgrom F., Kano K., et al.: Pemphigus-like antibodies in patients with skin burns. *Vox Sang.* 16:73, 1969.

71. Dobmeier J.L., Sams W.M. Jr., Beutner E.H.: Intercellular antibodies in a patient without clinical pemphigus. *Ann. NY Acad. Sci.* 177:218, 1971.

72. Farb R.N., Dykes R., Lazarus G.S.: Anti-epidermal cell surface pemphigus antibody detaches viable epidermal cells from culture plates by activation of proteinase. *Proc. Natl. Acad. Sci. USA* 75:459, 1978.

73. Anhalt G.J., Labib R.S., Voorhees J.J., et al.: Induction of pemphigus in neonatal mice by passive transfer of IgG from patients with the disease. *N. Engl. J. Med.* 306:1189, 1982.

74. Bean S.F., Waisman M., Michael B.: Cicatricial pemphigoid immunofluorescent studies. *Arch. Dermatol.* 106:195, 1972.

75. Beutner E.H., Chorzelski T.P., Bean S.M.: *Immunopathology of the Skin,* ed. 2. New York, A. Wiley Medical Publications, 1979, pp. 243–255.

76. Houlbar K., Wolff K., Konrad K., et al.: Ultrastructure localization of immunoglobulins in bullous pemphigoid skin. *J. Invest. Dermatol.* 64:220, 1975.

77. Anhalt G.J., Vahn C.F., Labib R.S., et al.: Pathogenic effect of bullous pemphigoid autoantibodies on rabbit corneal epithelium. *J. Clin. Invest.* 68:1097, 1981.

78. Katz A., Minto J.O., Toole J.W.P., et al.: Immunopathological study of herpes gestationis in mother and infant. *Arch. Dermatol.* 113:1069, 1977.

79. Katz S.I., Stroeber W.: The pathogenesis of dermatitis herpetiformis. *J. Invest. Dermatol.* 70:63, 1978.

80. Seah P.P., Fry L., Hoffbrand A.V., et al.: Tissue antibodies in dermatitis herpetiformis: An adult coeliac disease. *Lancet* 1:834, 1971.

81. Honeyman J.F., Honeyman A., Lobitz W.C.: The enigma of bullous pemphigoid and dermatitis herpetiformis. *Arch. Dermatol.* 106:22, 1973.

82. Esterly N.B., Furey N.L., Kirschner R.S.: Chronic bullous dermatitis of childhood. *Arch. Dermatol.* 113:42, 1977.

83. Grossman J., Callerami M.L., Condemi J.J.: Skin immunofluorescence studies in lupus erythematosus and other antinuclear antibody-positive diseases. *Ann. Intern. Med.* 80:496, 1974.

84. Ullman S., Spielvogel R.L., Kersey J.H.: Immunoglobulins and complement in skin in graft vs. host disease. *Ann. Intern. Med.* 85:205, 1976.

85. Mathison D.A., Arroyave C.M., Bahat K.N.: Hypocomplementemia in chronic idiopathic urticaria. *Ann. Intern. Med.* 86:534, 1977.

86. Provost T.T.: Lupus band test, in Beutner E.H., Chorzelski T.T., Bean S.F. (eds.): *Immunopathology of the Skin.* New York, A. Wiley Medical Publications, 1979, p. 399.

87. Gilliam J.M., Prystowsky S.D.: Mixed connective tissue disease syndrome: Cutaneous manifestations of patients with epidermal nuclear staining in high-titer serum antibody in ribonuclease-sensitive extractable nuclear antigen. *Arch. Dermatol.* 113:583, 1977.

88. Gilliam J.M.: The significance of cutaneous immunoglobulin deposits in SLE and NZB-NZW F1 hybrid mice. *J. Invest. Dermatol.* 65:154, 1975.

89. Waisman M., Dundon B.C., Michael B.: Immunofluorescent studies in lichen planus. *Arch. Dermatol.* 107:200, 1973.

90. Abel L.E.: The diagnostic significance of immunoglobulin and fibrin deposition in lichen planus. *Br. J. Dermatol.* 93:17, 1975.

91. Sobel S.: Lichen planus pemphigoides: Immunofluorescent findings. *Arch. Dermatol.* 112:1280, 1976.

92. Strickland R.G., Mackay I.R.: A reappraisal of the nature and significance of chronic atrophic gastritis. *Am. J. Dig. Dis.* 18:426, 1973.

93. Howitz J., Schwartz M.: Vitiligo, achlorhydria and pernicious anemia. *Lancet* 1:1331, 1971.

94. Irvine W.J., Cullen D.R., Mawhinne Y.H.: Natural history of autoimmune achlorhydric gastritis. *Lancet* 2:482, 1974.

95. Irvine W.J., Davies S.H., Titelbaum S., et al.: The clinical and pathological significance of gastric parietal cell antibody. *Ann. NY Acad. Sci.* 124:657, 1965.

96. Samloff I.M., Turner M.D.: Rabbit blocking and binding antibodies to human intrinsic factor and intrinsic factor B_{12} complex. *J. Immunol.* 101:578, 1968.

97. Samloff I.M., Kleinman M.S., Turner M.D., et al.: Blocking and binding antibody to intrinsic factor and parietal cell antibody in pernicious anemia. *Gastroenterology* 55:575, 1968.

98. Douglas S.D., Goldberg L.S., Fudenberg H.H., et al.: Agammaglobulinemia and coexistent pernicious anemia. *Clin. Exp. Immunol.* 6:181, 1970.

99. Glass G.B.J.: Immunology of atrophic gastritis. *NY State J. Med.* 77:1697, 1977.

100. Rose M.R., Hjort T., Rumke P., et al.: Techniques for detection of iso- and autoantibodies to human spermatozoa. *Clin. Exp. Immunol.* 23:175, 1976.

101. Boettcher B., Hjort T., Rumke P., et al.: Auto- and isoantibodies to antigens

of human reproductive system: Results of an international comparative study. *Clin. Exp. Immunol.* 30:173, 1977.

102. Rumke P., Hellinga G.: Autoantibodies against spermatozoa in sterile males. *Am. J. Clin. Pathol.* 32:357, 1959.

103. Isojina S., Tsuchiya K., Koyama K., et al.: Further studies on sperm immobilization antibody found in sera of unexplained cases of sterility in women. *Am. J. Obstet. Gynecol.* 112:199, 1972.

104. Jones W.R.: Immunological aspects of infertility, in Scott J.S., Jones W.R. (eds.): *Immunology of Human Reproduction.* New York, Academic Press, 1976, pp. 65–76.

105. Irvine W.J.: Adrenalitis, hypoparathyroidism and associated diseases, in Samter M. (ed.): *Immunological Diseases,* ed. 2. Boston, Little, Brown & Co., 1978, pp. 1278–1295.

106. Davis P., Read A.E.: Antibodies to double-stranded DNA in active chronic hepatitis. *Gut* 16:413, 1975.

107. Doniach D., Roitt I.M., Walker J.G., et al.: Tissue antibodies in primary biliary cirrhosis, active chronic hepatitis, cryptogenic cirrhosis, and other diseases and their clinical implications. *Clin. Exp. Immunol.* 1:237, 1966.

108. Holborow E.J., Hemsted E.H., Mead S.V.: Smooth muscle autoantibodies in infectious mononucleosis. *Br. Med. J.* 3:323, 1973.

109. Liedman K., Biberfield G., Fagraeus A., et al.: Anti-actin specificity of human smooth muscle antibodies in chronic active hepatitis. *Clin. Exp. Immunol.* 24:266, 1976.

110. Alacon-Segovia D., Diaz-Jounen E., Fishbein E.: Features of Sjögren's syndrome in primary biliary cirrhosis. *Ann. Intern. Med.* 79:31, 1973.

111. Reynolds T.B., Dennison E.K., Frankl H.D., et al.: Primary biliary cirrhosis with scleroderma, Raynaud's phenomena and telangiectasia. *Am. J. Med.* 50:302, 1971.

112. Klatskin G., Kantor F.S.: Mitochondrial antibody in primary biliary cirrhosis and other diseases. *Ann. Intern. Med.* 77:533, 1972.

113. Feizi T.: Immunoglobulins in chronic liver disease. *Gut* 9:193, 1968.

114. Wands J.R., Dienstag J.L., Bahn A.K., et al.: Circulating immune complexes and complement activation in primary biliary cirrhosis. *N. Engl. J. Med.* 289:233, 1978.

115. Paronetto F., Schaffner F., Popper H.: Immunocytochemical and serological observations in primary biliary cirrhosis. *N. Engl. J. Med.* 271:1123, 1964.

6

Interpretation of Complement and Immune Complex Assays

Stephen I. Rosenfeld, M.D.

THE COMPLEMENT SYSTEM consists of 14 serum glycoproteins and at least four inhibitory proteins that together comprise 2%–3% of the normal serum protein concentration. Originally described by several workers at the beginning of this century as the heat-labile serum factors required for lysis of specifically sensitized bacteria or erythrocytes, the complement system is now recognized as a major effector mechanism for many of the biologic activities of the humoral immune system, capable of producing many of the phlogistic elements of the inflammatory reaction. Although generally considered "nonspecific" in comparison with the exquisite recognition specificity of the antibodies that activate them, complement proteins interact with one another in a series of tightly controlled, highly specific biochemical reactions. This potent biologic effector system is important in amplifying the effects of specific antibodies in host defense against bacteria, viruses, and parasites, and through a less efficient alternative activation pathway, which phylogenetically antedates the specific antibody system, it can interact with certain microorganisms and provide a first line of defense before specific antibody is synthesized.

In addition to this important role in host defense, the complement system can be inappropriately activated by circulating immune complexes or autoantibodies, in which case its inflammatory properties can lead to tissue damage and clinical disease. Since complement can be activated in a variety of situations by a number of specific and nonspecific activating substances, assays designed to detect activation of the complement system do not give specific information about the activating stimulus. In order to request and interpret complement assays appropriately, it is necessary for the clinician to understand something about the biochemistry of the complement interactions and the biologic effects of these interactions. (For more detailed reviews, see Atkinson and Frank,[1] Gigli,[2] and Stroud et al.[3])

The terminology of the complement system appears intimidating but actually is reasonably straightforward. The proteins of the classical pathway are generally numbered in their order of interaction, from C1 through C9, with two exceptions. C1, long after its discovery as the first component to interact with antibody, was shown to be a calcium-dependent macromolecular complex of three independent proteins which were subsequently labeled C1q, C1r, and C1s. C4 was the fourth component to be discovered but subsequently was found to interact second in the classical pathway sequence; however, its historical enumeration as C4 was retained. Therefore, the reaction sequence in order of activation is C1q, C1r, C1s, C4, C2, C3, and C5 through C9. C3 is quantitatively the most abundant complement protein, with serum concentrations averaging approximately 1,400 µg/ml, and its very important biologic properties place it in a pivotal position in the complement sequence.

Two separate pathways leading to cleavage of C3 have evolved. The first to be recognized, although phylogenetically more recent, is the so-called classical pathway, consisting of C1, C4, and C2. Contact of the C1qrs calcium-dependent complex with complexes of IgM or IgG antibody, in combination with soluble or cellular or viral antigens, leads to the activation of C1s to a proteolytic enzyme capable of cleaving C4 and C2, the larger fragments of which can bind to the cell surface or complex and form a new magnesium-dependent enzyme (C4b,2a) capable of cleaving C3. Although the most important activating materials for this classical pathway system involve immunoglobulins, more recently a number of other substances (Table 6–1), such as C-reactive protein-phosphorylcholine complexes, polyanion-polycation complexes, and lipid A of certain bacterial endotoxins, as well as some circulating enzymes such as plasmin, have been recognized as capable of initiating C1 activation. C1 can also be activated by contact with certain viruses on cell surfaces, even in the absence of antibody. C1 activation in whole serum or plasma is kept under tight control by a natural inhibitor, called C1 inhibitor or C1 esterase inhibitor, which binds to and inactivates C1r and C1s and normally limits the cleavage of C4 and C2 to the local area where the C1 was initially activated.

TABLE 6–1.—SUBSTANCES CAPABLE OF INITIATING CLASSICAL
PATHWAY ACTIVATION

IgM or IgG subclasses 3>1>2, heat-aggregated or complexed with antigen (1 IgM or at least 2 IgG molecules required)
C-reactive protein complexed with C polysaccharide or phosphorylcholine
Polyanion-polycation complexes (e.g., heparin-protamine)
Certain RNA viruses
Lipid A of endotoxin
Some proteolytic enzymes (plasmin, kallikrein)

The alternative pathway[4] is phylogenetically older and less efficient because its initiation involves the formation of a fluid-phase complex of C3, perhaps chemically altered, with factor B. This leads to the formation of a labile magnesium-dependent enzyme, C3b,Bb, which can cleave more C3. This fluid-phase enzyme is very labile, and fluid-phase C3b is rapidly inactivated by the natural inhibitors, factor H (β 1H) and factor I (C3b inactivator). This system can become amplified only if the C3b binds to a so-called activator surface, such as certain polysaccharides or certain cell surfaces, which partially protects the C3b from the action of these inhibitors (Table 6–2). On such a surface C3b can complex with more factor B, which is cleaved by the proteolytic enzyme factor D to form a magnesium-dependent C3b,Bb enzyme which is stabilized by properdin and which is capable of cleaving more C3. C3b produced by classical pathway C3 convertase can also bind factor B and produce additional alternative pathway C3 convertase, thus generating a positive feedback or amplification circuit.

When C3 is cleaved by the C3-converting enzyme of either pathway, some of the major fragment C3b binds to the cell surface or complex surface in the vicinity of the C3-converting enzyme. These additional C3b molecules, bound in close proximity to alternative or classical pathway C3 convertase, provide binding sites for C5 and allow the convertases to cleave C5. Additional molecules of C3b may bind to cell membranes or immune complexes at sites not immediately adjacent to the activation enzymes. This excess bound C3b can interact with receptors on a number of cell types and markedly enhance opsonization for phagocytosis and perhaps interact with B lymphocytes to enhance antibody production.

The small cleavage fragment of C3, C3a, is an anaphylatoxin capable of degranulating mast cells and basophils and of contracting smooth muscle. The smaller fragment of C5 cleavage, C5a, is a potent chemotactic agent for neutrophils, monocytes, and eosinophils, causes neutrophil aggregation, and is also a potent anaphylatoxin. The serum enzyme carboxypeptidase B can cleave C5a and C3a to destroy or reduce their anaphylatoxin properties, but the cleaved fragment of C5a, C5a des-Arg, retains its chemotactic and neutrophil-stimulating activities.

TABLE 6–2.—Substances Capable of Supporting
or Enhancing Alternative Pathway Activation

Aggregated immunoglobulins (all classes)
Yeast cell walls (zymosan)
Bacterial cell walls
Polysaccharide portion of certain bacterial lipopolysaccharides
(deficient in sialic acid)
Rabbit erythrocytes
Renal dialysis membranes

C5b produced by the C5 cleaving enzymes of either activation pathway can bind to lipid membranes, a process that is facilitated and stabilized by the binding of uncleaved C6 and C7 to C5b. Membrane-bound C5b67 then binds C8 and C9, also without enzymatic cleavage, to form the C5b-9 membrane attack unit. The C5b-9 unit can penetrate the lipid bilayer and induce channels that allow leakage of ions and inflow of water, resulting in the lysis of the cell by an osmotic effect.[5] The biologic functions of the complement system are summarized in Table 6–3.

Activation of C components by immunologic or nonimmunologic means leads to their irreversible consumption, although in certain instances cleavage products of components such as C3 or factor B may be found in the circulation. The normal catabolism of most of the complement components that have been studied, including C3, C4, C5, and factor B, is much faster than that of other serum components such as albumin or γ-globulin, ranging from 1.5%–2.0% of the serum pool per hour.[6] The serum level of any individual complement component is the resultant of the rate of synthesis, the normal catabolic rate, and any enhanced removal rate that is triggered by activation. A number of complement proteins behave as acute-phase reactants (with increased synthesis and elevated levels during inflammatory processes). Thus, elevated complement levels are common findings of little diagnostic significance. Most of the clinical interest in complement component assays focuses on reduced serum levels due to increased consumption in disease processes or, more rarely, due to decreased synthesis in hereditary deficiency states. It must be appreciated that considerable excess consumption of a complement component can occur without a reduction in the serum level if the rate of synthesis is also increased. Measurements of the synthetic and catabolic rates of complement proteins are possible.[6] However, they involve the injection of radiolabeled, purified

TABLE 6–3.—Biologic Functions of the Complement System

COMPONENTS OR FRAGMENTS	FUNCTIONS
C2 kinin	Vascular permeability
C5a > C3a > C4a	Anaphylatoxins (mediator release from basophils and mast cells)
C5a des-Arg	Anaphylatoxin, chemotactic for phagocytes, enhance neutrophil aggregation and margination
C4b, C3b, iC3b, C3d	Opsonization for phagocytosis, viral neutralization
C3b, possibly iC3b and/or C3d	Immune complex solubilization; immune response modulation
C5b through C9	Membrane damage, cell lysis
Factor B	Macrophage activation and spreading

complement components into individuals and then following the component over a period of time, so they are not generally clinically applicable.

ASSAYS OF COMPLEMENT COMPONENTS

Complement assays in general use are divided into functional and immunoprecipitation tests, as described below.

Assays Depending on Functional Activity of Complement Proteins

Total Hemolytic Complement (CH$_{50}$) Assay

This is the most widely employed and generally useful of the functional complement assays, although it only measures the activity of the classical pathway components, C1–C9, and not the alternative pathway components. In this assay, which has several widely used modifications, sheep red blood cells (RBCs) optimally sensitized with rabbit IgM antibody are incubated with dilutions of test serum in a buffer containing the optimal concentrations of calcium and magnesium ions. The degree of lysis of the RBCs is measured by determining the amount of hemoglobin released from the lysed cells, and the dilution of serum required to lyse 50% of the standardized sheep RBC suspension in the standardized volume is determined. The reciprocal of this dilution is then called the CH$_{50}$ titer of this serum. For example, if 1 ml of a 1:100 dilution of patient's serum produced 50% lysis of the standardized sheep RBC suspension, the undiluted serum would be said to contain 100 CH$_{50}$ units/ml. This assay is most sensitive to the early components of the activation system, particularly C1 and C2, and, to some extent, C4 and C3. The later components, C5–C9, are much more efficient in their action. Very marked reductions in their concentrations are required to produce a reduction in CH$_{50}$ titer. The sensitivity of the CH$_{50}$ assay can vary with different batches of sheep RBCs and different batches of antibody, as well as with buffer composition and other factors. Therefore, it is important for the laboratory to run appropriate standards and maintain good quality control for these results to be clinically useful.

The tube dilution method for total hemolytic complement described in the previous paragraph is based on extensive work done by Mayer and is the most quantitative method available for assessing total hemolytic complement. Numerous modifications involving changes in reaction volume, buffers, indicator cells, and other reaction conditions have been utilized, and each modification produces a change in the hemolytic units found in normal serum. Some modifications have improved sensitivity over the original tube dilution method. Another method for assessment of total hemolytic complement in serum involves measuring the rate of hemolysis of a standard indicator cell suspension by a fixed serum dilution. This has been partially adapted to an automated method but has not yet achieved wide popularity. One commercial total hemolytic complement method in fairly wide use involves qualitative screening by hemolytic radial diffusion. In this assay, sensitized RBCs incorporated into agarose are poured into immunodiffusion plates. Wells are cut, and fresh serum added to these wells produces a circular zone of hemolysis as the complement components diffuse radially from the wells. The diameter of the zone of lysis is a qualitative measure of the amount of hemolytic complement present, which is generally scored as normal, low, or absent. This assay is rapid and simple to perform and is sometimes used as a screening procedure for laboratories interested in genetic complement deficiencies. It is not sufficiently quantitative to follow the course of lupus activity, however. Normal values for complement assays vary considerably from laboratory to laboratory.

Individual Hemolytic Complement Component Assays

These assays are based on modifications of the total hemolytic complement assay system. The lysis of sensitized sheep RBCs is measured in a system in which all of the required complement components are supplied in excess except for the component to be tested, which is provided by dilutions of the test serum. The assays are extremely sensitive and reasonably precise, but, because purified complement components or specifically deficient complement reagents are needed, such assays are not generally available outside of research laboratories. At least one commercial laboratory does offer hemolytic assays of the individual components of the classical pathway.

Hemolytic Assays of Alternative Pathway Function

Although they are not yet in wide clinical use, several screening assays for alternative pathway function have been devised,[7, 8] based on the observations (1) that unsensitized rabbit RBCs can serve as activators of the human alternative complement pathway and can be lysed by alternative pathway activation of complement on their surfaces, and (2) that the classical pathway depends on both calcium and magnesium, whereas the alternative pathway is only magnesium dependent. Therefore, the classical pathway can be blocked, but the alternative pathway can still be activated in the presence of the chelating agent EGTA, which binds calcium more strongly than magnesium. In these assays, dilutions of serum in Mg^{++}-EGTA buffer are incubated with unsensitized rabbit RBCs and the lysis of the rabbit RBCs is measured either as a function of time[8] or as a function of the dilution of serum supplied.[7] Because initiation of the alternative pathway is a fluid-phase diffusion-dependent process, high concentrations of serum are required and the serum dose-response for the assay is very steep, compared to the more gradual dose-response in the classical pathway assays.

Assays Depending on Analysis of Complement Proteins as Antigens

With the availability of specific antisera for most of the complement proteins, immunoprecipitation assays that have been used for other serum proteins have been adapted to measure individual complement proteins. These are most widely employed for C3, C4, factor B, and occasionally for C1q and C5. The other complement proteins are present in very low concentrations in serum, and special adaptations of immunoprecipitation assays are necessary to measure these protein levels reliably.

The most common immunoprecipitation assay is single radial immunodiffusion, wherein antiserum impregnates an agar gel and test sera and standards are placed in wells in the gel. Diffusion of antigen out of the well creates a ring of precipitation that can be measured, and the diameter of the ring can be related to the concentration of the protein in the well, using a standard curve (see Chap. 2).

Another commonly employed technique is nephelometry, which uses special instruments to measure the light-scattering property of antigen-antibody complexes in fluid-phase solutions. In this assay, small amounts of test sera are added to predetermined dilutions of monospecific antiserum in buffers designed to maximize the precipitation reaction. The amount of complement protein as antigen is then measured by comparing light scattering given by the test sera with that given by dilutions of a standard serum.

Another sensitive method is electroimmunodiffusion, or so-called rocket electrophoresis. In this technique specific antiserum is incorporated into agarose gels, and test serum and standards are placed in wells in the agarose. However, instead of allowing diffusion of the antigen to occur passively, antigen is electrophoresed out of the well in an electrical field so that the precipitation reaction develops in a rocket shape from the well, rather than in a ring, as in immunodiffusion. The height of the rocket is proportional to the concentration of antigen, and individual complement components can again be quantitated by comparing the rocket height from test sera with the rocket height from known standards.

It should be emphasized that these immunoprecipitation techniques detect complement proteins as antigens and do not distinguish between functional proteins and cleavage products of complement proteins. In fact, since the cleavage products are smaller than the native proteins and may be deficient in one or more determinants, cleavage of complement components can elevate the apparent concentration of the proteins, especially in radial immunodiffusion assays, since the smaller molecules diffuse more readily. This is most striking for C3, but probably is also significant with C4 and factor B. Nephelometry and rocket electrophoresis are somewhat less susceptible to this source of artifact, but they too can be affected by the presence of complement cleavage products.

Assays of Complement Cleavage Products

Because absolute levels of complement proteins do not always fall during activation owing to increased synthesis, some investigators have favored measuring the concentration of complement cleavage products, particularly C3d or C3c, or both, which are breakdown products of the action of C3b inactivator on C3b.[9, 10] The presence of complement breakdown products in carefully collected plasma can be taken as evidence of complement activation, but care must be taken to prevent in vitro cleavage of C3, which can occur to a variable extent during the clotting of blood. For assays of complement breakdown products, therefore, carefully collected EDTA plasma is commonly used, since the chelation of the calcium and magnesium prevents much of the in vitro cleavage of C3. For determination of C3 breakdown products, immunoprecipitation assays such as nephelometry or radioimmunodiffusion, using antisera that recognize only the breakdown product and not native C3, have been utilized.

Since the cleavage products of C3 and factor B have different electrophoretic mobilities from those of the native molecules, the relative concentrations of cleavage products versus the native molecules can be assessed by a technique known as crossed immunoelectrophoresis. Test plasma is electrophoresed in one direction in plain agarose, and a second electrophoresis at 90 degrees to the first dimension is done in agarose containing specific antiserum to C3 or factor B. This produces a double-humped pattern of precipitation arcs, the areas under which are proportional to the concentrations of the cleavage product and the native molecule. The arcs can be measured by planimetry and the results expressed as a proportion of C3 or factor B cleaved. Controls for uncleaved C3 (normal EDTA plasma) and cleaved C3 (inulin- or zymosan-treated normal serum) must be run in each assay.

Another proposed assay for classical pathway activation[11] takes advantage of the observation that, when C1 is activated in serum, C1 inhibitor binds to C1r and C1s, dissociating them from macromolecular C1 and blocking the antigenic reactivity of C1r but not C1s. Thus, the ratio of C1s to C1r (measured in radial immunodiffusion with commercially available antisera) increases when C1 is activated in the presence of C1-inhibitor. This ratio could presumably be used as a measure of C1 activation in vivo. A modification of this assay[12] has been used to measure the functional presence of C1 inhibitor in serum by activating C1 in vitro with aggregated IgG and measuring the change in C1r concentrations by radial immunodiffusion. For these assays, serum rather than EDTA plasma is used, although EDTA is added just before analysis of C1r and C1s by radial immunodiffusion.

Handling of Blood Samples for Complement Assays

Since a number of the complement proteins are quite labile to heat and proteolytic activity, careful handling of blood samples to be processed for complement assays is essential. For functional assays such as total hemolytic complement determinations, most laboratories prefer to use serum, as anticoagulants can interfere with the hemolytic assays. Heparin in particular interferes with complement function at several levels. EDTA and citrate anticoagulants do not irreversibly inactivate complement, and under a number of circumstances, blood plasma collected in EDTA may be quite useful for complement determinations. For assays of total hemolytic complement, in which high dilutions of serum are made in calcium- and magnesium-containing buffer, carefully collected EDTA plasma is usually satisfactory. Care should be taken that the correct amount of blood for the amount of EDTA in commercial collection tubes is drawn (i.e., the tubes are filled completely), the venipuncture is atraumatic, and the plasma is separated promptly. This is also the best sample for assays involving determination of complement split products. If serum is to be used, the blood must be delivered to the laboratory promptly, preferably within an hour of drawing. The serum should be separated from the clot as soon as possible, since proteolytic enzymes in white blood cells or platelets may be detrimental to the complement proteins. Serum or EDTA plasma for functional complement assays should be stored at −70 C in small aliquots if storage is to be prolonged. C3 and perhaps C4, when stored in an ordinary freezer at −20 C, tend to degrade over a period of weeks to months. In the refrigerator, degradation of C3 and C4 occurs in hours to days. Repeated freezing and thawing of the serum sample should also be avoided.

If cryoglobulins are suspected, the blood should be collected in a warm tube and transported immediately to the laboratory in a cup of warm water. Serum should be separated at 37 C and then flash-frozen in small aliquots at −70 C to prevent in vitro complement activation by the cryoglobulins.

Blood for immunochemical determination of complement proteins is somewhat less susceptible to these handling factors, but one must remember that in vitro cleavage of the complement proteins, particularly C3 and C4, can lead to false increases in the immunochemical estimates of their concentration, especially by radial immunodiffusion.

CLINICAL USE OF COMPLEMENT ASSAYS

As mentioned earlier, many complement proteins are acute-phase reactants. Therefore, elevated levels due to increased synthesis can be found in many inflammatory disease states. These observations are no more helpful diagnostically than other measurements of acute-phase reactants, such as sedimentation rate.

Most of the clinical interest in assays of serum complement component levels relates to reductions of these levels in various diseases. Serum levels of complement components can be reduced as a result of decreased synthesis or of increased consumption, usually related to activation.

Decreased or absent synthesis of individual complement components may be due to a genetic deficiency of the synthesis of the component. In some patients with membranoproliferative glomerulonephritis, reduced synthesis of C3 accompanies increased catabolism, possibly suggesting a negative feedback of high levels of complement breakdown products on the rate of synthesis. Reduced levels of serum hemolytic complement due to reduced synthesis of one or more components are sometimes seen in severe hepatic disease. Increased breakdown of complement proteins can occur through activation of the alternative or classical pathway, most often associated with circulating immune complexes; or increased catabolism of complement proteins may be secondary to a genetic deficiency of a regulatory protein such as C1 esterase inhibitor or C3b inactivator.

For most clinical purposes, a reasonable assessment of the status of the complement system can be achieved by combining a functional total hemolytic complement determination with immunochemical determinations of C3, C4, and factor B. Occasionally, assays for C1, C1q, C1 inhibitor, and C5 may be useful. As functional assays for alternative pathway activation become more widely available, they will probably be useful in screening for potential host defense deficiencies.

Genetic Deficiencies of Complement Proteins

We will first consider the genetic complement abnormalities because, despite their rarity, they have been quite informative about the role of the complement system in normal immunobiology.[13, 14] It is only in these primary complement abnormalities that laboratory assessment of the complement system can provide a definitive diagnosis of the disease state.

The most common and clinically the most important genetic defect of complement is hereditary angioedema.[15] This disease, first described by Osler in 1888, is marked by recurrent episodes of localized edema of subcutaneous tissue, the gastrointestinal tract, and upper airway mucosa. This edema is nonpruritic when it involves the skin but may produce severe abdominal pain and dehydration when it involves the gastrointestinal tract, as well as asphyxiation when it involves the upper airway structures. The disease is marked by an autosomal dominant genetic deficiency of the inhibitor of C1 esterase.[16] This serum α-globulin is also an inhibitor of other plasma proteases, including kallikrein, plasmin, Hageman factor, and clotting factor XI, but the most obvious serologic results of its absence are in the complement system. Since C1 esterase inhibitor deficiency is inherited as a dominant trait, affected individuals are heterozygous for the deficient gene, but 85%–90% of affected individuals have very low serum levels of C1 inhibitor (10%–15% of normal) measured either immunochemically or functionally. The remaining 10%–15% of affected individuals synthesize an abnormal C1 inhibitor protein which is detectable by immunochemical assays, but which is usually abnormal in electrophoretic mobility and is nonfunctional.

Clinical manifestations of hereditary angioedema usually do not begin until after puberty and often may begin later in life, although the biochemical defect can be detected much earlier. Affected individuals have activated C1 detectable in their circulation, and this active C1 cleaves its primary substrate, C4, such that virtually all untreated patients have low C4 levels even between attacks of edema. During attacks of angioedema, the total hemolytic complement and C4 levels fall to very low values. C2 also falls quite low. C1 and C3 levels remain normal.

The importance of diagnosing this potentially fatal and highly symptomatic disorder is highlighted by the fact that treatment with testosterone analogs is accompanied by increases in C1 inhibitor levels, C4 and C2 levels, and a marked decrease or cessation of attacks. The best screening assay for hereditary angioedema is a serum C4 level. If C4 is normal during an attack of angioedema, the diagnosis of hereditary angioedema is virtually eliminated. If the C4 level is low, especially with normal C3 levels, immunochemical determinations of C1 inhibitor, which are widely available, will confirm the diagnosis in a majority of instances. If the C1 inhibitor level is normal immunochemically and the disease cannot be detected in family members to confirm the diagnosis, functional assays[12, 16, 17] of C1 inhibitor levels can be done by a number of research laboratories but in practice are rarely required. A recently described method for assessing the functional activity of C1 inhibitor by immunochemical estimation of C1r and C1s after complement activation[12] may be more feasible for clinical laboratories than were previous assays.

An acquired form of C1 inhibitor deficiency has been reported in a number of patients. It is usually associated with lymphoproliferative disorders and often associated with low molecular weight (monomeric) IgM.[18] Patients may present with angioedema even before the lymphoproliferative disorder becomes clinically apparent. The complement profile resembles that of hereditary angioedema in that the total hemolytic complement, C4, and C1 inhibitor levels are markedly reduced, while the C3 level is normal. However, in the acquired form, the C1 level is low as opposed to normal levels in hereditary angioedema. This suggests that the reduced C1 inhibitor level is related to consumption of the inhibitor by C1 which has been activated by an unusual mechanism, perhaps related to the low molecular weight IgM or perhaps related to properties of the abnormal lymphocytes themselves. Angioedema in this acquired form has also been reported to be responsive to the administration of testosterone analogs.[19]

Genetic deficiency of C3b inactivator[20] has been reported. It was accompanied by severe hypercatabolism of C3 and alternative pathway components due to uncontrolled activation of the alternative pathway C3 convertase. The patient presented with a low CH_{50} titer, a low C3 level, circulating C3b in the serum, and C3b on the RBCs. The main clinical manifestations have been severe bacterial infections, presumably related to the very low C3 levels.

Genetic deficiencies of each of the individual complement components of the classical pathway have also been reported.[1, 2, 13, 14] These deficiencies are all inherited as autosomal co-dominant traits, with heterozygous individuals having roughly half-normal levels of the component in question. C2 deficiency is by far the most common, with an incidence possibly reaching 1 in 10,000. Only a few cases of deficiencies of each of the other components have been reported so far. Individuals homozygous for deficiency of any one of the classical components, with the exception of C9, have total hemolytic complement levels that are zero or exceptionally low. Because slow lysis of erythrocytes coated with C1–C8 can occur, C9-deficient individuals have reduced but not absent total hemolytic complement levels. Generally, the clinician should suspect a genetic complement deficiency if the CH_{50} titer is persistently and markedly reduced in carefully drawn serum specimens, despite normal C3 and C4 levels. Genetic deficiency of C3 or C4 is signaled by persistently absent levels of the relevant protein, in the absence of active disease, known to be associated with complement activation.

The probands in complement-deficient families are nearly always identified by absence of CH_{50} activity. Since complement levels are usually determined because of suspected immunologic disease, it is not surprising that a disproportionate number of probands with genetic complement deficiencies have had autoimmune or rheumatic diseases. The association is particularly striking in patients with deficiencies of the early acting components, including C1r, C1s, C4, and C2, as well as deficiency of C1 inhibitor. However, patients with deficiencies of C5, C7, and C8 have also been reported to have rheumatic diseases. The true magnitude of the association between the complement defects and autoimmune or rheumatic diseases is difficult to assess because of this potential ascertainment bias. However, it is of some interest because C2, C4, and factor B are known to be closely linked to the major histocompatibility complex of chromosome 6 in man, raising the possibility of linkage disequilibrium with immune response or immune regulatory genes (reviewed by Alper and Rosen[21]). Other speculations about this apparent association of genetic defects of the early acting complement components and rheumatic diseases have implicated reduced viral neutralization by complement, leading to the initiation or potentiation of the autoimmune response, or a reduced role of complement in enhancing clearance or solubilization of immune complexes.

The role of complement in host defense[22, 23] is underscored by the observations that homozygous deficiency of C3 is almost always associated with severe and frequent bacterial infections quite similar to those seen in agammaglobulinemia. Only a minority of C2-deficient individuals have increased infections, and some of these have in addition low levels of factor B, possibly reflecting the close genetic linkage of C2 and factor B.[24] It is quite striking that homozygous deficiency of the later-acting complement components C5, C6, C7, C8, and C9 appears to have a high association with disseminated *Neisseria* infections, either gonococcal or meningococcal. This observation has helped emphasize the importance of serum bactericidal activity, which depends on an intact C5b-9 membrane attack mechanism, in preventing dissemination of these organisms.[25]

Acquired Complement Abnormalities

The major clinical attention in the area of acquired serum complement abnormalities has focused on reduced levels of various complement components (implying complement activation) in the setting of diseases thought to be associated with antigen-antibody reactions occurring in the circulation or in tissues. Because antibody-directed complement activation can produce tissue injury rather efficiently with relatively little consumption of complement components in the presence of the natural serum inhibitors, there are a number of examples of complement involvement in autoantibody-induced tissue damage without reduction in serum complement titers. Examples of such diseases include Goodpasture's syndrome, several types of autoimmune hemolytic anemia, pemphigus, bullous pemphigoid, and myasthenia gravis. However, one occasionally does see reduced serum complement levels in individual patients with these diseases.

Patterns of Complement Reduction due to Activation

Diseases associated with intravascular formation of antigen-antibody reactions and soluble immune complexes are, however, commonly associated with complement activation and reduced serum complement levels. In contrast to the genetic deficiencies, in which a single component is absent, these usually involve reduced levels of more than one component. By assessing total hemolytic complement and by determining, immunochemically, C4, C3, and factor B levels in such disease states, one can form a reasonably accurate impression of the mode of activation of the complement system in the individual patient (Table 6–4). Patterns of complement reduction are called complement profiles and are not usually diagnostic for one particular disease, but they may be suggestive of certain groups of diseases.[26, 27] Furthermore, once the pattern of complement reduction has been established in an individual patient, the levels of the involved components often fluctuate with disease activity or response to therapy and can be useful guides to prognosis and therapy.[27, 28] The usual examples of circulating immune complex diseases, such as systemic lupus erythematosus, serum sickness, the serum sickness-like syndrome sometimes accompanying acute viral hepatitis, and bacterial endocarditis with nephritis, are associated with predominantly classical pathway activation. This is manifested by reduced levels of total hemolytic complement, C4, and C3, with normal or only minimally reduced factor B. In some individuals with marked classical pathway activation, the positive feedback loop through the alternative pathway is activated and factor B level may also be reduced.

Patients with poststreptococcal glomerulonephritis usually have evidence of activation of the classical pathway and the feedback loop initially, but later in the disease C4 levels may return to normal and C3 levels may be low for weeks, apparently due to reduced C3 synthesis.[26, 29]

Patients with endotoxemia during gram-negative sepsis may have evidence of direct activation of the alternative pathway with reduction in CH_{50}, C3, and factor B levels but a normal C4 level. Severe activation of the alternative pathway is often associated with endotoxin shock.[30] Many patients with membranoproliferative glomerulonephritis have a pattern of complement activation that resembles alternative pathway activation, with normal C4, reduced C3, and reduced factor B levels, which occurs in association with a circulating protein called C3 nephritic factor. This is an IgG antibody directed against neoantigens on the C3-converting enzyme, usually the alternative pathway enzyme, C3b,Bb, but occasionally the clas-

TABLE 6–4.—SERUM COMPLEMENT PROFILES RESULTING FROM VARIOUS MECHANISMS OF ACTIVATION*

ACTIVATION MECHANISM	CH$_{50}$	COMPLEMENT LEVELS				EXAMPLE
		C1q or C1	C4	C3	Factor B	
In vitro activation after blood drawn	↓	N, ↓	N	N, ↑	N	Poor sample handling or storage; cryoglobulinemia; some SLE with cold-reacting immune complexes; can mimic genetic C deficiency
Loss of classical pathway control (C1-inhibitor function reduced)	↓	N	→ or ↓↓	N	N	Hereditary angioedema
	↓ or ↓↓	↓	→ or ↓↓	N	N	Acquired C1 inhibitor deficiency; occasionally in cryoglobulinemia
Loss of alternative pathway control	↓	N	N	↓	↓	C3b inactivator deficiency
	↓	N	N	→ or ↓↓	↓ or ↓↓	C3 nephritic factor (membranoproliferative glomerulonephritis); some SLE
Classical pathway activation	↓	↓	↓	↓	N or ↓ (if feedback loop activated)	SLE; serum sickness; severe RA with vasculitis or extra-articular disease; other circulating immune complex diseases
Alternative pathway activation	↓	N	N	↓	↓	Endotoxemia; occasional SLE

*N, normal; SLE, systemic lupus erythematosus; RA, rheumatoid arthritis.

sical pathway enzyme, C4b,2a. The etiology of these unusual autoantibodies is not clear, but they stabilize the C3 convertase enzymes against dissociation decay and therefore lead to intense fluid-phase activation and cleavage of C3 with some associated consumption of factor B. This pattern of fluid-phase alternative pathway activation is also seen in genetic deficiency of C3b inactivator, although in this instance the reduction in factor B is profound.

Fluid-phase activation of the classical pathway, such as is seen in C1 inhibitor deficiency, does not permit efficient formation of C3 convertase, so one finds reduced total hemolytic complement, low C4, but normal C3 and factor B levels. This pattern is occasionally seen in patients with lupus or cryoglobulinemia.

INDICATIONS FOR COMPLEMENT ASSAYS

An assessment of the serum complement system can be useful in the evaluation and management of patients presenting with various clinical manifestations which may be produced by the generation of, or through the deficiency of, the various biologic activities inherent in the complement system. These include deficiencies in host defense mechanisms, particularly repeated or severe pyogenic infections or disseminated infections with *Neisseria*, either *N. gonorrhoeae* or *N. meningitidis*.[22, 23, 25] To evaluate the possible role of a complement abnormality in host defense, which may be manifested by deficiency of a single component, one must assay the total hemolytic complement to evaluate the classical pathway components. If possible, a functional screening assay of the alternative pathway should also be performed.

In patients presenting with clinical manifestations that may be related to inappropriate activation of the complement system, a complement screening profile consisting of CH_{50}, C3, C4, and, if available, factor B, may be useful. Clinical manifestations may include repeated angioedema, especially if it is associated with episodes of abdominal pain or if the family history suggests hereditary angioedema; chronic urticaria or palpable purpura, both of which may be manifestations of cutaneous vasculitis; arthritis, arthralgias; unexplained fever; or other symptoms suggestive of an immunologic disorder.[26-28] A similar complement screening profile may be useful in the evaluation and management of patients with various forms of nephritis.[29]

Serial determinations of complement components may be of value in the management of patients with chronic immune complex diseases, such as systemic lupus erythematosus, in which severe nephritis is almost always preceded or accompanied by reductions in serum levels of C4 or C3, or both.[28] Complement levels should not serve as the only guide for therapy in these immune complex–mediated disorders, but reduced complement levels should raise the clinician's level of concern about the patient and lead to an increased frequency of clinical assessment and an intensified search for internal organ involvement, particularly nephritis.[27, 28] A recent study suggested that patients with lupus nephritis whose serum CH_{50} could be kept normalized by therapy over a 5-year period had a more favorable renal outcome than those whose CH_{50} could not be so normalized, although normalization of anti-DNA antibody levels showed no such correlation.[31] Although rheumatoid arthritis is usually accompanied by normal or elevated complement levels, reductions in CH_{50}, C2, C4, and occasionally C3 levels are seen in severe disease, usually accompanied by vasculitis or other extra-articular manifestations.[32] Furthermore, circulating complement activation products (C3d) have been found in serum and synovial fluid of rheumatoid arthritis patients, and the C3d levels correlated with clinical activity and presence of extra-articular manifestations.[10] Thus, decreased complement levels or increased complement activation products may have some prognostic usefulness in rheumatoid arthritis, but it is not yet clear how useful they are as guides to therapy.

The demonstration of reduced complement levels in certain body fluids such as joint effusions or pleural or pericardial effusions has occasionally proved useful, but many laboratories do not have the necessary experience with normal body fluids to provide appropriate interpretation of these results. When joint or body space effusions are assayed, serum complement protein levels must be determined simultaneously, and complement levels corrected for total protein in the effusions should be compared to complement levels corrected for total protein in the serum. In osteoarthritis, joint effusions generally contain approximately one third of serum complement levels, so that reductions below those levels are taken as evidence of in situ complement fixation. Measurements of cerebrospinal fluid C4 by sensitive functional assays have been claimed to be useful in diagnosing CNS lupus, but, because of the extreme lability of C4 and very low levels in normal cerebrospinal fluid, these have not proved to be of practical importance.

When they become more widely available, measurements of complement breakdown products[9, 10] or other more direct assays of complement activation[11] will probably prove more useful than assays of native components in assessing the role of complement activation in disease states.

IMMUNE COMPLEX ASSAYS

The above-mentioned patterns of complement activation in a number of diseases in which immune reactants are found deposited in affected tissues have provided indirect evidence for the role of circulating immune complexes in the pathogenesis of these diseases, in analogy with well-defined animal models.[33] These and other observations have spurred a search for more direct assays of circulating immune complexes in the hope of improving the sensitivity or specificity of diagnosis in these disease states.[34–37]

Two general approaches have been taken to implicate the role of immune complexes in human diseases. The first involves the examination of sections of involved tissue for the presence of immune reactants by immunohistologic and electron microscopic techniques.[38] This approach has allowed the demonstration of immunoglobulin deposits, sometimes associated with complement components and occasionally associated with identified antigens, in tissue and vascular lesions in a pattern suggestive of the deposition of immune complexes. The second approach has been to analyze biologic fluids, mainly serum, for the presence of immune complexes and to correlate assay findings with the presence or activity of various disease states.[39]

Many assays intended to detect soluble immune complexes in blood and body fluids have been designed in the last 10 years. These have been employed in a wide variety of clinical conditions with somewhat variable results. The initial hope that some of these assay systems could be adapted to the isolation of circulating immune complexes in various presumed immune complex diseases in which the antigens are not known, thus facilitating the identification of the antigen, has proved more difficult to realize than was anticipated, and results have generally been disappointing.

Because no single immune complex assay has proved to be clearly superior to the others in specificity and sensitivity of detection of immune complexes in a variety of diseases, and because the different assays detect different types of immune complexes (as well as nonimmune reactants) with varying sensitivity,[39] most laboratories interested in immune complex detection utilize several assays. These assays are based on various characteristics of immune complexes, which are briefly outlined below (Table 6–5).

Assays Depending on Physical Characteristics of Immune Complexes

A number of techniques best suited to research laboratories, including analytic ultracentrifugation, sucrose density gradient ultracentrifugation, and gel filtration, have been used to demonstrate the presence of IgG or occasionally IgM or complement components in molecular weight ranges that suggest aggregation. These methods are too complex and too slow for clinical use.

An older assay that is still of considerable clinical usefulness—the cryo-

TABLE 6–5.—ASSAYS FOR SOLUBLE IMMUNE COMPLEXES IN SERA*

ASSAY	IMMUNE COMPLEX PROPERTY UTILIZED	SENSITIVITY	AVAILABILITY	COMMENT
Cryoglobulins	Reduced solubility in cold	Low	Wide	Careful blood handling; not all cryoglobulins represent immune complexes
Polyethylene glycol (PEG) precipitation	Reduced solubility of high molecular weight complexes	Low-moderate	Several reference labs	Usefulness depends on techniques used to analyze precipitate
^{125}I C1q binding	Binding C1q, precipitation by PEG	Moderate-high	Wide	Polyanionic substances ↑ slightly; bacterial products ↓, but minimal
C1q deviation tests	Compete with solid-phase aggregated Ig for C1q binding	Moderate-high	Limited	Sensitive to polyanions, DNA, CRP-complex, bacterial products; heating or dilution of serum required
Solid-phase C1q binding	Binding to C1q; detection of bound Ig with labeled anti-Ig	Moderate-high	Moderately wide	Interference by C1q in test serum, and by rheumatoid factors
Conglutinin-binding assays	Complexes containing iC3b bind to bovine conglutinin (Ca^{++} dependent)	Fair	Limited	Detects large complexes bearing C3 fragments; requires purified conglutinin
Solid-phase anti-C3 assays	Presence of C3 antigens in complex	Not fully assessed	Limited, may increase	Not widely tested, but seems attractive
Raji cell assay	Binding of ICs to Raji cells via C receptors, identification with labeled anti-Ig	High	Moderately wide, but decreasing	Antilymphocyte antibodies, common in SLE, give false positive results
Platelet aggregation	Interaction of ICs with platelet Fc receptors	Moderate	Limited	Increased by antiplatelet antibodies, some myxoviruses; decreased by RF, high C1q
Monoclonal rheumatoid factor assay (mRF)	Increased affinity of mRF for aggregated IgG over monomer IgG	Depends on RF used	Limited	Requires appropriate mRF; inhibited by free IgG, requires dilution to equal IgG concentration; potential inhibition by RF in sera

*IC, immune complex; mRF, monoclonal rheumatoid factor.

precipitation or cryoglobulin test—reflects the reduced solubility of many immune complexes under conditions of reduced temperature. This assay is performed by collecting blood into a warm tube, allowing a clot to form and separate at 37 C, and then allowing the supernatant serum to sit at refrigerator temperatures for several days. Any precipitate formed can be measured for protein concentration, analyzed for immunoglobulin and complement composition, or simply centrifuged and expressed as the percentage of the serum volume occupied by the packed precipitate (analogous to a hematocrit). Many such cold-induced serum precipitates consist of at least two different immunoglobulin classes and so are called mixed cryoglobulins. Mixed cryoglobulins often represent immune complexes of IgM rheumatoid factor and IgG, possibly complexed to a nonimmunoglobulin antigen. Certain myeloma proteins or other monoclonal immunoglobulins have structural abnormalities that cause reduced solubility in the cold. These monoclonal cryoprecipitates do not represent immune complexes. Cryoprecipitation assays are inexpensive and easy to perform, and so are useful in following patients in whom an assay has been found to be positive. However, cryoprecipitation assays are of relatively low sensitivity, requiring large amounts of immune complexes before they become positive. The reduced solubility of antigen-antibody complexes in the cold can be enhanced by adding polyethylene glycol, a water-soluble uncharged linear polymer, to serum. This reduces the available water content of the serum and will precipitate proteins generally in the order of their molecular weight. If the conditions of precipitation are carefully controlled, it is possible to precipitate immune complexes from serum somewhat selectively. The precipitate can then be washed and analyzed for the cryoglobulin.[40] This method also lacks sensitivity and specificity, so a number of assays reflecting the biologic properties of immune complexes have been devised.

Assays Reflecting Biologic Properties of Immune Complexes

Assays Utilizing C1q Binding Properties of Immune Complexes

One of the more popular assays is the ^{125}I-C1q binding assay, which was originally described by Nydegger et al.[41] and subsequently modified.[42] It is based on the ability of purified human C1q to bind to aggregated γ-globulin or immune complexes containing IgG1, IgG2, IgG3, or IgM with much higher affinity than it binds to the monomeric immunoglobulins. In this assay human serum is mixed with EDTA, which dissociates the native C1 into C1q, C1r, and C1s, presumably to facilitate the exchange of the radiolabeled C1q added in the assay with any native C1q already bound to the immune complexes in test serum. After the radiolabeled C1q is added, the immune complexes are precipitated with polyethylene glycol at a concentration that does not precipitate free C1q. The results are either expressed as percentage of the radiolabeled C1q precipitated or can be referred to a standard curve generated by varying amounts of heat-aggregated γ-globulin (AHG), then expressed as microgram equivalents of AHG. Several substances that may occur in serum, such as DNA, can bind to C1q. Most of these complexes are soluble in the concentrations of polyethylene glycol used and do not interfere. C-reactive protein complexes that might bind to C1q tend to be dissociated by the EDTA used in the serum. Some polyanionic substances can still give false positive results, and serum containing bacterial products may give reduced levels of C1q binding.

Other assays involving the interaction of C1q with immune complexes have been devised. These include solid-phase C1q assays. In these systems purified C1q is bound to a solid-phase substance such as a plastic test tube and incubated with the serum containing immune complexes, and the immune complexes that remain bound to the solid-phase C1q after washing are identified with radiolabeled antisera to IgG or other components. Alternatively, the immune complexes in the test sera can be assayed by their ability to interfere with the binding of radiolabeled aggregated IgG to the solid-phase C1q.

Assays based on the ability of immune complexes to interfere with the binding of C1q in the fluid phase to solid-phase IgG aggregates have also been devised. These latter types of inhibition assays are sometimes called C1q deviation tests.

Assays Detecting Immune Complex–Bound C3 Breakdown Products

When certain immune complexes activate complement in plasma, C3b is covalently bound to the complex, either to the antigen or the antibody. This C3b is rapidly acted on by C3b-inactivator in the presence of β 1H to form the initial product, iC3b. Subsequent proteolytic activity cleaves iC3b into C3c, which enters the fluid phase, and C3d, which remains bound to the immune complex. The C3 cleavage products that remain attached to the complexes (C3b, iC3b, and/or C3d) can be detected by several assays.

Conglutinin-binding assays utilize a high molecular weight protein found in most bovine sera which, in the presence of calcium, can bind to breakdown products of human C3 (most probably iC3b). This protein (bovine conglutinin) is purified from appropriate bovine sera and can be radiolabeled and used in a fluid-phase assay analogous to the C1q binding assay except that EDTA is not used.[43] A solid-phase conglutinin binding assay is performed by fixing the conglutinin to polypropylene tubes, adding test serum, washing the tubes and then assaying bound immune complexes with radiolabeled or enzyme-conjugated anti-immunoglobulin antibodies.[44]

A recently described assay for complex-bound C3 fragments which appears to have promise employs F(ab')$_2$ anti-human C3 bound to a solid-phase matrix.[45] A dilution of the test serum is incubated with the solid-phase anti-C3, followed by washing. Radiolabeled anti-human IgG is added, and the amount of antibody bound is taken as an indication of the amount of C3-containing circulating immune complexes. The developing antibody can either be polyspecific for all immunoglobulins or monospecific for various immunoglobulin classes.

Assays Based on Interaction With Cell Surface Receptors

The most common of these assays uses a B cell tissue culture line, called Raji cells, which originated from a patient with Burkitt's lymphoma.[46] The cells contain surface receptors for C3 breakdown products, probably iC3b or C3d, or both, as well as some receptors for the Fc region of IgG and some receptors for C1q. Test sera are incubated with the Raji cells, which are then washed, and the presence of immunoglobulin bound to the Raji cells via any of the above-mentioned receptors is detected with radiolabeled anti-immunoglobulin serum. One disadvantage of this assay is that the serum of many patients with SLE contains warm-reactive antilymphocyte antibodies that can bind to antigenic determinants on the surface of Raji cells and subsequently can be detected by the radiolabeled anti-immunoglobulin antiserum.[47]

Immune complexes can also aggregate human platelets in an energy-dependent reaction, probably by interaction with Fc receptors on the platelet surface. Immune complex assays have been devised based on the highest dilution of either native or heat-inactivated serum that is capable of reducing platelet aggregation. This assay is sensitive for large (19s or greater) immune complexes, but false positive results can be given by anti-platelet antibodies, viruses, aggregated γ-globulin, heparin, and thrombin, or other proteolytic enzymes.[37]

Tests Depending on Antigenic Characteristics
of Immune Complexes

A number of tests employ either monoclonal or polyclonal rheumatoid factors, which react with antigenic determinants on IgG. Monoclonal rheumatoid factors, particularly 7S rheumatoid factors, have approximately 50 times greater affinity for aggregated IgG than for monomer IgG. In these assays, test sera are diluted to equivalent IgG concentrations to cancel out the interference by monomer IgG, and the binding of immune complexes to the rheumatoid factors is measured in solid-phase or fluid-phase assays.

CLINICAL APPLICATIONS OF IMMUNE COMPLEX ASSAYS

As might be expected, application of various immune complex assays in many laboratories has detected immune complexes in a number of rheumatic, infectious, and other idiopathic diseases. In many of these diseases, no clear immunopathologic role has been demonstrated for the immune complexes. Certain assays appear to have greater sensitivity than others for detecting immune complexes in specific diseases. For example, tests utilizing monoclonal rheumatoid factors and, to some extent, C1q binding assays detect immune complexes in sera from patients with rheumatoid arthritis more frequently than does the Raji cell assay. On the other hand, the Raji cell assay is more often positive in systemic lupus, but part of this distinction may relate to the presence of antilymphocyte antibodies in lupus sera.[39]

In general, immune complex assays such as the Raji cell assay and the C1q binding assay tend to detect higher levels of complexes in patients whose rheumatic disease, particularly systemic lupus, is active, but there does not appear to be any particular correlation between these assays for immune complexes and renal disease in lupus.

At the present state of technology in detecting immune complexes by these various assays, their direct applicability in diagnosis and management of most presumably immune complex–mediated diseases is still somewhat limited. We have noticed, for example, that the C1q binding assay is frequently positive in patients with cutaneous vasculitis of varying etiologies, but the level of circulating complexes detected by this assay does not appear to correlate with the presence or absence of vasculitis in other organs or with response to various therapeutic measures. However, certain empirical observations in some disease states may, if confirmed, provide useful therapeutic or prognostic information. For example, Dreisin et al.[48] found that the Raji cell assay demonstrated elevated levels in patients with idiopathic interstitial pneumonitis with active cellular infiltrates in their lungs, whereas patients with predominantly fibrosis did not have abnormal Raji cell assays. These workers found that the response to corticosteroid therapy was better in patients with elevated Raji cell assays prior to therapy. In another study, Hardin et al.[49] found that persistent positivity of the C1q binding assay in patients with Lyme arthritis was associated with a higher incidence of neurologic or cardiac complications and that persistent inflammatory arthritis was associated with high titers of C1q binding materials in the synovial fluid. Thus, peristent immune complexes in patients with Lyme arthritis might identify a group of patients for whom more aggressive therapy would be beneficial.

In some patients with severe systemic vasculitis associated with circulating immune complexes and in whom plasmapheresis therapy is contemplated, the levels of complexes detected by these assays may serve as a useful guide to the efficacy and extent of plasmapheresis required.

In summary, in recent years a large number of different assays for circulating immune complexes have been developed, but these are not yet well standardized from laboratory to laboratory. Except for a few specific clinical examples such as those cited, the clinical usefulness of immune complex assays is not entirely clear at the present time. Although positive results in such assays should lead the clinician to suspect a pathogenetic role for immune complexes and to search for involvement in organs most commonly affected in these diseases, namely, blood vessels and kidneys, I believe there is insufficient experience at this point to justify basing major therapeutic decisions on the results of these assays.

On the other hand, negative results in immune complex assays in conjunction with negative tests for autoantibodies and normal complement levels may be very helpful in eliminating humoral immunologic reactions as the cause of undiagnosed multisystem disease.

REFERENCES

1. Atkinson J.P., Frank M.: Complement, in Parker C.W. (ed.): *Clinical Immunology*. Philadelphia, W.B. Saunders Co., 1980, vol. 1, pp. 219–271.
2. Gigli I.: The complement system: Mechanisms of action, biology, and participation in dermatological diseases, in Safai B., Good R.A. (eds.): *Immunodermatology of Comprehensive Immunology*. New York, Plenum Publishing Corp. 1981, vol. 7, pp. 65–100.
3. Stroud R.M., Volonakis J.E., Nagasawa S., et al.: Biochemistry and biological reactions of complement proteins, in Atassi M.Z. (ed.): *Immunochemistry of Proteins*. New York, Plenum Publishing Corp., 1979, vol. 3, pp. 167–221.
4. Fearon D.T., Austen K.F.: Current concepts in immunology: The alternative pathway of complement—a system for host resistance to microbial infections. *N. Engl. J. Med.* 303:259, 1980.
5. Mayer M.M., Michaels D.W., Ramm L.E., et al.: Membrane damage by complement. *Crit. Rev. Immunol.* 2:133, 1981.
6. Ruddy S., Carpenter G.B., Chin K.W., et al.: Human complement metabolism: An analysis of 144 studies. *Medicine* 54:165, 1975.
7. Platts-Mills T.A.E., Ishizaka K.: Activation of the alternate pathway of human complement by rabbit cells. *J. Immunol.* 113:348, 1974.
8. Polhill R.B., Pruitt K.M., Johnston R.B.: Kinetic assessment of alternative complement pathway in a hemolytic system. *J. Immunol.* 121:303, 1970.
9. Perrin L.H., Lambert P.H., Miescher P.A.: Complement breakdown products in patients with systemic lupus erythematosus and patients with membranoproliferative or other glomerulonephritis. *J. Clin. Invest.* 56:165, 1975.
10. Nydegger U.E., Zubler R.H., Gabay R., et al.: Circulating complement breakdown products in patients with rheumatoid arthritis: Correlations between plasma C3d, circulating immune complexes and clinical activity. *J. Clin. Invest.* 59:862, 1977.
11. Ziccardi R.J., Cooper N.R.: Demonstration and quantitation of activation of the first component of complement in human serum. *J. Exp. Med.* 147:385, 1978.

12. Ziccardi R.J., Cooper N.R.: Development of an immunochemical test to assess C1 inactivator function in human serum and its use for the diagnosis of hereditary angioedema. *Clin. Immunol. Immunopathol.* 15:465, 1980.

13. Day N.K., Moncada B., Good R.A.: Inherited deficiencies of the complement system, in Good R.A., Day N.K. (eds.): *Biological Amplification Systems in Immunology,* vol. 2 in *Comprehensive Immunology.* New York, Plenum Publishing Corp., 1977, pp. 229–246.

14. Agnello V.: Complement deficiency states. *Medicine* 57:1, 1978.

15. Frank M.E., Gelfand J.A., Atkinson J.P.: Hereditary angioedema: The clinical syndrome and its management. *Ann. Intern. Med.* 84:580, 1976.

16. Donaldson V.H., Evans R.R.: A biochemical abnormality in hereditary angioneurotic edema: Absence of serum inhibitor of C1 esterase. *Am. J. Med.* 35:37, 1963.

17. Gigli J., Ruddy S., Austen K.F.: The stoichiometric measurement of the serum inhibitor of the first component of complement by inhibition of immune hemolysis. *J. Immunol.* 100:1154, 1968.

18. Caldwell R.J., Ruddy S., Schur P.H., et al.: C1 inhibitor deficiency in lymphosarcoma. *Clin. Immunol. Immunopathol.* 1:39, 1972.

19. Cohen S.H., Koethe S.M., et al.: Acquired angioedema associated with rectal carcinoma and its response to danazol therapy. *J. Allergy Clin. Immunol.* 62:217, 1978.

20. Abramson N., Alper C.A., Lachmann P.J., et al.: Deficiency of C3 inactivator in man. *J. Immunol.* 107:19, 1971.

21. Alper C.A., Rosen F.S.: Genetics of the complement system. *Adv. Hum. Genet.* 7:141, 1976.

22. Rosen F.S.: The complement system and increased susceptibility to infection. *Semin. Hematol.* 8:221, 1971.

23. Goldstein I.M.: *Complement in Infectious Diseases.* Kalamazoo, Mich., Upjohn Co., 1980.

24. Neuman S.L., Vogler L.B., Feigin R.D., et al.: Recurrent septicemia associated with congenital deficiency of C2 and partial deficiency of factor B and the alternative complement pathway. *N. Engl. J. Med.* 299:290, 1978.

25. Leddy J.P., Steigbigel R.T.: Complement, serum bactericidal activity and disseminated gram-negative infection, editorial. *Ann. Intern. Med.* 90:984, 1979.

26. Alper C.A., Rosen F.S.: Clinical applications of complement assays. *Adv. Intern. Med.* 20:61, 1975.

27. Schur P.H.: Complement testing in the diagnosis of immune and autoimmune diseases. *Am. J. Clin. Pathol.* 68:647, 1977.

28. Lloyd W., Schur P.H.: Immune complexes, complement, and anti-DNA in exacerbations of systemic lupus erythematosus (SLE). *Medicine* 60:208, 1981.

29. Lewis E.J., Carpenter C.B., Schur P.H.: Serum complement component levels in human glomerulonephritis. *Ann. Intern. Med.* 75:555, 1971.

30. Fearon D.T., Ruddy S., Schur P.H., et al.: Activation of the properdin pathway of complement in patients with gram-negative bacteremia. *N. Engl. J. Med.* 292:937, 1975.

31. Jarrett M.P., Sablay L.B., Walter L., et al.: The effect of continuous normalization of serum hemolytic complement on the course of lupus nephritis: A five-year prospective study. *Am. J. Med.* 70:1067, 1981.

32. Hunder G.G., McDuffie F.C.: Hypocomplementemia in rheumatoid arthritis. *Am. J. Med.* 54:461, 1973.

33. Dixon F.J.: The role of antigen-antibody complexes in disease. *Harvey Lect.* 58:21, 1963.
34. Zubler R.H., Lambert P.H.: Detection of immune complexes in human diseases. *Prog. Allergy* 24:1, 1978.
35. Barnett E.V. (moderator): Circulating immune complexes: Their immunochemistry, detection, and importance. *Ann. Intern. Med.* 91:430, 1979.
36. Inman R.D., Day N.K.: Immunologic and clinical aspects of immune complex disease. *Am. J. Med.* 70:1097, 1981.
37. Lawley T.J.: Methods of detection of circulating immune complexes. *Clin. Immunol. Allergy* 1:383, 1981.
38. Wilson C.B., Dixon F.J.: Diagnosis of immunopathological renal disease. *Kidney Int.* 5:389, 1974.
39. Lambert P.H., et al.: A WHO collaborative study for the evaluation of eighteen methods for detecting immune complexes in serum. *J. Clin. Lab. Immunol.* 1:1, 1978.
40. Chia D., Barnett E.V., Yamagata J., et al.: Quantitation and characterization of soluble immune complexes precipitated from sera by polyethylene glycol (PEG). *Clin. Exp. Immunol.* 37:399, 1979.
41. Nydegger U.E., Lambert P.H., Gerber H., et al.: Circulating immune complexes in the serum in systemic lupus erythematosus and in carriers of hepatitis B antigen. *J. Clin. Invest.* 54:297, 1974.
42. Zubler R.H., Lange G., Lambert P.H., et al.: Detection of immune complexes in unheated sera by a modified ^{125}I-Clq binding test: Effect of heating on the binding of Clq by immune complexes and application of the test to systemic lupus erythematosus. *J. Immunol.* 116:232, 1976.
43. Macanovic M., Lachmann P.J.: Conglutinin binding polyethylene glycol precipitation assay for immune complexes. *Clin. Exp. Immunol.* 38:274, 1979.
44. Casali P., Bossus A., Carpentier N.A., et al.: Solid-phase enzyme immunoassay or radioimmunoassay for the detection of immune complexes based on their recognition by conglutinin. Conglutinin-binding test. *Clin. Exp. Immunol.* 29:342, 1977.
45. Pereira A.B., Theophilopoulos A.N., Dixon F.J.: Detection and partial characterization of circulating immune complexes with solid-phase anti-C3. *J. Immunol.* 125:763, 1980.
46. Theophilopoulos A.N., Wilson C.B, Dixon F.J: The Raji cell radioimmune assay for detecting immune complexes in human sera. *J. Clin. Invest.* 57:169, 1976.
47. Anderson C.L., Stillman W.S.: Raji cell assay for immune complexes: Evidence for detection of Raji-directed immunoglobulin G antibody in sera from patients with systemic lupus erythematosus. *J. Clin. Invest.* 66:353, 1980.
48. Dreisin R.B., Schwarz M.I., Theophilopoulos A.N., et al.: Circulating immune complexes in the idiopathic interstitial pneumonias. *N. Engl. J. Med.* 298:353, 1978.
49. Hardin J.A., Steere A.C., Malawista S.E.: Immune complexes and the evolution of Lyme arthritis. *N. Engl. J. Med.* 301:1358, 1979.

7

Immunohematology

Klaus Mayer, M.D.

THE CLINICAL FIELD of hematology lends itself to immunologic testing because of its very nature. The cellular components of blood contain antigens that are usually but not always recognized by the immunocompetent cells as "self." In disease states this recognition process may fail, resulting in autoimmune disease. Immune destruction of red blood cells (RBCs) is manifested as an acquired hemolytic anemia, autoimmune destruction of granulocytes results in neutropenia, and analogous destruction of platelets is the etiology of idiopathic thrombocytopenic purpura. Cell lysis may be intravascular or may require participation of organs of the reticuloendothelial system, especially the spleen. Correct localization of the site of destruction may be of importance in developing a strategy for effective therapy. When antibody-coated cells are destroyed in a normally functioning spleen it may prove helpful to remove the spleen, since the cells not trapped in this organ might otherwise survive. Diagnosis of these cytopenias, therefore, includes identification of antibody and the role of complement, determination of cell survival, and the quantification and localization of cell sequestration and destruction. The latter depends on macrophage function. Understanding the etiology of these diseases has a direct bearing on management.

HEMOLYTIC ANEMIA

The diagnosis of anemia follows a well-defined algorithm. Hemoglobin or hematocrit levels lower than normal define anemia, provided hypervolemia of plasma can be excluded, and mean corpuscular volume determines RBC size. Hemolytic anemias usually are normocytic, but if there is very active random destruction of cells there may be a skewing of the cell population in favor of younger cells, leading to a moderate macrocytosis. Microcytosis is characteristic of iron deficiency but it is also found in the thalassemias, hemolytic states due to a hereditary hemoglobin defect. When hemolysis is active, especially in microangiopathic hemolytic anemia, RBCs will be fragmented, some having the appearance of helmet cells, as shown in Figure 7–1. Concurrently with hemolysis there may be an increase in granulocytes and platelets unless these cells are also destroyed in the disease process.

An increase in circulating reticulocytes due to increased erythropoiesis and earlier release from the marrow frequently but not always accompanies peripheral hemolysis. If erythropoiesis is also suppressed the reticulocyte count may be low or even zero. There are individuals with active autoimmune hemolytic anemia (AIHA) who stop producing RBCs altogether, as reflected in the marrow. Such patients do not have reticulocytosis. In most hemolytic anemias there is an erythroid hyperplasia of the bone marrow that is normoblastic. This reflects a compensatory mechanism in which RBC production is stimulated by tissue anoxia. In autoimmune hemolytic processes there may be an increase in morphologically normal marrow plasma cells.

Autoimmune hemolytic anemia is most often (about 80% of the time) associated with "warm" antibodies that react best at 37 C. The condition may be idiopathic but is often associated with malignant neoplasms such as lymphoma, chronic lymphocytic leukemia, and ovarian and thymic tumors.

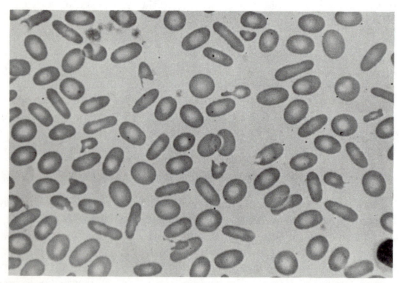

Fig 7–1.—Helmet cells and schistocytes as seen in microangiopathic hemolytic anemia.

About 1% of patients with Hodgkin's disease develop warm AIHA, and lupus erythematosus and other connective tissue diseases are also frequently associated.[1] Autoimmune gastrointestinal, muscular, and thyroid conditions are occasionally accompanied by a warm-reacting RBC antibody.

The antibodies associated with AIHA coat the RBC and may or may not fix complement. They do not react with Rh null cells, suggesting that there is specificity directed against the Rh antigen. Specificity or lack thereof may be determined by reacting the serum and the eluate from cells against a panel of cells, each of which includes different antigens. The presence of one or more specific antibodies is determined by exclusion of cells that do not react with the unknown antibody.

The Antiglobulin (Coombs) Test (AGT)

The diagnosis of AIHA is based on finding characteristic serologic abnormalities in a patient with clinical evidence of hemolysis. The direct antiglobulin test (DAGT) is most helpful in this regard. It is an antiglobulin test that determines whether a patient's RBCs are coated with IgG, complement components, or both. An indirect AGT (IAGT) test may be performed to identify antibody in serum or in RBC eluates. Both tests are a type of agglutination test (see Chap. 2). Antisera to IgG and a complement component, C3d, are used. It is generally not helpful to perform this assay with other monospecific antisera. IgM antibody is difficult to detect with the AGT, and when this antibody is present, complement is almost always also detectable.

The AGT test does not by itself determine the presence or absence of hemolysis. In interpreting the results of the direct Coombs test, the pattern of reactivity with IgG and/or C3 is noted. Various diagnostic entities are thereby suggested or excluded. Table 7–1 lists conditions associated with various reactivity patterns of the DAGT.

Titrations may be performed by diluting the antiglobulin sera in order to assess the relative strength of positive reactions. The result may be reported as a specific titer or graded descriptively from weak to very strong. A titer does not necessarily determine the presence or absence of hemolysis, nor do titers necessarily decrease when a patient who is hemolyzing goes into remission.

In a small percentage of patients with AIHA the DAGT result will be negative because of a lower concentration of antibody on the RBC than can be detected by antiglobulin serum. Performing the indirect Coombs test to look for antibody in the serum or in RBC eluates of such a patient may be helpful. The IAGT is positive in 57% of patients with warm antibody

TABLE 7–1.—INTERPRETATION OF THE DIRECT AGT (COOMBS TEST)

Positive to both IgG and C3d:
  67% of warm antibody AIHA
  SLE with warm antibody AIHA
  Hemolytic disease of the newborn (anti-A or -B)
  Chronic lymphocytic leukemia
Positive to C3d only:
  13% of warm antibody AIHA
  SLE without hemolytic anemia
  Cold agglutinin syndrome
  Paroxysmal cold hemoglobinuria (may be only weakly positive)
  Some drug-induced hemolytic anemias ("innocent bystander" type)
Positive to IgG only:
  20% of warm antibody AIHA
  Chronic lymphocytic leukemia
  Hemolytic disease of the newborn (anti-Rh, anti-A or -B)
  Hemolytic anemia induced by penicillin, methyldopa, procainamide, hydralazine, or
    cephalothin (occasionally also associated with positive C3d test)

AIHA. A positive test result in patients previously transfused or who are pregnant may be due to these events rather than to AIHA. The IAGT is usually negative in patients with cold agglutinin syndrome or paroxysmal cold hemoglobinuria (PCH).

An agglutination test utilizing enzyme-treated RBCs is also practical to perform in the clinical laboratory and may be positive in AIHA when the DAGT is negative. Other assays that might be used to find small amounts of antibody in AIHA, such as agglutination augmentation by polyvinylpyrrolidone or a complement fixation consumption test, are limited to research or reference laboratories.

Immune hemolytic anemia induced by drugs is usually related to methyldopa or penicillin. Fifteen percent of patients taking methyldopa will have a positive DAGT result, although most of these do not develop hemolytic anemia.[2] Once the test is positive, it may remain so for 1 month to 2 years after the drug is discontinued. About 3% of patients taking massive doses of parenteral penicillin will have a positive direct Coombs test. Only a small percentage of these will manifest hemolytic anemia.[3]

Cold Agglutinins

Antibodies that react at lower temperatures are generally of the IgM class. These antibodies are usually specific for the I antigen on RBCs of most adults and sometimes to the i antigen, usually found on cord cells and in the fetus. Cold-reacting antibodies (cold agglutinins, saline agglutinins) will agglutinate normal erythrocytes at 20 C or lower. Increased titers of cold agglutinins are found in the serum of 18% of patients with AIHA;

however, increased titers are also found in a variety of other diseases (Table 7–2). Titers at 4 C in AIHA are often very high (> 1,024). Values may be considerably lower in other diseases, and there is no clear correlation between titer and cold-induced symptoms. Sequential titers frequently provide more information.

In *Mycoplasma pneumoniae* infections, rises in titer usually occur toward the end of the first week of illness. To avoid false negative results on cold agglutinin tests, serum should be separated from erythrocytes before refrigeration.

Cold Hemolysins

The Donath-Landsteiner antibody, a hemolytic antibody of the IgG class, can be detected by a biphasic hemolysis test known as the Donath-Landsteiner test.[4, 5] A positive result is essentially diagnostic of PCH; a negative result excludes the diagnosis. Paroxysmal cold hemoglobinuria occurs in association with some viral infections, some autoimmune vasculitides, congenital or tertiary syphilis, and as a primary entity. The PCH syndrome is rare; however, the Donath-Landsteiner test is easy to perform, and Petz believes that the test is indicated in any patient with hemoglobinuria, patients with a history of hemolysis exacerbated by cold, and all patients with AIHA with atypical findings.[6]

RED BLOOD CELL SURVIVAL

Red blood cell survival can be measured by labeling cells or otherwise differentiating transfused cells from those of the host. A method was first developed at the turn of the century in which O cells were transfused to type A, B, or AB recipients and samples were periodically exposed to he-

TABLE 7–2.—ILLNESSES ASSOCIATED
WITH INCREASED TITERS OF COLD
AGGLUTININS

Autoimmune hemolytic anemia
Waldenström's macroglobulinemia
Lymphomas
Some adenocarcinomas
Polycythemia vera
Systemic lupus erythematosus
Idiopathic cold agglutinin disease
Mycoplasma pneumoniae infection
Cytomegalovirus infection
Infectious mononucleosis
Infectious hepatitis
Bronchiectasis
Tropical eosinophilia

TABLE 7–3.—METHODS OF DETERMINING RED BLOOD CELL SURVIVAL

METHOD	ELUTION	NORMAL	REINCORPORATION OF LABEL
Random label of peripheral blood			
Differential hemolysis	No	Linear	No
Differential agglutination	No	Linear	No
[32]P-labeled diisopropylfluorophosphate	No	Linear	No
Chromate-31	Yes	Curvilinear	No
Cohort label of young, newly formed cells			
[13]N-glycine	No	Life span plateau	Minimal
[14]C-glycine	No	Life span plateau	Minimal
Sulfate-35	No	Life span plateau	Moderate
[75]Se-selenomethionine	No	Life span plateau	Minimal
[59]Fe-iron	No	Life span plateau	Maximal

molytic anti-A or anti-B antibody and complement. The hemoglobin of the O cells then was a measure of the survival of transfused cells.[7] In 1919 Ashby developed an alternative method whereby the recipient's cells were agglutinated and the transfused type O cells were counted.[8] Either approach gave a valid indication of the survival of transfused RBCs. Survival

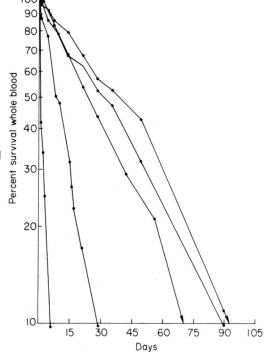

Fig 7–2.—Red blood cell survival studies using ^{51}Cr show normal to very shortened survival.

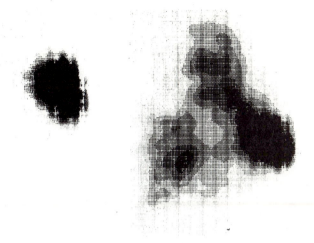

Patient with autoimmune hemolytic anemia due to warm anitbody (IgG) with red cell sequestration mainly in the spleen.

Patient with cold agglutinin disease due to IgM with red cell sequestration in the spleen and to a lesser extent in the liver.

Fig 7–3.—Radiograms *(left)* from patient with autoimmune hemolytic anemia due to warm antibody (IgG), with RBC sequestration mainly in the spleen, and *(right)* from patient with cold agglutinin disease due to IgM, with RBC sequestration in the spleen and, to a lesser extent, in the liver.

studies using isotope-labeled amino acids were found generally to apply only to measurement of autologous cell survival. A cohort population was labeled at the time of cell production, and amino acids were incorporated into globin or, in the case of glycine, also heme. Initially nonradioactive isotopes were used, but their detection and measurement required a mass spectrograph. When ^{14}C became available, radioactive techniques were applied. Table 7–3 lists the characteristics of each of these methodologies.

Chromate-51-labeled RBC survival studies have now become the standard procedure. The method is simple to perform and accurate. A major drawback, which complicates interpretation of data, is that about 1% of the ^{51}Cr elutes from RBCs each day. A sampling of typical ^{51}Cr survival studies is shown in Figure 7–2. [51]Cr, being a gamma emitter, can also be counted externally, permitting determination of the site of RBC sequestration and destruction. Using a high-energy gamma counter with dual collimation, it is possible to determine ^{51}Cr concentration in the spleen and or liver (Fig 7–3). By quantifying the role played by these organs of the reticuloendothelial system it is possible to predict the usefulness of splenectomy in hemolytic anemia.[9]

TRANSFUSION REACTIONS

The most severe and potentially life-threatening transfusion reactions are those associated with hemolysis.[10] Transfusion of ABO-incompatible cells usually causes immediate intravascular hemolysis. This event may trigger disseminated intravascular coagulation, leading to massive thrombosis, embolization, and, with consumption of platelets and coagulation factors, renal shutdown and death.[11] IgG antibodies, such as those directed against the Rh system, coat RBCs and are manifested by a positive direct Coombs test. Hemolysis may initially produce hemoglobinemia and hemoglobinuria, followed by a rise in methemalbumin and a drop in haptoglobin levels. When jaundice occurs the bilirubin will be mainly indirect and therefore will not be excreted in the urine. Workup of all transfusion reactions is essential. The following procedure is prescribed by the Standards of the American Association of Blood Banks:[12]

1. Any adverse reaction of the patient associated with a transfusion is a suspected transfusion reaction. Circulatory overload or allergic reactions need not be evaluated as possible hemolytic transfusion reactions.
2. The following must be done immediately for investigation of patients with symptoms or findings suggestive of a hemolytic transfusion reaction:
   a. The label on the container of blood and all other records must be examined to detect whether there has been an error in identifying the patient or the blood.
   b. A new suitable, properly labeled blood sample must be obtained from the patient, avoiding hemolysis, and must be sent promptly to the blood bank. In addition, the blood container, whether or not it contains any unused blood, should be sent to the blood bank with the attached transfusion set and intravenous solutions.
   c. The patient's postreaction serum or plasma must be inspected for hemolysis and icterus. A prereaction sample may be used for comparison.
   d. A direct antiglobulin test must be performed on a postreaction specimen of recipient RBCs.
3. Based on evaluation of clinical findings, review of accuracy of records, and results of laboratory tests, additional tests may be indicated, such as:
   a. Determination of ABO and Rh types on prereaction and postreaction blood specimens from the patient and from the blood container and/or attached segment.
   b. Repeat test for recipient unexpected antibodies and/or crossmatch using the immediate prereaction and postreaction blood samples and donor blood from an attached sealed segment and/or from the container.
   c. Examination of postreaction urine for hemoglobin and its metabolites.
   d. Determination of bilirubin concentration on serum preferably obtained 5–7 hours after the transfusion.
   e. Examination of stained smear of plasma and culture of contents of blood container for bacteria.
4. Interpretation of the evaluation must be recorded in the patient's chart and, if possible, must be reported immediately to the patient's physician.

Some patients have weak antibodies to specific RBCs that are not detectable by standard methods for antibody detection and compatibility testing. Under these circumstances, which usually represent an anamnestic reaction to previous sensitization, a delayed reaction occurs a few days after transfusion. Although such reactions are usually mild, severe reactions have been reported.

In any transfusion reaction, it is highly desirable to identify the relevant antibody through the use of a panel of cells with known antigenicity. The antibody is detected in the serum and will also be found on elution from antibody-coated RBCs.

AUTOIMMUNE THROMBOCYTOPENIA

Autoimmune thrombocytopenia, or idiopathic thrombocytopenic purpura (ITP), is due to immune destruction of platelets and so is analogous to Coombs-positive AIHA. Characteristically the bone marrow is rich in megakaryocytes, but the platelets do not survive in circulation. It was long known that splenectomy was sometimes effective in raising the platelet count, often to normal levels. It was also known that platelet survival improved empirically on immunosuppressive therapy. From these two observations it was concluded that the humoral factor constituted an autoimmune response manifested by elaboration of an immunoglobulin. Since platelets exert their primary function of preventing bleeding by aggregation and adhesion, their agglutination was inapplicable as an indicator of an immune response.

The antiglobulin (Coombs) test, applicable to determination and identification of RBC antibodies, also was inapplicable. Direct agglutination and complement fixation tests were developed, but these tests are rarely useful.[13–15] Cumbersome antiglobulin consumption tests were devised[16, 17] and were further refined by labeling anti-human IgG antibody with radioactive materials, enzymes, or fluorescent materials.[18, 19] These tests are considered to be indicators of the presence of antiplatelet antibody. Serotonin release measured by determining the exchange of ^{14}C-labeled serotonin is another test advocated by Hirschman and Shulman, among others.[13, 20, 21] Similarly, ^{51}Cr release from paroxysmal nocturnal hemoglobinuria (PNH) platelets damaged by immunoglobulin has also been proposed as an indicator of disease.[22] These tests have not proved to be sufficiently precise or reproducible for routine clinical use.

Brand et al. suggested the combined use of lymphocytotoxicity and platelet fluorescence tests to determine platelet donor compatibility with proposed thrombocytopenic recipients.[23] They were able to predict successful transfusion some of the time, but the test is far from reliable.

Much work continues to be done to develop laboratory tests for the presence of autoantibodies or alloantibodies to platelets. To date none of these is very useful clinically because of practical drawbacks.

Measuring the survival of homologous platelets may be complicated by the presence of alloantibodies. When platelets are labeled in vivo there is damage to the platelets, and even under the best conditions, about one third of the platelets do not circulate and are taken up by the spleen. The radiolabels employed for determining platelet survival and organ sequestration have included ^{35}S (sulfate), ^{32}P (diisopropylfluorophosphate [DFP]), ^{51}Cr (sodium chromate), ^{111}In (indium oxine), and ^{75}Se (selenomethionine).[24–26]

Alloantibodies from the mother may be transmitted via placenta to the child, causing an immune thrombocytopenia. The mechanism is analogous to hemolytic disease of the newborn due to RBC alloantibodies from the mother. Platelet-specific antibodies have been identified.[27]

Sudden development of severe thrombocytopenia with transfusion of RBCs and whole blood has been observed. The first concern must be the exclusion of disseminated intravascular coagulation due to transfusion of incompatible blood and intravascular hemolysis. Once this mechanism is excluded, it is also possible that passive transfer of antibodies to platelets may have occurred, since an apparently normal blood donor could have autoantibodies or alloantibodies to platelets.[28]

In general, tests for platelet antibodies are still the province of specialized or reference laboratories. In the case of ITP, results of clinical value can be obtained by assaying the patient's platelets for membrane-bound antibody. An immunofluorescent technique can be used and the results assessed by fluorescence microscopy or microfluorometry. Another assay, used by the Scripps-Miles reference laboratory, measures platelet-associated IgG by determining the amount of radiolabeled IgG bound to the patient's platelets.

CIRCULATING ANTICOAGULANTS

In health, circulating blood is prevented from clotting by the elaboration of inhibitors to each coagulation factor playing a role in the coagulation cascade (Fig 7–4). What the inhibitors of the clotting factors cannot accomplish may then be done by antithrombin, especially antithrombin III. Even after clot formation plasminogen is activated to plasmin, if it is not counteracted by antiplasmin, which lyses the formed clot.

Although clotting inhibitors generally exert their action enzymatically, immunoglobulins with specificity for coagulation factors may appear on transfusion of homologous plasma or factor concentrates in patients with congenital clotting deficiencies. Hemophiliacs repeatedly treated either for bleeding episodes or prophylactically are likely to develop antibodies to

CLOTTING, ANTITHROMBIN, FIBRINOLYSIS

XII → XII a
XI → XI a
IX → IX a   ⟶   ⟵ ——— FACTOR INHIBITORS
VIII → VIII a   ⟶   ⟵
VII → VII a   ⟶   ⟵
X → X a

PROTHROMBIN → THROMBIN ← ANTITHROMBINS (AT III)
FIBRINOGEN → FIBRIN ← PLASMIN ← PLASMINOGEN
Simplified coagulation cascade, clot inhibitors and clot lysis
Fig 7–4.—Coagulation cascade.

factor VIII. About 20% of these individuals will respond inadequately to administration of factor VIII. Antibody activity to factor VIII is usually determined by ascertaining the partial thromboplastin time (PTT) with a mixture of the patient's plasma and normal plasma. Instead of the normal plasma correcting the defect, the circulating anticoagulant in the patient's plasma will inactivate the added factor VIII, resulting in a prolonged PTT. Antibodies to factor IX and factor V have been observed but with much less frequency than antibodies to factor VIII.

Disseminated lupus erythematosus has been associated with abnormal coagulation not corrected by normal plasma. Patients with this condition may have normal coagulation function, may bleed, or may have a tendency to thrombosis. The circulating anticoagulant in systemic lupus erythematosus may be detected by utilizing the PTT with equal parts of the patient's and normal plasma. Circulating anticoagulants have also been reported during drug therapy (especially with INH, penicillin, and streptomycin) and post partum.

IMMUNE NEUTROPENIA

Antibodies directed against neutrophils have been implicated in the following conditions:

1. Autoimmune neutropenia (IgG mediated).
2. Isoimmune neutropenia of the newborn.
3. Drug-induced immune neutropenia (especially semisynthetic penicillins).
4. Neutropenia associated with systemic lupus erythematosus or Felty's syndrome. In the proper clinical setting, if neutropenia appears to be re-

lated to increased destruction of neutrophils, a search for antineutrophil antibodies may be helpful. This will probably require the help of a specialized laboratory.

Initially, the only test available for antineutrophil antibodies was an agglutination assay. This assay was subject to inaccuracy because a patient's serum would not necessarily agglutinate the neutrophils employed and spontaneous agglutination was common. More recently, a simplified agglutination test that precludes nonspecific agglutination has been used, with more success. A useful test employing membrane-associated immunofluorescence of neutrophils has also been developed.

ACKNOWLEDGMENT

Photographs were provided through the courtesy of Ms. Susan McKenzie, Supervisor, Bone Marrow Laboratory, Memorial Sloan-Kettering Cancer Center, New York.

REFERENCES

1. Eisner E., Ley A.B., Mayer K.: Coombs positive hemolytic anemia in Hodgkin's disease. *Ann. Intern. Med.* 66:258, 1967.
2. Worlledge S.M.: Immune drug-induced hemolytic anemias. *Semin. Hematol.* 10:327, 1973.
3. Petz L.D., Garratty G.: *Acquired Immune Hemolytic Anemias.* New York, Churchill Livingstone, 1980.
4. Ries C.A., Garratty G., Petz L.D., et al.: Paroxysmal cold hemoglobinuria. *Blood* 38:491, 1971.
5. Weiner W., Gordon E.G., Rowe D.: A Donath-Landsteiner antibody (nonsyphilitic type). *Vox Sang.* 9:684, 1964.
6. Petz L.D.: Autoimmune and drug-induced hemolytic anemias, in Rose N.R., Friedman H. (eds.): *Manual of Clinical Immunology.* Washington, D.C., American Society for Microbiology, 1980, p. 726.
7. Mayer K., D'Amaro J.: Improvement of methods of differential haemolysis by haemoglobinometry. *Scand. J. Haematol.* 1:331, 1964.
8. Ashby W.: The determination of the length of life of transfused blood corpuscles in man. *J. Exp. Med.* 29:267, 1919.
9. Laughlin J.S., Ritter F.W., Dwyer A.J., et al.: Development and applications of quantitative and computer-analyzed counting and scanning. *Cancer* 25:395, 1970.
10. Pineda A., Brizica S.M. Jr., Taswell H.F.: Hemolytic transfusion reaction: Recent experience in a large blood bank. *Mayo Clin. Proc.* 53:378, 1978.
11. Goldfinger D.: Acute hemolytic transfusion reactions: A fresh look at pathogenesis and considerations regarding therapy. *Transfusion* 17:85, 1977.
12. *Standards for Blood Banks and Transfusion Services,* ed. 10. Washington, D.C., American Association of Blood Banks, 1981, pp. 35–36.
13. Hirschman R.J., Shulman N.R.: The use of platelet serotonin release as a sensitive method for detecting anti-platelet antibodies and a plasma anti-platelet

factor in patients with idiopathic thrombocytopenic purpura. *Br. J. Haematol.* 24:793, 1973.

14. Cines D.B., Schreiber A.D.: Immune thrombocytopenia: Use of a Coombs antiglobulin test to detect IgG and C3 on platelets. *N. Engl. J. Med.* 300:106, 1979.
15. Helmerhorst F.M., Bossers B., deBruin H.G., et al.: Detection of platelet antibodies: A comparison of three techniques. *Vox Sang.* 39:83, 1980.
16. Soulier J.P., Patereau C., Drouet J.: Platelet indirect radioactive Coombs test: Its utilization for PLa$_1$ grouping. *Vox Sang.* 29:253, 1975.
17. Orsini F., Gregory S., Dale M., et al.: A quantitative determination for the detection of immunoglobulin (IgG) on the surface of platelets. *Hum. Immunol.* 3:153, 1981.
18. Gudino M., Miller W.V.: Application of the enzyme linked immunospecific assay (ELISA) for the detection of platelet antibodies. *Blood* 57:32, 1981.
19. Engvall E., Perlmann P.: Enzyme-linked immunosorbent assay, ELISA: III. Quantitation of specific antibodies by enzyme-labeled anti-immunoglobulin in antigen-coated tubes. *J. Immunol.* 109:129, 1972.
20. Gockerman J.P., Bowman R.P., Conrad M.E.: Detection of platelet isoantibodies by (^{3}H) serotonin: Platelet release and its clinical application to the problem of platelet matching. *J. Clin. Invest.* 55:75, 1975.
21. Heinrich D., Gutschank S., Mueller-Eckhardt C.: HLA-antibody-induced ^{14}C-serotonin release from platelets: A methodological analysis. *Vox Sang.* 33:65, 1977.
22. Aster R.H., Enright S.E.: A platelet and granulocyte membrane defect in paroxysmal nocturnal hemoglobinuria: Usefulness for the detection of platelet antibodies. *J. Clin. Invest.* 48:1199, 1969.
23. Brand A., van Leeuwen A., Eernisse J.C., et al.: Platelet transfusion therapy: Optimal donor selection with a combination of lymphocytotoxicity and platelet fluorescence tests. *Blood* 51:781, 1978.
24. Leeksma C.V.W., Cohen J.A.: Determination of the life span of human blood platelets using diisopropylfluorophosphate. *J. Clin. Invest.* 35:964, 1956.
25. Zucker M.B., Ley A.B., Mayer K.: Studies on platelet life span and platelet depots by use of DFP.^{32} *J. Lab. Clin. Med.* 58:405, 1961.
26. Joist J.H., Baker R.K., Thakur M.L., et al.: Indium ^{111}-labeled human platelets. *J. Lab. Clin. Med.* 92:829, 1978.
27. von dem Borne A.E.G.K., von Riesz E., Verheugt F.W.A., et al.: Bak^a, a new platelet-specific antigen involved in neonatal allo-immune thrombocytopenia. *Vox Sang.* 39:113, 1980.
28. Mollison P.L.: *Blood Transfusion in Clinical Medicine*, ed. 6. Oxford, Blackwell Scientific Publications, 1979, pp. 603–605.

8

Allergic Disorders

Richard Evans III, M.D., COL. M.C.

Richard J. Summers, M.D., LT. C. M.C.

IMMUNOGLOBULIN E

In 1966 Ishizaka and Ishizaka described a new class of immunoglobulins responsible for mediating allergic reactions to foreign antigens.[1] They called the new protein immunoglobulin E (IgE). IgE is present in sera of both normal and allergic subjects. It is present in very small amounts (nanograms per milliliter), and detection and quantitation methods must be very sensitive. In most laboratories today immunoassays are done using radioisotope- or enzyme-labeled antisera to achieve this degree of sensitivity.

The human IgE molecule contains three antigens in its heavy chain structure that are different from antigens contained in the other classes of immunoglobulins. These antigens, $D_\epsilon 0$, $D_\epsilon 1$, and $D_\epsilon 2$, are recognized by other animal species (e.g., goats, rabbits, and sheep) when they are immunized with IgE. Anti-IgE antibodies raised in these animals are used in immunoassays to detect IgE in human serum. Antibody to the $D_\epsilon 2$ antigen of human IgE is preferable because it is the most specific. This antibody is tagged with an isotope, usually iodine[125], or an enzyme, usually alkaline phosphatase. The isotope or enzyme label provides an indicator system for the presence of IgE in human sera because the samples can be quantitated in a gamma counter or a fluorometer, respectively (see Chap. 2). The methods appear to be comparable in sensitivity. Iodine[125] decays rapidly, and ^{125}I-labeled antibody expires in 6 months. The enzyme-linked assay is limited only by the quantity of reagents prepared. Because radioisotopes must be handled by experienced technicians and according to Nuclear Regulatory Agency guidelines, radioimmunoassays are not practical in the office setting.

Measurement of Total Serum IgE

In commercial laboratories the most frequently used assay for the measurement of total IgE levels is the PRIST assay (Pharmacia, Piscataway, N.J.). The most recent survey of total serum IgE levels in normal sera using the PRIST assay was conducted by the Sloan Kettering Institute, New York.[2] The values listed in Table 8–1 are for sera obtained from a normal U.S. population. Immunologic assays for the measurement of total serum IgE must be standardized in order for different laboratories to obtain the same results with the same serum samples; consequently, the availability of a standard reference serum to all laboratories performing the test is important. The American Academy of Allergy has recently prepared a new reference serum, which is available from the NIAID Research Reagents Branch.[3]

Total serum IgE level varies with age (see Table 8–1). IgE is synthesized in the fetus as early as the first trimester and is present in newborn serum in small amounts (< 2 IU/ml). Total IgE in normal sera is highest after age 5 years. Rapid rises of total serum IgE in the first year of life, with higher concentrations than normal at age 1 year, are associated with a considerably increased risk of allergy in later years.[4]

Because IgE mediates allergic reactions, it was initially hoped that the measurement of total serum IgE in a patient's serum would be a definitive test for the presence or absence of allergy. Johansson et al.,[5] in a comparison of normal and allergic subjects, found that 1% of the healthy individuals had a serum IgE level higher than 100 IU/ml, and 2% of the allergic subjects had a total IgE less than 20 IU/ml (1 IU $\simeq$ 2.4 ng of protein). There was considerable overlap of total IgE levels at the mid-range in sera from healthy and allergic individuals. The total serum IgE level, therefore, does not precisely correlate with the presence or absence of allergy in a patient. A low or normal IgE level is not incompatible with the diagnosis. This observation has been confirmed by Yunginger and Gleich.[6]

TABLE 8–1.—EXPECTED PHADEBAS IgE PRIST LEVELS: POOLED DATA, U.S. POPULATION STUDY[2]

| | | | GEOMETRIC MEAN | |
AGE	N	IgE IU/ml	IgE IU/ml, ± 1SD	IgE IU/ml, ± 2SD
Newborn	37	0.53	(0.27–1.04)	(0.14–2.05)
1–11 mo.	51	2.45	(0.51–11.75)	(0.11–56.28)
1 yr	22	2.74	(0.50–15.08)	(0.09–83.02)
2–4 yr	86	8.40	(2.13–33.00)	(0.54–129.80)
5–80 yr	484	19.62	(4.54–84.80)	(1.05–366.90)

The highest levels of total serum IgE have been reported in patients with parasitic infections, including ascariasis, toxocariasis, necatoriasis, capillariasis, echinococcosis, trichinosis, and filariasis.[7] Elevated serum IgE levels are demonstrable 3–4 weeks after the parasitic infection occurs. The IgE level often reaches 10,000 ng/ml and remains elevated throughout the disease. A very high IgE level, particularly in the context of eosinophilia, should prompt a thorough search for a parasitic infection. By contrast, a normal serum IgE level in a patient being evaluated for eosinophilia makes the diagnosis of tissue-invasive parasitism unlikely.

Several immunodeficiency states in addition to atopy are associated with high levels of IgE.[8] These include the Wiskott-Aldrich syndrome with eczema, the hyper-IgE syndrome of Job and Buckley, thymic hypoplasia, and IgA deficiency.

Measurement of total serum IgE is most helpful in the diagnosis and subsequent management of asthmatic patients who develop allergic bronchopulmonary aspergillosis. This disease, if untreated, can lead to bronchiectasis and pulmonary fibrosis. An elevated serum IgE level is an important criterion in the diagnosis. Table 8–2 summarizes clinical indications for the measurement of total serum IgE.

Other conditions that have been reported in association with elevated levels of total serum IgE are Wegener's granulomatosis, IgE myeloma, bullous pemphigoid, leprosy, and the Guillain-Barré syndrome.

In Vivo Assays for Specific IgE Antibody

Measurements of specific antibodies of the IgE class provide more information on the nature of a patient's allergic sensitivities. Indications for diagnostic tests in allergic patients are listed in Table 8–3. These tests can be done in vivo, by direct or passive transfer skin tests, or in vitro, using

TABLE 8–2.—CLINICAL USEFULNESS OF
TOTAL SERUM IgE DETERMINATIONS

POSSIBLE USEFULNESS
  Atopic disorders (allergic rhinitis, asthma, eczema)
    Prediction
    Detection
  Evaluation of skin disorders
PROBABLE USEFULNESS
  Tissue-invasive parasitism
  Bronchopulmonary aspergillosis
  Immunodeficiency disorders
    Wiskott-Aldrich syndrome
    Hyper-IgE syndrome
  Eosinophilia

TABLE 8–3.—INDICATIONS
FOR DIAGNOSTIC TESTS

Allergic rhinitis
  Refractory to antihistamines
Allergic asthma
  Refractory to bronchodilators
Insect sting allergy
  Generalized reaction
  Increasingly large local reaction
Food allergy
  When the food is uncertain
Penicillin allergy
  When patient needs penicillin

serum or white blood cells. It should be emphasized that diagnostic tests should be done to confirm the physical examination findings and the clinical history, not as a substitute for them.

Direct Skin Tests

Direct skin tests are the most commonly employed of all tests in clinical allergy. In direct skin tests, an attempt is made to reproduce the allergic reaction by introducing a small amount of suspected allergen into the patient's skin (see Chap. 3). The direct skin test is much safer than the direct challenge of other organ systems, such as the respiratory system or the intestinal tract. When the results are positive, a large wheal and flare reaction occurs within 15 minutes at the site where an extract of a relevant allergen has been introduced. This reaction closely resembles the allergic reaction to allergens that cause symptoms in other tissues.

Direct skin tests require the availability of the allergenic molecule to which the patient is sensitive. A number of drugs—cephalosporins and sulfonamides, for example—are allergenic only after they have been metabolized and perhaps bound to protein. Other agents, such as morphine, meperidine, and tubocurare, elicit a skin test response by direct stimulation of histamine release from skin mast cells and not by an IgE-mediated reaction.

There are other conditions in which direct skin tests may not be possible. Since direct skin tests can be affected by antihistamines, the patient should be instructed not to take such drugs for 48 hours prior to testing. Hydroxyzine can inhibit the skin test response for 72 hours.[9] Dermographism and skin disorders such as eczema may prevent good skin test results.

Skin tests are indicated when there is any reasonable suspicion that a patient's symptoms may be allergic. They are most helpful as confirmatory tests in allergic rhinitis, allergic asthma, insect sting allergy, and penicillin allergy. The choice of skin test material is dictated by the patient's history of sensitivity, as well as by the physician's knowledge of allergens that may be relevant to the patient's symptoms. This is an important concept and implies that the physician knows what materials are allergenic and what allergens are prevalent in the patient's environment.

Passive Transfer Tests

Prior to its identification as a distinct immunoglobulin, IgE was termed "reagin," characterized by the ability to sensitize tissue of nonallergic patients. The phenomenon of sensitization of homologous tissue was the basis for the classic experiments of Prausnitz and Küstner in 1921.[10] Prausnitz passively sensitized an area of his forearm skin by intracutaneous injection of the serum of Küstner, who was allergic to fish. On challenge with fish antigen 24 hours later, the skin sites gave an immediate 15-minute wheal and flare reaction. This classic test for reaginic, or IgE, antibody is antigen specific. That is, only antigens to which the atopic serum donor is allergic will elict the wheal and flare response. The P-K reaction of Prausnitz and Küstner was for decades the ultimate method for determining reaginic activity in allergic sera. Today, the test is a valuable tool in the evaluation of difficult allergic problems. P-K tests are indicated when the patient's life may be endangered by exposure to an allergen and there is no suitable alternative test. Serum collected from the allergic patient should first be tested for hepatitis-associated antigen. Spouses and other close relatives are suitable recipients. In 24 hours, significant allergic sensitivities to a variety of antigens can be determined in an allergic patient.

In Vitro Assays for Specific IgE Antibody

Radioallergosorbent Test

A number of new in vitro approaches to confirming allergy in a sensitive patient have been developed in the past 10 years. The most widely accepted of these tests is the radioallergosorbent test (RAST). The RAST is a radioimmunoassay that uses serum from the allergic patient. The test quantitates the amount of serum IgE antibody to a relevant allergen.

The RAST test was first introduced in 1968 by Wide, Bennich, and Johansson of Sweden.[11] The technique has been described in detail in Chapter 2. Briefly, allergen-coated cellulose particles or cellulose disks are incubated with the patient's serum. The particles are washed and a second incubation is performed with radiolabeled, highly specific, anti-IgE FcD2 antibody. The allergens and the anti-IgE antibodies are added in excess. The radioactivity count is then directly proportional to the serum level of the specific IgE antibody. The results are compared with a reference serum value and are semiquantitated. The RAST is a very sensitive test capable of measuring picogram quantities of IgE antibody; furthermore, the test correlates well with results achieved by the classic Prausnitz-Küstner technique.[12]

In ragweed-allergic patients, a good correlation has been found between symptom index score during the ragweed pollenation season and RAST titer.[13] Similarly, there is a good correlation between direct skin test results and RAST titer. In studies performed at Johns Hopkins University a purified ragweed antigen was used and skin sensitivity was measured by titration to a predetermined end point.

The RAST is less sensitive than direct skin tests using standard whole allergenic extracts, and so it will not provide additional information in the evaluation of patients who have a negative skin test result.

Berg et al. of Sweden have compared provocation responses in sensitive patients to a variety of common inhalant allergens with circulating IgE antibody levels as measured by RAST.[14] The average correlation between RAST and provocation test results was 80%–90%. The degree of correlation increased with the increase in challenge titer (Table 8–4).

Because of simplicity, safety, and generally good correlations with results achieved by other diagnostic procedures in allergy, the RAST has promise of becoming a standard diagnostic test. Currently the RAST result is interpreted according to a reference serum that is different in every laboratory. For clinical use, therefore, each laboratory should provide the reference data necessary for clinical interpretation of the results of every allergen tested in the RAST. A relatively large amount of antibody to one antigen may be equivalent in clinical significance to relatively small amounts against an independent antigen. RAST results, therefore, are very depen-

TABLE 8–4.—OCCURRENCE OF CIRCULATING IgE ANTIBODY, AS MEASURED BY RAST, TO COMMON INHALANT ALLERGENS, IN CHILDREN WITH ASTHMA OR HAY FEVER: CORRELATION BETWEEN RAST AND PROVOCATION TEST (PT)*

PT ALLERGEN DILUTION (W/V)	RAST NO. OF TESTS +	RAST NO. OF TESTS −	CORRELATION (%)
Negative	44	328	88
Positive			
>1/10	348	112	76
1/10	94	82	53
1/100	118	26	82
1/1,000	136	4	97

*Data from Berg et al.[14]

dent on interpretation for clinical significance. The advantages and disadvantages of the RAST are compared in Table 8–5.

Clinical interpretation of the RAST is complicated by the use of different methods, among laboratories performing this assay, for defining a clinically positive result. Some laboratories define positivity in reference to dilutions of serum with a high titer of birch pollen–specific IgE. A test serum resulting in radioactive counts per minute (cpm) above that achieved with the second most diluted solution of this reference serum is considered positive. In this instance the definition is not linked to a baseline value with normal control sera.

Another method defines clinically significant positivity as radioactive binding by test serum of 200% or greater of cpm bound utilizing normal control sera. Since control nonallergic serum induces binding by anti-IgE which varies with different antigens, ideally a separate antigen control should be run for each antigen tested.

A third system defines the end point of counting as 25,000 cpm measured in a tube containing 25 μg of IgE and anti-IgE antibody bound to cellulose. Under these conditions, a cpm of 500 is usual for normal control serum, a cpm of 720–1,600 is considered equivocal, and a higher cpm is defined as positive. The equivocal area usually falls in the range of 150%–300% of the cpm of labeled anti-IgE resulting after first stage incubation with normal nonallergic serum.

Still another method uses pooled cord sera as a control. The percent bound of the total cpm of anti-IgE added to each tube is analyzed. Clinical positivity is defined as a percent binding with the test serum of the total cpm added that is greater than twice the percent binding of the total cpm

TABLE 8–5.—ADVANTAGES AND DISADVANTAGES OF RAST

Advantages
  Serum can be used
  Useful in patients with dermographism and other severe skin diseases such as atopic
    dermatitis
  Less traumatic for children
  Skin testing with potentially hazardous allergens (seeds, danders, fish, drugs) is avoided
  Test materials that liberate histamine in the skin do not affect the RAST
  Serum samples can be saved for follow-up studies
  Potential for standardization of extracts
  Possible use for studying industrial chemicals such as isocyanates
Disadvantages
  Not as sensitive as intradermal tests
  Non-IgE antibody can interfere
  Requires a laboratory with a trained technician and a gamma counter
  Requires proper controls for handling radioactivity
  Not a complete substitute for skin tests
  Expensive

added to pooled control cord sera. To be accurate, binding by control sera must be less than 1.5% for any antigen utilized. To date, there is no agreement on which of the various ways to define positivity is best for clinical use.

Leukocyte Histamine Release

In 1968 Osler et al. confirmed that histamine was released from peripheral blood leukocytes of allergic patients when these cells were challenged by the antigen to which patients were sensitive.[15] The basophil is believed to be the most important cell in this reaction.[16] This in vitro test is comparable to the direct skin test, its in vivo counterpart. The results of both tests compare very well with the symptom index score, a quantitation of the patient's symptom response to inhaled antigens.[12] The in vitro leukocyte histamine release procedure is time-consuming and requires an expert laboratory technician. The number of allergens that can be tested is limited by the amount of whole blood that must be collected from an allergic patient. This disadvantage has recently been mitigated by Siraganian and Hook, who have adapted the technique to small amounts of blood.[17] Even with this adaptation the procedure is time-consuming and requires expensive equipment, and so it is not practical as a routine diagnostic procedure. It is, however, an excellent method for evaluating allergic diseases in the research laboratory setting and can be used to test the capacity of pharmacologic agents to modulate the allergic reaction. And if a particular allergen is believed responsible for the allergic reaction in an affected patient, and there is probable risk to the patient from direct skin testing, the histamine release assay is a reasonable alternative.

The leukocyte histamine release assay is primarily a research tool. The advantages to the patient are safety and the opportunity for evaluation of newer pharmacologic modalities and identification of new antigens. Advantages and disadvantages of the leukocyte histamine release assay are listed in Table 8–6.

SERUM PRECIPITINS IN PULMONARY DISORDERS

Measurement of the antigen-antibody interaction by precipitin methods is the only in vitro technique for estimating antibody concentration in serum or other fluids in absolute weight units. This procedure was developed by Heidelberger and Kendall in 1929.[18] Among the numerous modifications of their original method for measuring antibody-antigen interaction are (1) the interfacial ring test, (2) the Swift-Wilson-Lancefield capillary tube test, (3) agar diffusion methods, (4) dilution for ascertaining optimal proportions, (5) phosphorus[80] analysis, and (6) turbidimetric anal-

TABLE 8–6.—LEUKOCYTE HISTAMINE RELEASE ASSAY:
ADVANTAGES AND DISADVANTAGES

Advantages
  No risk of anaphylaxis to the patient
  No risk of sensitizing a patient to an antigen
  Test not dependent on reactivity or normal state of patient's skin
  Unpurified antigens or antigens unproved for clinical use can be employed
  Better approximates biologic sensitivity of allergic patient
  Appropriately modified, assay can detect non-IgE antibodies that might protect the
    patient from an allergic reaction
Disadvantages
  Time-consuming
  Larger volumes of blood required
  Experienced technician and expensive equipment required

---

ysis.[19] These methods usually entail placing a specific allergen into a solid or liquid phase, followed by introduction of serum with suspected IgG or IgM antibody directed toward the antigen; the serum is obtained from a patient with a clinical disorder suggesting a possible antigen-antibody mechanism as its etiology. The antibody and antigen then combine and form a precipitate, if in the liquid phase, or a precipitin ring or arc in the solid phase.

The classic precipitin reaction occurs when antigen is added to an antiserum containing specific antibodies. The amount of precipitate formed varies, depending on the antigen and its size and the species making the antibody. As can be seen in Figure 8–1, when small amounts of antigen are added to large amounts of antibody (antibody excess), the complexes formed are insoluble and do not form a precipitate. However, an estimate of antigen valency is best made in these reaction tubes. As increasing amounts of antigen are added an optimum level is reached, beyond which less and less formation of precipitate occurs.

The double diffusion method of Ouchterlony can be used to visualize the antigen-antibody reaction. The antigen and antibody are placed in wells cut into agar gel (see Chap. 2). The antigen and antibody diffuse toward each other, and an opaque line (precipitate) forms when the zone of optimal proportions is reached. There may be single or multiple lines, depending on the number of antigens and specificity of the antiserum used.

The formation of precipitin rings or arcs may be useful in confirming or ruling out the diagnosis in disorders associated with the development of precipitating antibodies, such as eosinophilic pneumonias, disorders with pulmonary fibrosis, hypersensitivity pneumonitis (extrinsic allergic alveolitis), occupational lung diseases, and pulmonary alveolar proteinosis.[20] A detailed list of these disorders is given in Table 8–7.

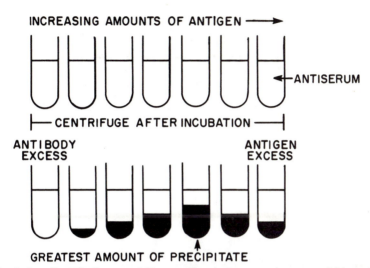

INCREASING AMOUNTS OF ANTIGEN ⟶

←ANTISERUM

⊢—CENTRIFUGE AFTER INCUBATION—⊣

ANTIBODY
EXCESS

ANTIGEN
EXCESS

GREATEST AMOUNT OF PRECIPITATE

Fig 8–1.—Quantitative precipitin reaction between a known soluble antigen and a specific antibody. The "zone of optimal proportions" between antigen and antibody is reached in the 5th tube. Addition of increasing amounts of antigen results in less and less precipitate.

PLASMA AND URINARY HISTAMINE DETERMINATION

Histamine was discovered by Windaus and Vogt in 1907,[21] and its actions were further described by Dale and Dixon in 1909.[22] Histamine is clearly an important mediator in IgE-mediated allergic reactions. It also serves a physiologic role in regulating gastric acid secretion.[23]

Several methods are available for measuring histamine in various body fluids, including (1) guinea pig ileum bioassay,[24] (2) fluorometric methods (manual and automated),[25–27] (3) enzymatic isotopic techniques,[28] (4) high-pressure liquid chromatography (HPLC),[26] and (5) COOF (cation-exchange chromatography, organic solvent extraction, o-phthalaldehyde condensation, and fluorescence measurement) of urine.[29]

Each of the various histamine assays has certain advantages. The enzyme isotope method has been useful in the experimental study of urticarias. Measurements of urinary histamine by the COOF method reveals relatively stable levels, and the method has the definite advantage of easy accessibility of urine for sampling, which obviates venipuncture; and provides the opportunity for retrospective analysis. Finally, the fluorometric method can be automated, which permits processing multiple samples efficiently; it is relatively specific; and the results obtained can be compared with those from published normal groups.

TABLE 8–7.—PULMONARY DISORDERS
ASSOCIATED WITH THE DEVELOPMENT OF
PRECIPITATING ANTIBODIES

Eosinophilic pneumonias
　Allergic bronchopulmonary aspergillosis
　Drug reactions
　Eosinophilic granuloma
　Hypereosinophilic syndrome
　Infection and infestation
　Tropical eosinophilia
Disorders with pulmonary fibrosis
　Goodpasture's syndrome
　Idiopathic fibrosing alveolitis
　Pansystemic sclerosis
　Polymyositis
　Rheumatoid arthritis
　Systemic lupus erythematosus
Hypersensitivity pneumonitis
　Farmer's lung
　Pigeon breeder's disease
　Maple bark stripper's disease
　Bagassosis
　Mushroom grower's disease
　Sequoiosis
Occupational lung diseases
　Anthracosis
　Asbestosis
　Berylliosis
　Silicosis
Miscellaneous
　Pulmonary alveolar proteinosis

However, the various techniques for histamine measurement have individual shortcomings. For instance, the enzyme isotope method requires venous samples from sites draining the reacting site at the exact time of histamine release, whereas the serum methods for histamine determination are relatively unstable.[30] In addition, histamine release from washed leukocytes requires large amounts of blood and the methods are quite time-consuming and technically complicated.[30] Finally, the serum of allergic patients contains blocking antibody (IgG), which increases as a result of immunotherapy. This blocking antibody competes for antigen and prevents it from reaching the IgE-sensitized basophils, causing further technical difficulties in interpreting results of these tests.

Determination of serum or urine histamine levels may be indicated in any disorder associated with abnormal histamine levels, such as (1) IgE-mediated allergic diseases (allergic rhinitis, insect sting allergy, anaphylaxis, allergic asthma, atopic dermatitis, urticaria, food allergy, drug allergy), (2) diseases in which complement is activated via either the alternative or classical pathway, with the resultant production of the histamine-releasing anaphylatoxins C3a, C4a, and C5a, and (3) anaphylactoid reactions, in which histamine may be released from mast cells or basophils by the direct nonimmunologic action of a chemical or physical agent. In addition, these methods may be especially helpful in determining the effects of various H_1 and H_2 antagonists (antihistamines) on histamine receptors.[31]

PROVOCATION TESTS

Provocation challenge tests are utilized to directly stimulate the tissue or end organ involved in the IgE-mediated reaction in an attempt to elicit clinical symptoms of allergy or hyperreactivity in response to a specific allergen, chemical, or physical agent. This abnormal response can be either of an immunologic or nonimmunologic nature. Agents used in nonimmunologic provocation tests include aspirin, tartrazine (FD and C yellow No. 5) dye, methacholine, and histamine; exercise challenges are also used. Immunologic provocation tests include antigen challenge by the ocular, nasal, respiratory, or gastrointestinal route.

Nonimmunologic Provocation Tests

Aspirin Challenge

Facial and laryngeal edema following aspirin ingestion was first described in Germany in 1902.[32] Cooke later described aspirin-induced asthma,[33] and since then diverse mechanisms for this reaction have been proposed. Although the exact nature of the aspirin idiosyncratic response (i.e., aspirin sensitivity, nasal polyps, and severe asthma—the "aspirin triad") is still controversial, it is clearly not an IgE-mediated disorder.[34] The most widely discussed current hypothesis is that aspirin-induced bronchospasm is due to a disturbance in the homeostatic balance between prostaglandin E_2 (PGE_2) and prostaglandin $F_{2\alpha}$ ($PGF_{2\alpha}$).[35]

Definitive diagnosis of aspirin-induced asthma can only be made by *cautious* oral challenge. A detailed protocol for aspirin challenge has been devised and used successfully by Farr et al.[36] Patients with suspected aspirin sensitivity are grouped according to history of aspirin use and asthma and challenged with placebo or aspirin according to the protocol in Table 8–8. Although this procedure is a controlled method for confirming the diagnosis of aspirin sensitivity, it is potentially life-threatening and should not be undertaken without appropriate resuscitative measures readily at hand.

The presence of a positive (>20% decrease in forced expiratory volume in [$FEV_{1.0}$]) response to oral aspirin challenge occurs in as many as 18% of

TABLE 8–8.—SELECTION AND CHALLENGE OF PATIENTS
WITH SUSPECTED ASPIRIN SENSITIVITY*

GROUP	CHALLENGE PROCEDURE†
I—No history of ASA idiosyncrasy and recent ASA usage II—No history of ASA idiosyncrasy and no ASA within one month	Placebo or 75, 325, or 650 mg of ASA on different days
III—History uncertain of ASA and asthma interrelation IV—History of asthma within 24 hours after ASA	Placebo or 15, 37.5, 75, 150, 325, or 650 mg of ASA on different days

*Modified from Farr et al.[36] ASA, acetylsalicylic acid.
†All medications (except steroids) withheld 6–12 hours before test. Positive response to challenge consists of a fall in $FEV_{1.0} \geq 20\%$ by 4 hours after ASA ingestion.

adult asthmatics and 26% of children with chronic asthma. There is no difference between male or female asthmatics in response to aspirin.

Aspirin challenge is not recommended as a routine diagnostic procedure and should be performed with extreme caution in a patient clearly reactive by history. It should be used to assist in the etiologic diagnosis of chronic asthma and to direct appropriate avoidance measures. It may also be used to determine the safety of using aspirin in the patient who requires aspirin or other nonsteroidal anti-inflammatory medications for rheumatoid arthritis or other inflammatory processes.

One must always warn the patient with aspirin sensitivity to avoid not only aspirin, but also other nonsteroidal anti-inflammatory agents (Table 8–9) and tartrazine as well. Although it has been said that sodium salicylate or acetaminophen may be used with impunity in aspirin-sensitive individuals, Farr has demonstrated that 2.2% of these persons may be sensitive to sodium salicylate and that 2.9% overreact to acetaminophen.[36] One must always caution aspirin-sensitive patients no matter what anti-inflammatory agent is prescribed.

Tartrazine Challenge

In 1967 Samter and Beers demonstrated that 3 of 40 aspirin-sensitive patients could not tolerate the yellow azobenzene, tartrazine (FD and C yellow No. 5) dye.[37] The mechanism for this reaction does not appear to involve prostaglandin synthetase.[38] Because of the ubiquitous use of this substance in many prescriptions and over-the-counter preparations,[39] tartrazine should always be considered a possible culprit in the patient with chronic asthma. Such widely differing products as Premarin and Tang Breakfast Drink contain large amounts of tartrazine.

TABLE 8–9.—Drugs That May
Cause Adverse Reactions in
Aspirin-Sensitive Individuals

Aspirin
Aminopyrine
Fenoprofen
Flufenamic acid
Ibuprofen
Indomethacin
Ketoprofen
Meclofenamate sodium
Mefenamic acid
Naproxen
Phenylbutazone
Sodium benzoate
Sulindac
Tartrazine
Tolmetin

Cautious oral challenge with tartrazine is the only definitive way to establish tartrazine sensitivity. The same basic procedure used for aspirin challenge is followed (Table 8–10). Tartrazine sensitivity, as demonstrated by this method, occurs in as many as one third of patients with aspirin-induced asthma, wherein the response is elicited by as little as 1 mg of tartrazine. In Farr's series, 11 of 277 asthmatics (4%) had a positive response to tartrazine challenge.[36] All 11 of these patients also had positive responses on oral challenge with aspirin. Oral tartrazine challenge should be initiated only by experienced individuals, it is best used to confirm or rule out tartrazine-induced asthma in a patient with a history suggestive of aspirin-induced or tartrazine-induced asthma. Tartrazine challenge may also be used to delineate a possible exacerbating factor in the asthmatic that is difficult to control.

TABLE 8–10.—Selection and Challenge of Patients With
Suspected Tartrazine Sensitivity*

GROUP	CHALLENGE PROCEDURE†
I—No history of tartrazine idiosyncrasy and recent tartrazine usage	Double-blind oral challenge with placebo or 50 mg of tartrazine
II—No history of tartrazine idiosyncrasy and no tartrazine within 1 month	
III—Uncertain history of tartrazine and asthma interrelation	Double-blind oral challenge with placebo or 1, 5, 15, 25 or 50 mg of tartrazine sequentially
IV—History of asthma within 24 hours after tartrazine ingestion	

*Modified from Farr et al.[36]
†All medications (except steroids) withheld 6–12 hours before test. Positive response to challenge consists of a fall in $FEV_{1.0} \geqq 20\%$ by 4 hours after oral tartrazine administration.

Methacholine Challenge

Methacholine inhalation challenge was described by Herxheimer in 1951,[40] was further refined by Townley et al.[41] in 1961, and was standardized by Chai et al.[42] in 1975. The method has since been used to define asthma and to determine the existence of a genetic marker (i.e., hyperreactivity of bronchial smooth muscle to methacholine).[43]

There are two methods for performing the methacholine provocation test: the constant breath-volume procedure[42] and the constant concentration-variable inhalation technique. Since the standardized constant breath-volume method has gained wide acceptance throughout many institutions, the technique is outlined in Table 8–11.

The methacholine challenge is an outpatient procedure. It is reliable,

TABLE 8–11.—Methacholine Inhalation
Challenge Procedure

1. Withhold medications as described for allergen challenge in appendix to Chapter 8.
2. Proceed if baseline $FEV_{1.0} \geqq 80\%$ of previous high.
3. Proceed if $FEV_{1.0} \geqq 90\%$ of baseline 10 minutes after 5 breaths of diluent control delivered by dosimeter.
4. Begin with 5 breaths of 0.075 mg methacholine/ml and increase according to the following table if $FEV_{1.0}$ 3 minutes after each 5 breaths is not $\leqq 90\%$ of baseline.

METHACHOLINE CONCENTRATION (mg/ml)	CUMULATIVE NO. OF BREATHS	UNITS/ BREATH*	UNITS/5 BREATHS	CUMULATIVE UNITS/5 BREATHS†
0.075	5	0.075	0.375	0.375
0.15	10	0.15	0.750	1.125
0.31	15	0.31	1.55	2.68
0.62	20	0.62	3.10	5.78
1.25	25	1.25	6.25	12.0
2.50	30	2.50	12.50	24.5
5.00	35	5.00	25.00	49.5
10.00	40	10.00	50.00	99.5
25.00	45	25.00	125.00	225.00

*One breath unit = 1 inhalation of 1 mg/ml.
†If final $FEV_{1.0}$ is determined at other than 5 breaths, cumulative units are calculated by multiplying additional number of breaths times methacholine concentration and adding to final $FEV_{1.0}$ for 5 breaths (e.g., for 8 breaths of 0.62 mg/ml: 3 × 0.62 = 1.86, added to 5.78 = 7.64).
Modified from Chai et al.[42]

5. Positive response is indicated by a drop in $FEV_{1.0} \geqq 20\%$ below baseline.
6. As this positive end point is approached, less than 5 breaths of the next higher concentration should be given.
7. Wait 2 hours after methacholine challenge before another procedure. Then proceed only if patient is back to baseline.

reproducible, and does not vary with sex of the patient, but does vary with age.[44] All results should be corrected for age. In most series more than 90% of asthmatics are sensitive to methacholine whereas less than 5% of patients with allergic rhinitis or normal controls have a positive response.[44]

The methacholine inhalation challenge test may be used to define the natural history of airways hyperreactivity. However, it is primarily used to confirm or rule out the existence of reversible obstructive hyperreactive airway disease (e.g., asthma) when other diagnostic criteria are inadequate.[14]

Histamine Challenge

Direct application of suspected allergen has been used in a diagnostic manner for over 5 decades.[45] Inhalation of histamine by an asthmatic individual causes bronchoconstriction and marked changes in lung volume similar to the changes that occur during a spontaneous attack of asthma.[46] Since Herxheimer studied the effects of bronchoprovocation in 1951,[40] many modifications to the technique have been developed. Most investigators now use either the constant breath-volume method or the constant concentration-variable inhalation procedure.[41] A positive response on the constant breath-volume method consists of a 20% or greater fall in $FEV_{1.0}$ at 5 or more breaths of 10 mg histamine base/ml (Table 8–12). (A decrease of 20% or more in $FEV_{1.0}$ at 10 mg of histamine base/ml is considered a positive response in the constant concentration-variable inhalation test.) Casterline and Evans have found this test to be a reliable and reproducible method for demonstrating hyperreactivity of the airways.[47]

Although the histamine bronchoprovocation test may also be used to define the natural course of hyperreactive airways disease and to confirm or rule out reversible obstructive airways disease, it has been largely supplanted by the methacholine inhalation challenge test for these two purposes. With either method, there may be variation that does not correlate with the individual patient history.

Exercise Challenge

Exercise-induced bronchospasm is a natural response to strenuous exercise in a patient with hyperreactive airways disease. Although there is no consensus on the actual mechanism of exercise-induced bronchoconstriction, many different hypotheses have been investigated, including (1) increased inhalation of antigen, (2) mediator release, (3) respiratory skeletal muscle fatigue, and (4) changes in thermal and humidity gradients that elicit reflex bronchospasm through irritant receptors.[48]

Many different types of exercise, including swimming, free running,

TABLE 8–12.—Histamine Inhalation Challenge Procedure

1. Withhold medications as described for allergen inhalation challenge in appendix to Chapter 8.
2. Proceed if baseline $FEV_{1.0} \geqq 80\%$ of previous high.
3. Proceed if the $FEV_{1.0} \geqq 90\%$ of baseline 10 minutes after 5 breaths of diluent control delivered by dosimeter.
4. Begin with 5 breaths of 0.03 mg of histamine base/ml and increase according to the following table if $FEV_{1.0}$ 3 minutes after each 5 breaths is not $\leqq 90\%$ of baseline.

HISTAMINE BASE CONCENTRATIONS (mg/ml)	CUMULATIVE NO. OF BREATHS	UNITS/ BREATH*	UNITS/5 BREATHS	CUMULATIVE UNITS/5 BREATHS†
0.03	5	0.03	0.15	0.15
0.06	10	0.06	0.30	0.45
0.12	15	0.12	0.60	1.05
0.25	20	0.25	1.25	2.30
0.50	25	0.50	2.50	4.80
1.00	30	1.00	5.00	9.80
2.50	35	2.50	12.50	22.30
5.00	40	5.00	25.00	47.30
10.00	45	10.00	50.00	97.30

*One breath unit = 1 inhalation of 1 mg/ml histamine base.
†If final $FEV_{1.0}$ is determined at other than 5 breaths, cumulative units are calculated by multiplying additional number of breaths times histamine concentration and adding to final $FEV_{1.0}$ for 5 breaths (e.g., for 8 breaths of 0.25 mg/ml, $3 \times 0.25 = 0.75$, added to $2.30 = 3.05$. Modified from Chai et al.[42]

jumping, kayaking, canoeing, treadmill running, stationary cycling, and rope jumping, have been used to elicit exercise-induced bronchospasm. Because of the great variability in performing these different methods, it is important to standardize the method of exercise challenge used in any group of patients with hyperreactive airways disease.

Eggleston and Guerrant have proposed a standardized exercise challenge that has been accepted by many investigators as an excellent means of approaching this clinical problem in a systematic fashion.[49] The protocol is outlined in Table 8–13.

Exercise challenge should be done only when the physician is certain that the patient being studied has a normal cardiovascular and cerebrovascular status, to avoid an obvious potential hazardous complication. A positive response consists of a 20% or more decrease in $FEV_{1.0}$, which usually occurs 10–30 minutes after a 4- to 6-minute exercise period. Obviously, the extent of exercise required and the outcome depend on many variables, among them the ambient temperature, humidity, and possibly barometric pressure; prior training; type and intensity of exercise; duration of exercise; and age.

The exercise provocation test, when performed according to the protocol

TABLE 8–13.—EXERCISE CHALLENGE PROCEDURE

1. Do *NOT* proceed unless cardiovascular and cerebrovascular status of the subject are adequate to withstand the stress.
2. Resuscitation equipment must be immediately available.
3. Withhold medications, as outlined in the appendix to this chapter.
4. Place chest electrodes for continuous monitoring.
5. Determine resting heart rate and calculate 90% of maximum heart rate for age.
6. Proceed only if baseline $FEV_{1.0}$ ≧80% of previous high.
7. Subject should stand on treadmill while speed and incline are slowly increased. Challenge is stopped when heart rate has been 90% of predicted maximum for 2–5 minutes.[19]
8. $FEV_{1.0}$ is determined before exercise and 1, 5, 10, 15, 30, 45, and 60 minutes after exercise.
9. Positive response is indicated by a drop in $FEV_{1.0}$ ≧20% below baseline.

outlined in Table 8–13, elicits a positive response for hyperreactive airways disease in as many as 71% of asthmatics.[49] Instillation of chemicals is not necessary. The method also may be adapted to free running, which obviates the need for expensive equipment and facilities. Again, the physician must use caution in exercising individuals with a questionable cardiovascular or cerebrovascular status, especially in the uncontrolled environment that is used for free running. Exercise challenge is especially useful for determining not only the presence and severity of bronchospasm, but also the efficacy and duration of effect of preexercise bronchodilators or mediator release inhibitors (e.g., cromolyn sodium) in running enthusiasts, athletes, or military personnel, for whom endurance and stamina are important.

Immunologic Provocation Tests

Direct application of a suspected allergen to the airways of asthmatic patients has been in use since 1934.[45] Over the years the procedure has been modified and adapted to its present form, as outlined in the appendix to this chapter. The techniques applied are quite similar to those followed in the methacholine and histamine provocation tests. Again, a positive inhalation antigen challenge is defined as a decrease in $FEV_{1.0}$ 20% or more below baseline.

The incidence of positive reactivity to antigen inhalation challenge varies from patient to patient and largely depends on individual sensitivity to a given allergen. Although skin tests are less time-consuming and easier to perform, evidence exists to support the use of bronchial inhalation challenges with allergens to provide information beyond that derived from a skin test or in vitro test.[50]

Antigen inhalation challenge can be clinically useful (Table 8–14) and should be considered for the following purposes: (1) to determine the effect

TABLE 8–14.—INDICATIONS AND CONTRAINDICATIONS
FOR THE PERFORMANCE OF ANTIGEN
INHALATION CHALLENGES*

Indications
To determine role of specific allergen in asthma
To evaluate new or specific allergens in pulmonary disease
To compare therapeutic efficacy of various treatment modalities
To convince patient or parents of cause-and-effect relationship
To compare other tests (e.g., in vivo or in vitro tests)
When skin tests are not possible
To evaluate immunotherapy efficacy in asthma
Contraindications
Unstable asthmatic patient
Individual reacts to control challenge
Patient has upper respiratory or other infection
Insufficient pulmonary reserve
History of cardiovascular or cerebrovascular disease

*Modified from Farr et al.[36]

of a specific allergen in asthma; (2) to differentiate the relative value of history, skin tests, or in vitro tests that reveal conflicting results; (3) in patients with severe atopic dermatitis or burns with insufficient normal skin to perform skin tests; (4) to evaluate the therapeutic efficacy of immunotherapy, especially in asthmatics; (5) to determine the therapeutic efficacy of bronchodilators and other agents that block antigen-induced bronchoconstriction; (6) to convince the patient or the patient's parents about cause-and-effect relationships; and (7) to evaluate new or specific allergens in pulmonary disease. Bronchoprovocation testing should not be done in the unstable asthmatic or the individual with a history of cardiovascular or cerebrovascular disease, for whom the transient hypoxia may be devastating. For similar reasons, individuals with inadequate pulmonary reserve should not undergo bronchoprovocation challenge. Finally, inhalation challenge with allergen should not be attempted in the individual who reacts to challenge with the control solution or in a patient with an upper respiratory tract or other infectious process.

APPENDIX

ANTIGEN INHALATION CHALLENGE PROCEDURE

1. Skin test patient intradermally (ID) with serial dilutions of the antigen to be studied using 1:100,000, 1:10,000, and 1:1,000 w/v and read wheal as follows:

1–2 mm>control ±	Continue to next higher concentration
3–5 mm>control +	
6–8 mm>control + +	Stop at 2+ reaction and, if greater, titrate back to 2+
9–11 mm>control + + +	
≥ 12 mm>control + + + +	

Histamine control should be > 10 mm.

2. Withhold medications prior to challenge, as follows:

MEDICATION	HOURS WITHHELD
α-Adrenergic	8
Anticholinergic	8
β-Adrenergic, inhaled or injected	8
β-Adrenergic, sustained release	12
Theophylline, short acting	12
Theophylline, sustained release	24
Cromolyn sodium	24
Antihistamine	48
Hydroxyzine hydrochloride	120

3. Proceed only if baseline $FEV_{1.0}$ ≧80% of previous high.
4. Proceed if $FEV_{1.0}$ ≧90% of baseline 10 minutes after 5 breaths of diluent control delivered by dosimeter.
5. Antigen challenge: begin with 5 breaths of the antigen concentration that gave a 2+ ID skin test and proceed with 5 breaths of each successive concentration, according to the following table, as long as the $FEV_{1.0}$ 10 minutes after a dose has not decreased >15% below baseline.

ANTIGEN CONCENTRATION (w/v)	CUMULATIVE NO. OF BREATHS	UNITS/ BREATH*	UNITS/5 BREATHS	CUMULATIVE UNITS/5 BREATHS†
1:1,000,000	5	0.005	0.025	0.025
1:500,000	10	0.01	0.05	0.075
1:100,000	15	0.05	0.25	0.325
1:50,000	20	0.1	0.5	0.825
1:10,000	25	0.5	2.5	3.32
1:5,000	30	1.0	5.0	8.32
1:1,000	35	5.0	25.0	33.3
1:500	40	10.0	50.0	83.3

*1 Breath unit = 1 inhalation of 1 mg/ml.
†If final $FEV_{1.0}$ is determined at other than 5 breaths, cumulative units are calculated by multiplying additional number of breaths times antigen concentration and adding to 5-breath value (e.g., for 8 breaths at 1:50,000, 3 × .01 = .03, added to 0.825 = 1.825).
Modified from Chai et al.[42]

6. Positive response is indicated by a drop in $FEV_{1.0}$ ≧20% below baseline.
7. As this positive end point is approached fewer than 5 breaths of the next higher concentration should be used.
8. Once the positive end point is reached, check the $FEV_{1.0}$ hourly for 10 hours or until it returns to baseline. Warn the patient about late reactions.
9. Do not perform another challenge for at least 24 hours.

REFERENCES

1. Ishizaka K., Ishizaka T., Hornbrook M.M.: Physico-chemical properties of human reaginic antibody: IV. Presence of a unique immunoglobulin as a carrier of reaginic activity. *J. Immunol.* 97:75, 1966.

2. Bhalla R., Rappaport I., Schwartz M.: Personal communication, Sloan-Kettering Institution, New York City.

3. Evans R., III: Committee report: A U.S. reference for human immunoglobulin E. *J. Allergy Clin. Immunol.* 68:79, 1981.

4. Hamburger R.N., Orgel H.A., Bazaral M.: Genetics of human serum IgE levels, in Goodfriend L., Sehon A.H., Orange R.P., (eds.): *Mechanisms in Allergy: Reagin-Mediated Hypersensitivity.* New York, Marcel Dekker, 1973, pp. 131–139.

5. Johansson S.G.O., Strandberg K., Uvnäs B.: Molecular and Biological Aspects of the Acute Allergic Reaction. New York: Plenum Publishing Corp., 1976, p. 179.

6. Yunginger J.W., Gleich G.J.: The impact of the discovery of IgE on the practice of allergy, in Ellis E.F. (ed.): *The Pediatric Clinics of North America Symposium on Pediatric Allergy.* Philadelphia, W.B. Saunders Co., 1975, pp. 3–15.

7. Johansson S.G.O., Foucard T.: IgE in immunity and disease, in Middleton E., Reed C., Ellis E.F. (eds.): *Allergy: Principles and Practice.* St. Louis, C.V. Mosby Co., 1978, vol. 2, p. 551.

8. Buckley R.H.: Immunologic deficiency and allergic disease, in Middleton E., Reed C., Ellis E.F. (eds.): *Allergy: Principles and Practice.* St. Louis, C.V. Mosby Co., 1978, vol. 1, chap. 13.

9. Cook T.J., MacQueen D.M., Wittig H.J., et al.: Degree and duration of skin test suppression and side effects with antihistamines. *J. Allergy Clin. Immunol.* 51:71, 1977.

10. Prausnitz C., Küstner H.: Studien über die Überemfindlichkeit. *Zentralbl. Bakteriol.* [A] 86:160, 1921.

11. Wide L., Bennich H., Johansson S.G.O.: Diagnosis of allergy by an in vitro test for allergen antibodies. *Lancet* 2:1105, 1967.

12. Evans R., Reisman R.E., Wypych J.I., et al.: An immunologic evaluation of ragweed-sensitive patients by newer techniques. *J. Allergy Clin. Immunol.* 49:285, 1972.

13. Bruce C.A., Rosenthal R.R., Lichtenstein L.M., et al.: Diagnostic tests in ragweed-allergic asthma: A comparison of direct skin tests, leukocyte histamine release and quantitative bronchial challenge. *J. Allergy Clin. Immunol.* 53:230, 1974.

14. Berg T., Bennich H., Johansson S.G.O.: In vitro diagnosis of atopic allergy: I. A comparison between provocation tests and the radioallergosorbent test. *Int. Arch. Allergy Appl. Immunol.* 40:770, 1971.

15. Osler A.G., Lichtenstein L.M., Levy D.A.: In vitro studies of human reaginic allergy. *Adv. Immunol.* 8:183, 1968.

16. Ishizaka T., Soto C., Ishizaka K.: Mechanisms of passive sensitization: 3. Number of IgE molecules and its receptor sites on human basophil granulocytes. *J. Immunol.* 111:500, 1973.

17. Siraganian R.P., Hook W.A.: Histamine release and assay methods for the study of human allergy, in Rose N.R., Friedman H. (eds.): *Manual of Clinical Immunology,* ed. 2. Washington, D.C., American Society for Microbiology, 1980, chap. 108.

18. Heidelberger M., Kendall F.E.: A quantitative study of the precipitin reaction between type III pneumococcus polysaccharide and purified homologous antibody. *J. Exp. Med.* 50:300, 1929.

19. Maurer P.: Precipitation reactions, in Williams C.A., Chase M.W. (eds.): *Methods in Immunology and Immunochemistry.* New York, Academic Press, 1971, vol. 3, p. 37.
20. Parker C.: Infiltrative hypersensitivity disease of the lung, in *Clinical Immunology.* 1980, vol. 2, chap. 44.
21. Windaus A., Vogt W.: Synthese des imidazolylethylamines. *Ber. Dtsch. Chem. Ges.* 40:3691, 1907.
22. Dale H.H., Dixon W.E.: The action of pressor amines produced by putrefaction. *J. Physiol.* 39:25, 1909.
23. Beaven M.A.: Histamine: Its role in physiological and pathological processes. *Monogr. Allergy* 13:1, 1978.
24. Austen K.F.: Assay of histamine, in Williams C.A., Chase M.W. (eds.): *Methods in Immunology and Immunochemistry.* New York, Academic Press, 1976, vol. 5, p. 126.
25. Davis T.P., Gehrke C.W. Jr., Cunningham T.D., et al.: High-performance liquid-chromatographic separation and fluorescence measurement of biogenic amines in plasma, urine and tissue. *Clin. Chem.* 24:317, 1978.
26. Mell L.D. Jr., Hawkins R.N., Thompson R.S.: Fluorometric determination of histamine in biological fluids and tissue by high-performance liquid chromatography. *J. Liquid. Chromatogr.* 2:1393, 1979.
27. Siraganian R.P., Hook W.A.: Histamine release and assay methods for the study of human allergy, in Rose N.R., Friedman H. (eds.): *Manual of Clinical Immunology.* Washington, D.C., American Society for Microbiology, 1980, pp. 808–821.
28. Horakova Z., Keiser H.R., Beaven M.A.: Blood and urine histamine levels in normal and pathological states as measured by a radiochemical assay. *Clin. Chim. Acta* 79:447, 1977.
29. Myers G., Donon M., Kaliner M.: Measurement of urinary histamine: Development of methodology and normal values. *J. Allergy Clin. Immunol.* 67:305, 1981.
30. Kapeller-Ader R., Renwick R.: On the enzymic breakdown of histamine and cadaverine in human serum and urine. *Clin. Chim. Acta* 1:197, 1956.
31. Summers R., Kaliner M.: Current concepts of histamine actions through H_1 and H_2 receptors on humans, unpublished manuscript.
32. Hirchberg V.G.S.R.: Mittheilung über eine Fall von Nebenwirkung des Aspirin. *Dtsch. Med. Wochenschr.* 27:416, 1902.
33. Cooke R.A.: Allergy in drug idiosyncrasy. *JAMA* 73:759, 1919.
34. Smith A.P.: Response of aspirin-allergic patients to challenge by some analgesics in common use. *Br. Med. J.* 1:494, 1971.
35. Szczeklik A., Gryglewski R.J., Czerniawska-Mysik G.: Relationship of inhibition of prostaglandin biosynthesis by analgesics to asthma attacks in aspirin-sensitive patients. *Br. Med. J.* 1:67, 1975.
36. Farr R.S., Spector S.L., Wangaard C.H.: Evaluation of aspirin and tartrazine idiosyncrasy. *J. Allergy Clin. Immunol.* 64:667, 1979.
37. Samter M., Beers R.F.: Concerning the nature of intolerance to aspirin. *J. Allergy* 40:281, 1967.
38. Gerber J.G., Payner N.A., Osward O., et al.: Tartrazine and the prostaglandin system. *J. Allergy Clin. Immunol.* 63:289, 1979.
39. Smith L., Slavin R.G.: Drugs containing tartrazine dye. *J. Allergy Clin. Immunol.* 57:456, 1976.

40. Herxheimer H.: Bronchial obstruction induced by allergens, histamine and acetyl-beta-methylcholine chloride. *Int. Arch. Allergy Appl. Immunol.* 2:27, 1951.
41. Townley R.G., Dennis M., Itkin I.H.: Comparative action of acetyl-beta-methylcholine, histamine and pollen antigens in subjects with hay fever and patients with bronchial asthma. *J. Allergy* 36:121, 1965.
42. Chai H., Farr R.S., Froehlich L.A., et al.: Standardization of inhalation challenge. *J. Allergy Clin. Immunol.* 56:323, 1975.
43. Reed C.E., Townley R.G.: Asthma: Classification and pathogenesis, in Middleton E., Reed C.E., Ellis E.F. (eds.): *Allergy: Principles and Practice.* St. Louis, C.V. Mosby Co., 1978, pp. 659–677.
44. Townley R.G., Bewtra A.K., Nair N.M., et al.: Methacholine inhalation challenge studies. *J. Allergy Clin. Immunol.* 64:569, 1974.
45. Stevens F.A.: A comparison of pulmonary and dermal sensitivity to inhaled substances. *J. Allergy* 5:285, 1934.
46. Bleecker E.R., Rosenthal R.R., Menkes H.A., et al.: Physiologic effects of inhaled histamine in asthma: Reversible changes in pulmonary mechanics and total lung capacity. *J. Allergy Clin. Immunol.* 64:597, 1979.
47. Casterline C.L., Evans R.: Further studies on the mechanism of human histamine-induced asthma. *J. Allergy Clin. Immunol.* 59:420, 1977.
48. Deal E.C., McFadden E.R. Jr., Ingram R.H. Jr., et al.: Airway responsiveness to cold air and hyperpnea in normal subjects and in those with hay fever and asthma. *Am. Rev. Respir. Dis.* 121:621, 1980.
49. Eggleston P.A., Guerrant J.L.: A standardized method of evaluating exercise-induced asthma. *J. Allergy Clin. Immunol.* 58:414, 1976.
50. Pepys J., Hutchcroft B.J.: Bronchial inhalation challenges with antigens. *J. Allergy Clin. Immunol.* 64:580, 1979.

9

Bacterial Immunology

Michael W. Rytel, M.D.

APPLICATION OF IMMUNOLOGIC METHODS to the diagnosis of bacterial infections was, until the 1970s, rather limited. The techniques were of four kinds: "febrile agglutinin" reactions, neutralization techniques, serologic tests, and fluorescence microscopy. In febrile agglutinin reactions, antibodies induced in the course of certain infections agglutinated whole organisms or their antigens. This assay is still used in infections due to *Salmonella, Leptospira, Brucella,* and *Francisella* organisms and in some forms of rickettsia (Weil-Felix test). The specificity of these reactions varies, and their role in the diagnosis of salmonellosis is mainly ancillary. The febrile agglutinin test is of greater value in diagnosing brucellosis, tularemia, and rickettsial infections. Various neutralization techniques to detect antibodies to exotoxins were developed for diphtheria, tetanus, and cholera. Serologic tests played an important role in the diagnosis of group A streptococcal infections and their sequelae, such as rheumatic fever and glomerulonephritis. These tests consist of antibody assays to various streptococcal products such as streptolysin, streptokinase, streptodornase, and deoxyribonuclease-B. Serologic tests also proved useful in diagnosing infections due to *Mycoplasma pneumoniae.* These tests include such nonspecific reactions as the cold agglutinin determination, which depends on agglutination of human type O erythrocytes at 4 C, and agglutination of *Streptococcus* MG. The sensitivity of these serologic tests is on the order of 50% and 25%, respectively. (Of course, the more specific assay for *M. pneumoniae* infection is the complement fixation [CF] antibody test.) Finally, fluorescence microscopy was used for the direct detection of such bacterial organisms as group A streptococci, *Yersinia pestis, Legionella pneumophila,* and others.

In the last decade the immunologic approach to the diagnosis of bacterial infections has been widely expanded. This chapter will briefly summarize the methodology of some of the more useful procedures currently employed (Table 9–1), with emphasis on the newer procedures. However, older, still useful methods will also be discussed. The most important characteristic distinguishing the newer from the older immunodiagnostic methods is the emphasis on antigen detection.

The chapter is divided into three sections. Following the introductory section, various current immunodiagnostic techniques of general applicability are described and their main uses listed. In the third section bacterial infections in which immunodiagnosis plays an important role are discussed. In selecting material for discussion, I was guided by what is already available in the literature. Topics that have been the subject of recent reviews are mentioned briefly and appropriate references are provided. Other topics for which thorough discussion is not available, or which are not easily accessible in the literature, are covered more completely.

METHODS

Detection of Microbial Metabolites in Body Fluids: Gas-Liquid Chromatography

Gas-liquid chromatography (GLC) is used in many laboratories to identify anaerobic bacteria isolated from clinical specimens. Products of microbial metabolism that are volatile or that can be volatilized give specific elution patterns on a gas chromatogram. This approach was initially used for identification of anaerobic organisms isolated in vitro.[1, 2] Several reports indicate that GLC can also be used in the diagnosis of streptococcal, staphylococcal, and gonococcal infections, among others, by direct identification of metabolites in body fluids.[3] More recently GLC has also been used to identify *L. pneumophila* metabolites. Best results have been achieved in infections in a closed space, such as septic arthritis, meningitis, and empyema.[4] Mitruka and Bonner have co-authored an exhaustive monograph describing GLC and its application.[5]

Newer Methods of Detection of Antigens and Antibodies in Body Fluids

Coagglutination of Staphylococcus aureus

Certain strains of coagulase-positive staphylococci bind the Fc fragment of antibody immunoglobulin to the A protein located on their outer surface. The Fab fragment thus faces outward and is free to combine with homologous antigen.[6] Coagglutination of *S. aureus* (COAG) has been used to identify and type several bacterial species from broth cultures and directly on the primary isolation plates, thus making it possible to give presumptive identification within hours after receiving the specimen.[7, 8] The method can also be used to detect microbial antigens in body fluids,[9] where it has

TABLE 9–1.—IMMUNOLOGIC PROCEDURES IN THE
DIAGNOSIS OF BACTERIAL INFECTIONS*

APPROACH	TECHNIQUE
Detection of microbial metabolites in body fluids	GLC

Detection of microbial antigens in body fluids	COAG
	CIE
	DID
	EIA
	  ELISA
	    Competitive
	    Double antibody (sandwich)
	    Inhibition
	  EMIT
	  Fluorescence microscopy
	    Direct
	    Indirect
	  LA

Detection of antibodies	COAG
	CIE
	DID
	EIA
	  ELISA: indirect method
	  Fluorescence microscopy: indirect
	  Indirect Hemagglutination

*GLC, gas-liquid chromatography; COAG, coagglutination of *Staphylococcus aureus;* CIE, counterimmunoelectrophoresis; DID, double immunodiffusion; EIA, enzyme immunoassay; LA, latex agglutination.

been reported to be more sensitive than counterimmunoelectrophoresis (CIE) and latex agglutination (LA).[10] It appears promising in the diagnosis of pneumococcal pneumonia by detection of *Streptococcus pneumoniae* capsular antigens in sputum, in which application it may have greater sensitivity than CIE.[11] It has also been used to detect *Salmonella* antigens in stool, either on direct examination or following 20-hour culture in enriched media,[12] and to detect pneumococcal and *Hemophilus* antigens in blood cultures that become nonviable in 20 hours.[13]

Latex Agglutination

Agglutination testing using latex particles coated with specific antibodies was first reported by Bloomfield et al. in the detection of cryptococcal antigen in cases of meningitis.[14] Other investigators (Bennett et al.,[15] Gordon and Vedder,[16] Goodman et al.[17]) confirmed and expanded these findings. Bennett et al., in an extensive study involving 49 patients, detected cryptococcal antigen in body fluids of 66% of patients with meningitis and 25%

of those with nonmeningeal cryptococcosis.[15] Body fluids of 110 control subjects were negative.

The LA test has been used by Newman et al.[18] in *H. influenzae* infections. *Hemophilus influenzae* type b antigen was detected in the cerebrospinal fluid (CSF) in 27 of 29 patients with *Hemophilus* meningitis. Some false positive reactions (2.3%) were observed. These were thought to be due to heat-labile factors, as heating of the specimens at 100 C for 15 minutes abolished the LA reaction. Severin reported LA useful in the diagnosis of meningococcal meningitis.[19]

Coonrod and Drennan reported using the LA test to detect type 7 pneumococcal polysaccharide, which, because of its poor anodal mobility, is difficult to detect by CIE.[20] Latex particles covered with type-specific pneumococcal antibody were agglutinated by antigen present in the specimens. The sensitivity of the method was comparable to that of CIE.

CIE

Counterimmunoelectrophoresis combines the features of gel immunodiffusion (Ouchterlony technique) plus electrophoresis (see Chap. 2). Body fluids thought to contain microbial antigens are placed in separate wells punched out of a buffered diffusion mechanism (e.g., agarose). Wells spaced 2–3 mm apart in a row are filled with antibodies. On application of electric current, polysaccharide antigens, which tend to be negatively charged at neutral or alkaline pH, migrate toward the anode, whereas antibodies that are less negatively charged will, as a result of endosmotic flow (as well as passive diffusion), migrate in the opposite or "counter" direction toward the cathode. In a short time (30–60 minutes) antigens and antibodies complex at equilibrium concentration, forming a distinct precipitin line. CIE may be used to identify unknown antigens or antibodies. Some of its diagnostic uses are listed in Table 9–2 and discussed below.

The most useful application of CIE has been in the detection of antigens in CSF. In most reported studies[21] antigen was detected in the majority of bacteriologically proved cases of meningitis caused by the three most common causative agents: *S. pneumoniae* (pneumococcus), 79%; *H. influenzae* type b, 84%; and *Neisseria meningitidis*, 75%.[22] Thus, CIE is not as sensitive as culture. This is because a certain minimal concentration of microorganisms in the CSF is required before enough antigen is released for detection by CIE. Generally, a concentration of microorganisms of 10^5 colony-forming units per milliliter is required.[23] The test is quite specific, however, and cross reactions have been seen only when a very large antigenic load was present ($\geq 10^8$ organisms/ml). Also, antigen cross reactions

TABLE 9–2.—CIE Diagnostic Panels Currently Employed at the Medical College of Wisconsin

| INFECTION | DETECTION OF | |
	ANTIGEN	ANTIBODY
Meningitis		
Community-acquired	*Streptococcus pneumoniae* (all types)	
	Hemophilus influenzae type b	
	Neisseria meningitidis (all types except B)	
Hospital-acquired	*Staphylococcus aureus* (teichoic acid)	
	Pseudomonas aeruginosa	
	Klebsiella pneumoniae (types 1–6)	
Neonates	*Escherichia coli* K1	
	Streptococcus group B	
Pneumonia	*S. pneumoniae*	*S. aureus*
	K. pneumoniae	
"Compromised host"	*P. aeruginosa*	*Candida albicans*
infections	*Pneumocystis carinii*	*S. aureus*
		P. aeruginosa
Endocarditis		*S. aureus*
		C. albicans
Parasitic infections		*Entamoeba histolytica*
Septic arthritis	*S. pneumoniae*	
	H. influenzae type b	
	S. aureus (teichoic acid)	

are more apt to occur with certain organisms, e.g., between *N. meningitidis* group B and *E. coli* K1, and between *E. coli* and *H. influenzae* type b and *S. aureus*.[22]

In pneumococcal pneumonia, the rate of antigen detection in serum is lower than that in CSF in cases of meningitis, but in most studies 50% of bacteremic cases were positive for antigen. If concentrated urine as well as serum is employed for antigen detection, antigen may be detected in as many as 70% of the patients. Pneumococcal antigen has been detected in sputum of patients with bacteremic pneumococcal pneumonia; sputa are generally treated with *N*-acetylcysteine.* Antigen detection in the sputum correlated with the presence of pneumococcal pneumonia in 80%–100% of reported cases.[24–26] In one study, the predictive value of CIE was twice as great as that of culture.[22] One problem with using CIE for antigen detection was that pneumococcal antigen was detected in approximately 20% of patients with bacterial bronchitis.[26] Chest roentgenograms should help to distinguish patients with bronchitis from those with pneumonia.

Other infections in which bacterial antigens have been detected by CIE

---

*Mucomist; Mead Johnson, Evansville, Ind.

include those caused by *Klebsiella pneumoniae, Pseudomonas* sp., and *Streptococcus* group B, and in *E. coli* K1 meningitis.[27] These latter infections occur most commonly in neonates.

Unfortunately, no antisera against *Pseudomonas* and *E. coli* K1 are commercially available. For detection of *K. pneumoniae* antigen, we have used polyvalent serum consisting of a pool of six type-specific antisera (types 1–6), as well as the same six individual type-specific antisera.* Types 1–6 are the most common types responsible for *Klebsiella* pneumonias.

Antigen detection may also be of aid in determining a patient's prognosis, because the severity of infection as well as the incidence of certain complications are higher in antigen-positive patients[28]; this is particularly true if the amount of the detected antigen is large.

One additional advantage of CIE (as well as of COAG and LA) over cultures is that an etiologic diagnosis can be established even in patients who have been partially treated with antibiotics and whose body fluids will therefore yield sterile cultures.

Although less specific than the detection of microbial antigens, CIE can be used for antibody detection when the amount of antigen in body fluids is below the sensitivity of the available methods. The best known example is the diagnosis of *S. aureus* infections. We have also found it helpful to use antibody detection to confirm the systemic nature of bacterial infections. Antigens are generally crude extracts of the organism, for example, *S. epidermidis, Serratia marcescens, Pseudomonas aeruginosa,* and *H. parahaemolyticus* (unpublished data).

Double Immunodiffusion

The double immunodiffusion test of Ouchterlony depends on the fact that antigens and antibodies will diffuse in a gel matrix and will form a precipitin line, if they are specific for each other (see Chap. 2).[29] The gel remains permeable to all other antigens and antibodies that are dissimilar to the precipitating pair. Wells, which may be of different size and distance from each other, are punched in the gel layer. Antigen and antibody are placed in opposite wells and diffuse through the gel. When the optimal antigen-antibody ratio is achieved (zone of equivalence), a precipitin line will form. Double immunodiffusion is approximately 10 times less sensitive than CIE; moreover, the reactions may require 1–3 days to develop, in contrast to the 30–60 minutes required for CIE. Thus, the only role for double immunodiffusion in modern immunodiagnostic tests for bacter-

---

*Available from Difco Laboratories, Detroit, Mich. Antiserum to *Streptococcus* group B can also be obtained from Difco Laboratories.

ial infections is in the detection and titration of antibodies to staphylococ-cal teichoic acid,[30] although even in this situation some investigators pre-fer CIE.

Enzyme Immunoassay

In enzyme immunoassay (EIA), enzyme-tagged reagents, either antigens or antibodies, are employed. EIA is as sensitive as radioimmunoassay (RIA) but has a number of advantages, such as lack of radioactivity, the lower cost of reagents and equipment, and relatively greater simplicity in per-forming the test. EIA actually refers to two different kinds of assays: en-zyme-linked immunoassay (ELISA) and enzyme-multiplied immunoassay (EMIT).[31] Because ELISA has been used for the diagnostic detection of antigens and antibodies in infectious diseases, while EMIT has generally been used in drug assays, only ELISA will be discussed here.

EIA studies can also be discussed in terms of the heterogeneous assay and the homogeneous assay. In the heterogeneous assay, antigen and an-tibody are separated physically (one of the two is usually attached to a solid carrier, such as a well in a microtiter plate or a bead). The antigen-antibody reaction does not affect the activity of the label (enzyme). ELISA is a het-erogeneous system. In the homogeneous assay the reactants are not sepa-rated and the activity of the label is inhibited. EMIT is a homogeneous assay.

Four main techniques have been employed in ELISA for detecting an-tigens and antibodies: (1) Double antibody sandwich method (for antigen detection), in which specific antibody is adsorbed onto a solid-phase sup-port (e.g., microplate, bead), the patient's specimen putatively containing the antigen is added, and then enzyme-labeled specific antibody is added. The sensitivity of this assay can be increased if the second antibody is not labeled, but the label is attached instead to a third antibody (modified dou-ble antibody sandwich method). This technique permits wider usage of the conjugated antibody, which may be specific for an immunoglobulin instead of bacterial antigen. (2) Competitive assay (for antigen detection). Here, specific antibody is attached to a solid-phase support and a mixture of the patient's specimen plus an enzyme-labeled antigen is added. For control, enzyme-labeled antigen alone is added to a parallel solid-phase support. Then enzyme substrate is added. The difference in the amount of substrate hydrolyzed indicates the antigen content of the patient's serum. (This ap-proach is also widely used in RIA.) (3) Inhibition assay (for antigen detec-tion). Antigen is coupled to a solid-phase support (plate) and a mixture of the patient's specimen plus a standard amount of specific antibody is added. This is followed by addition of enzyme antiglobulin conjugate. The plate is washed and enzyme substrate is added. If antigen was present in patient's specimen, there will be no enzymatic activity mixture (fixed antigen, antibody, antiglobulin conjugate) in the final reaction and thus no substrate degradation. (4) Indirect method (for antibody detection). Antigen is attached to a solid-phase support, the specimen is added, and then enzyme-labeled antiglobulin is added.

The two most commonly used enzyme tags are peroxidase and alkaline phosphatase. These two enzymes are active at the pH of antigen-antibody binding. The substrates, *o*-phenylenediamine (OPD) or 5-aminosalicylic acid, change color when acted on by peroxidase. A common substrate for alkaline phosphatase is *p*-nitrophenyl phosphate. The colorimetric reaction, which indicates that an antigen-antibody reaction has taken place, can be measured spectrophotometrically or read visually.

To date, ELISA has been applied in the diagnosis of a number of bacterial infections, either by detection of antigens or antibodies (Table 9–3).[32–61] Most of these assays have been experimental and none, unlike CIE, has yet been widely established in diagnostic laboratories. There are, as yet, no diagnostic kits available commercially for diagnosis of bacterial infections, as there are for viral infections and toxoplasmosis. Most commercial assays depend not only on detection of antibodies (e.g., rubella, herpes simplex, cytomegalovirus), but also of antigens (rotaviruses).

Fluorescent Antibody (FA) Techniques

Fluorescence microscopy methods can be divided into direct techniques, in which the label (fluorochrome) is linked to the specific antibody, and indirect (also called double sandwich), in which the label is attached to the antiglobulin antibody. Direct procedures require only one incubation step, the interaction of antigen and antibody. Indirect procedures require two incubation steps; however, a single labeled antiglobulin antibody can be used for a number of procedures (same as in double sandwich ELISA). The indirect procedure may also be used for the detection and titration of unknown antibodies. The union of labeled antibody and antigen results in a product that fluoresces when ultraviolet light passes through it, and the reaction can be observed in a specially equipped microscope (see Chap. 2).

The most common current applications of direct FA are in presumptive identification of group A streptococci[62] and *L. pneumophila*.[63] Specimens are either smears prepared from infected body fluids or tissue sections. Other bacteria that can be indentified by FA in some laboratories include *H. influenzae, Leptospira, Neisseria gonorrhoeae* and *meningitidis, Bacteroides fragilis* and other *Bacteroides* species, *Brucella, Listeria, Bordetella pertussis, Yersinia pestis*, and *Francisella tularensis*.[64, 65] Detection of *B*.

TABLE 9–3.—APPLICATION OF ELISA IN
DIAGNOSIS OF BACTERIAL INFECTIONS:
ANTIBODY & ANTIGEN DETECTION

ANTIBODY DETECTION	REFERENCES
Salmonella sp.	32, 33
Hemophilus influenzae	34
Brucella abortus	35, 36
Bordetella pertussis	37
Escherichia coli	38
Yersinia enterocolitica	35
Treponema pallidum	39
Clostridium tetani	40
Tuberculosis	41
Neisseria meningitidis	42, 43
Rickettsia prowazekii and typhi	44
Rochalimaea (Rickettsia) quintana	45
Vibrio cholerae	32, 46
Neisseria gonorrhoeae	47
Chlamydia psittaci	48
Klebsiella pneumoniae	49
Legionella pneumophila	50
Streptococcal (M protein)	51
Corynebacterium diphtheriae	52
Francisella tularensis	53

ANTIGEN DETECTION	REFERENCES
Y. enterocolitica	35
E. coli enterotoxin	54
N. meningitidis	55
Streptococcus pneumoniae	55
Hemophilus influenzae	55, 56
L. pneumophila	57, 58
B. abortus	35
S. typhi	59
Staphylococcus enterotoxin A	60
V. cholera	61

fragilis is one of the more important current uses of indirect FA, as it may help in antibiotic selection.[64]

The most widely employed FA method for antibody detection in bacteriology is the Fluorescent Treponemal Antibody-Absorbed Test (FTA-ABS) for syphilis[66] and the indirect FA test for Legionnaires' disease.[63]

RIA

Radioimmunoassay is based on the competitive binding of radiolabeled antigen (ligand) and various dilutions of nonreactive test antigen for a limited number of antibody binding sites. Since the amount of labeled antigen in the mixture is known, the amount of test antigen present may be calculated. This method is similar to competitive ELISA. A number of variants of RIA exist, including an inhibition method, in which antibody is labeled and bound competitively by ligands fixed to a solid-phase substrate and by test antigen. This variant is similar to indirect or inhibition ELISA. There are also radiometric assays for detecting antibody. These may be competitive or direct.

RIA has received its widest application in studies of hepatitis B antigens and their corresponding antibodies.[67] RIA has been used in the diagnosis of the following bacterial infections: *Vibrio cholerae*, streptococcal, *P. aeruginosa*, *M. tuberculosis*, *E. coli*, *Fusobacterium polymorphum*, *N. gonorrhoeae* and *meningitidis*, *Staphylococcus*, and clostridial.[68]

For reasons of convenience and economy, RIA is rapidly giving way to ELISA in the diagnosis of infections.

Immune Adherence Hemagglutination Test

Even though it was initially described by Japanese workers as early as the 1960s,[69, 70] the immune adherence hemagglutination (IAHA) test has only recently been applied to detection of antigens and antibodies in the United States. IAHA is based on the principle that in the presence of homologous antigens and antibodies, immune complexes form, complement is activated, and the complexes are bound via C3b receptors to primate (including human type O) erythrocytes.[71] After an incubation period of 1–2 hours at room temperature, the resulting hemagglutination pattern is scored (1+ to 4+). Agglutination of 3+ or greater is considered positive. The test is simpler to perform than the traditional CF test, it is 4 to 20 times more sensitive for antibody detection, without suffering in specificity, and results are available in 4 hours, as opposed to the 20 hours or more required for the CF test.

To date, IAHA has been employed in the diagnosis of a number of viral infections, *M. pneumoniae* and *Chlamydia psittaci*.[72] It has not been widely used for direct detection of antigens in body fluids but appears to offer great promise in this regard.

Hemagglutination Inhibition

In this technique, which is somewhat more complex, erythrocytes (frequently pretreated with tannic acid) are coated with an antigen. A homologous antibody is added to the test system. In a positive control reaction, hemagglutination results due to the interaction of specific antibody and antigen-coated erythrocytes. However, if an unknown body fluid containing homologous antigen is added to the reaction mixture, the free antigen will bind the antibodies, and hemagglutination will be diminished or abolished. This is an extremely sensitive technique and has been utilized by Weiner and Young[73] in detection of *Candida* cell wall mannan polysaccharide antigen. Antigenemia was detected in the course of infection in 6 of 19 patients with significant candidiasis. This is encouraging, but the diagnostic yield was low. More recently, ELISA has been successfully used in *Candida* antigen detection.[74]

More Traditional Serologic Methods in Bacteriology

Agglutination and Flocculation

The agglutination test is used to measure antibodies to microorganisms either directly, when whole organisms are agglutinated, or indirectly, when soluble antigens are adsorbed onto inert particulate matter such as charcoal, carmine, bentonite, (tanned) erythrocytes, or latex particles.[75]

The test for agglutinating antibodies is used for two purposes: (1) to screen sera for rapid detection of antibodies in suspected but not proved infections, and (2) to test sera when isolation of the suspected organism is difficult or impossible because of too few organisms in the sample, overgrowth by contaminating organisms, influence of prior therapy, or because the causative agent is generally difficult to culture.

Agglutinating antibody tests have been used in the diagnosis of brucellosis, leptospirosis, tularemia, rickettsia (Weil-Felix reactions, in which strains of *Proteus*, e.g., OX-19, K, 2, have been used as agglutinogens) and salmonellosis. Diagnosis of salmonellosis will be discussed in a separate section. Other than in leptospirosis, where antibody titers may peak in 1–2 weeks, the time to peak antibody titer is generally 3–5 weeks. In most cases, a single titer of 1:80 or 1:160 is considered indicative of infection, but as in all serologic tests, a fourfold or greater change in titer between acute and convalescent specimens is more diagnostic. Because of similarity in antigens, cross reactions may occur, but the antibody titers tend to be highest to the infecting organism.

The flocculation method is similar to agglutination. In this test, antibody causes suspended particles or bacteria to aggregate in relatively large masses, called "floccules."

Neutralization Assay

The neutralization assay is based on the principle that an antibody binding with a toxin (antigen) will prevent its deleterious effect on a living indicator system. Neutralization has been employed for detection of antibodies to toxins as well as for detection of toxins themselves.[75] Because they require living host systems (eggs, animals, cell cultures), are time-consuming, and often yield imprecise results, these assays are not popular and have gradually been replaced by more efficient techniques (CIE, RIA, ELISA). Examples of diseases diagnosed by neutralization of toxins include tetanus, cholera, diphtheria, staphylococcal infections, and, more recently, enterotoxinogenic *E. coli*[76] and *Clostridium difficile*. *Clostridium difficile* diagnosis will be discussed separately.[77]

SPECIFIC APPLICATIONS

Serologic studies have become standard in diagnosing a number of bacterial infections. These are discussed below. In some instances it will be necessary to introduce additional immunodiagnostic methods as they apply specifically to the conditions discussed.

Salmonellosis

Classically, the febrile agglutinin reaction of Widal has been employed in the serological diagnosis of salmonellosis.[78] H and O *Salmonella* antigens are used in an agglutination reaction in a test tube or on a slide to detect agglutinating antibodies. Improvements in techniques for isolating the organisms, as well as a number of variables that have always plagued the test, make this procedure less than optimal. Some of these variables are (1) confusing nomenclature; (2) physicians' lack of understanding of the makeup and interpretation of the test; (3) serofastness and cross reactivity of antibodies (effect of immunization with typhoid vaccine and of unrelated febrile illness, respectively); (4) the test's inherent inability to specifically identify pathogenic strains, for example, *S. typhimurium*, the strain responsible for most cases of salmonella gastroenteritis in the United States; and (5) antibiotic therapy, which may suppress or modify antibody response.

A recent vaccination may affect the antibody level. Particularly influenced is the titer to the H or flagellar antigen. Typical serologic reactions in various clinical conditions associated with salmonellosis are listed in Ta-

TABLE 9–4.—Typhoidal Serologic Reactions

REACTION	O TITER*	H TITER†
Normal	< 1:80	< 1:80
Present infection	≥ 1:80 (4+) and	≥ 1:80 (4+)
Past infection	< 1:80	≥ 1:80 (4+)
Recent vaccination	< 1:80	≥ 1:80 (4+)
Carrier	< 1:80	≥ 1:80 (4+)

*On serology slip generally referred to as "*Salmonella* group D."
†On serology slip generally referred to as "Typhoid H."

ble 9–4. Generally, a single titer of 1:160 to the O or somatic antigen, or a fourfold or greater rise in titer indicates acute infection. The Widal reaction lacks specificity. Both the O and H antigens, as employed in commercially available kits, are shared by a number of strains of *Salmonella*. Cross reactions can therefore occur not only between strains of *Salmonella*, but also between *Salmonella* and *Brucella* or *F. tularensis*. ELISA and COAG assays that use antibody (IgM) and antigen detection are being developed for the diagnosis of *Salmonella* infections, and they (or similar newer techniques) will undoubtedly replace the agglutinin reaction.

Syphilis

The serologic diagnosis of syphilis has traditionally depended on detection of reaginic antibodies to mammalian cardiolipin, followed by a confirmatory test of specific antitreponemal antibodies. Various assays had been used over the years, and many, such as the Wasserman and Kahn assays, are of historical interest only. Assays in current use are the Venereal Disease Research Laboratory (VDRL) test and the FTA-ABS for reaginic and antitreponemal antibodies, respectively. Much clinical and epidemiologic information about the natural course of syphilis has accrued based on the results of serologic assays, and most of the material presented in this section is based on results of the VDRL and FTA-ABS. It should be pointed out, however, that many laboratories have switched to another set of assays because of greater simplicity and lower costs without loss of specificity and sensitivity. These are the Rapid Reagin (RPR) card test,[79, 80] which replaces VDRL, and the microhemagglutination test for *Treponema pallidum* (MHA-TP), which replaces the FTA-ABS.[81]

In the RPR test, serum is mixed on a card with a suspension of specifically prepared RPR antigen-charcoal particles. After the mixture is rotated for 8 minutes, the resulting macroscopic coagglutination is read immediately and graded as reactive, minimally reactive, or nonreactive. By contrast, VDRL requires venous blood, a heat inactivation period of 30 minutes, antigen dilution, and microscopic visualization of clumping. The agreement between the two tests is 98.5%; however, the RPR is slightly more sensitive. In one study, the overall reactivity of RPR on 63,803 specimens was 7.9% whereas the overall reactivity of VDRL was 6.6%.[82] Thus, RPR would detect more cases, particularly of the late latent type. If results are reported in terms of titers, RPR titers are twofold to fourfold higher than comparable VDRL titers. These differences must be kept in mind when interpreting results of serum titers obtained longitudinally and which initially were reported in terms of the VDRL and subsequently in terms of the RPR. A spurious rise in titer could be misinterpreted as indicating relapse, reactivation, or reinfection of syphilis.

The MHA-TP is based on agglutination of sensitized sheep erythrocytes by antibodies to *T. pallidum*. Before the test is performed, the serum sample is mixed with absorbing diluent (Reiter treponeme protein) to remove most nonspecific reactants. Serum containing the specific antibody will react with the sensitized sheep RBCs, which are coated with *T. pallidum* antigen (Nichol's strain) to form a smooth mat of agglutinated cells in the well of the microtitration tray. Negative reactions are characterized by a ringlike pattern formed by the settling of nonagglutinated cells. Even though the overall agreement between FTA-ABS and MHA-TP has been reported to be between 96.1% and 99%, MHA-TP may be less sensitive in cases of untreated primary syphilis.[81, 83] As with the FTA-ABS, sera from patients with conditions characterized by dysgammaglobulinemia (autoimmune diseases, infectious mononucleosis, drug addiction) may give false positive results. These false positives due to heterophile antibodies can be resolved by determining whether a serum's titer against sensitized cells is at least two doubling dilutions higher than its titer against unsensitized cells. Overall, however, MHA-TP may be slightly less specific for syphilis than the FTA-ABS test.[84]

In some cases there may be reason to suspect that both the reaginic and treponemal antibody test results are false positive. An accurate diagnosis can then be made by using the standard test of specificity in syphilis serology, the *T. pallidum* immobilization (TPI) test. Because the TPI requires detection of antibodies that decrease the motility of live *T. pallidum,* it is available in only a few research laboratories.[85]

One of the most frequent queries received by infectious disease specialists is what to do with a patient who has positive serologic test results for syphilis. It may be worthwhile, therefore, to review the clinical course of syphilis in relation to the reaginic and antitreponemal tests for syphilis. Figure 9–1 correlates the natural course of untreated syphilis with serologic findings. During the early stages of primary syphilis, the VDRL may be negative. However, toward the end of the fourth week of primary syphilis or in the early stage of secondary (disseminated) syphilis, the VDRL will be positive in virtually 100% of the cases. Because of time lag between onset of disease and serologic test confirmation, the most important diagnostic tool in early syphilis is the darkfield examination for *T. pallidum.*[85] During the secondary stage, or at about 4–6 weeks following the primary stage, the VDRL should reach its peak titer—somewhere between 1:64 and 1:256. The late stage, both clinical (neurologic, cardiovascular) and latent, starts 1 year after infection. The diagnosis is made by serologic studies and a history of primary or secondary syphilis.

It is important to note that in approximately one third of untreated patients, the VDRL will eventually become negative, in one third it will re-

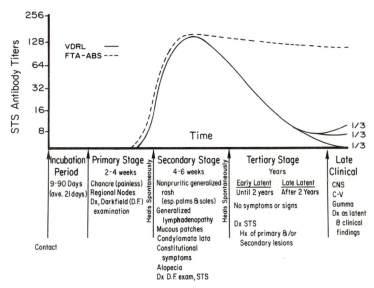

CLINICAL COURSE OF UNTREATED SYPHILIS

Fig 9–1.—Relationship of serologic studies to clinical course of untreated syphilis. (Reproduced by permission, from Crespo J.H., Rytel M.W.: Venereal Diseases. *American Family Physician,* August, 1978.)

main positive, but at a low titer or in undiluted serum samples only, and in one third it may remain elevated. The FTA-ABS will remain positive for a lifetime, despite adequate early therapy, and therefore it need not be repeated.

What happens to the VDRL reaction in adequately treated syphilis? If syphilis is treated in the primary stage, more than 95% of the patients become seronegative in 6–18 months. If treatment is instituted during the secondary stage, the percentage of seronegative patients will be somewhat lower—76%, and it may take up to 2 years for the titers to drop. However, if syphilis is treated in the late stage, less than one half of the patients will become seronegative. These patients are referred to as being "serofast." The VDRL titer, however, should remain quite low (≤1:8). An elevated titer or a rise in titer suggests disease activity; this may be due to reinfection, reactivation, or inadequate therapy.

Table 9–5 summarizes recommendations as to whether to treat patients or not, depending on the results of VDRL and the specific FTA-ABS tests, as well as the history of previous therapy.

Spinal tap is always recommended in late syphilis (because serum-CSF dissociation in reaginic activity is known in neurosyphilis). It should be

TABLE 9–5.—DECISIONS ON THERAPY FOR PATIENTS WITH POSITIVE SEROLOGIC
TESTS FOR SYPHILIS

VDRL (SERUM)	FTA-ABS	VDRL TITER	PREVIOUS THERAPY	THERAPY
Positive	Positive	≥ 1:8	None or unknown	Yes
			Documented; > 6 mo. previously	Yes
			Documented; < 6 mo. previously	No*
Positive	Positive	< 1:8	None or unknown	Yes
			Documented; any time	No†
Positive	Negative	Any	Irrelevant	No

*VDRL should be repeated every 3 to 6 months; if there is no fall in titer in 6 to 12 months, the patient should be retreated.
†Spinal tap should be done since the cerebrospinal fluid may be positive.

mentioned, however, that in some 60 pairs of CSF and serum samples from patients with late latent syphilis and low serum VDRL levels, we have to date found none with positive CSF VDRL (data to be reported). The last condition listed in Table 9–5, in which the VDRL is positive and FTA-ABS negative, represents a biologic false positive reaction. This is associated with conditions accompanied by dysgammaglobulinemias, such as collagen diseases.

Finally, it should be pointed out that although reaginic antibody tests should be done first, and only if they are positive should the confirmatory treponemal antibody test be requested, there are two situations in which if the index of suspicion for syphilis is high enough, one should request the treponemal antibody test even if the reaginic antibody tests were negative. These are early syphilis, in which treponemal antibodies may be elevated before reaginic ones are, and late syphilis, in which reaginic antibodies may fall to a level undetectable by VDRL but the antitreponemal antibody test is still positive.[83]

Staphylococcal Infections

Staphyloccus aureus continues to account for a significant proportion of infections in hospitalized patients. The spectrum of staphylococcal disease varies from the usually uncomplicated, superficial, suppurative infection to deep tissue infection of various organ systems. The latter is frequently associated with high morbidity and mortality. Diagnosis of staphylococcal infection may be difficult to establish, particularly in partially treated patients. Also, the seriousness of infection, which may vary between endocarditis and transient bacteremia, may be impossible to assess with certainty. Detection of precipitin antibodies against staphylococcal cell wall component teichoic acid in patients with staphylococcal endocarditis has been reported utilizing double immunodiffusion techniques and CIE[86, 87] and may be of diagnostic aid.

Although less specific than when they are used to detect microbial antigens, double immunodiffusion and CIE can be applied in situations where the amount of antigen in body fluids is below the sensitivity of the methods, or where other methods of antibody determination (such as CF) are not available. Wheat and White have summarized results of a number of diagnostic studies employing double immunodiffusion and CIE (Table 9–6).[88] It is obvious that there is much overlap in antibody detection rates. In a study by Jackson et al., titration of staphylococcal antibodies by CIE was of help in differentiating deep-seated staphylococcal infections, including endocarditis, from less serious infections.[89] All patients with staphylococcal endocarditis (5/5) and with deep tissue infection (pneumonia, abscesses; 22/22) tested by CIE had antistaphylococcal antibodies. All patients with endocarditis had antibodies in their initial specimens, which were obtained within a few days of admission, whereas only 18/22 patients (82%) with deep tissue infections had antibodies detected in their initial specimens. In the 4 remaining patients, sera which were negative on the initial examination were positive by the tenth hospital day. Thus, in most cases in these groups, there was suggestive evidence of a staphylococcal infection on the basis of the initial CIE study. In the group with endocarditis, all patients had an antibody titer of 1:4 or higher, whereas in the group with deep tissue infection, 88% of the patients had such a titer. Thus, it is impossible to distinguish patients with these two conditions on the basis of CIE results, even when titers are obtained.

In the other groups of patients, such as those with superficial infections or transient bacteremia, a smaller percentage had detectable antistaphylococcal antibody; titers of these antibodies were almost uniformly less than

TABLE 9–6.—TEICHOIC ACID ANTIBODY DETECTION RATES BY DID AND CIE IN VARIOUS STAPHYLOCOCCAL CONDITIONS*

	DID		CIE	
CONDITION	No. Tested	% Positive	No. Tested	% Positive
Endocarditis	144	88	70	98
Bacteremia without endocarditis	210	41	111	59
Infections without bacteremia	68	26	25	48
Bone and joint infections	93	38	. . .	. . .
Subjects without infection	389	5	249	5
Subjects with nonstaphylococcal infections	241	6	113	4

*DID, double immunodiffusion; CIE, counterimmunoelectrophoresis. Table adapted from Wheat and White.[88]

1:4. Only 4 of 90 control subjects (without staphylococcal infections) had detectable antibodies of low titers (< 1:4).

Based on observations such as these, Tuazon and Sheagren[90] devised an algorithm to help in therapeutic decision-making in patients with *S. aureus* bacteremia. Briefly, in patients with no clinical evidence of endocarditis and no detectable teichoic acid antibodies on admission and at 2 weeks, therapy should be terminated at 2 weeks, particularly if the source of bacteremia, such as an infected intravenous catheter, can be identified and removed. By contrast, in patients with a high titer or a rise in titer, therapy should be continued for 4 weeks (no metastatic foci) or 6 weeks (metastatic foci present). In our own experience, we have seen a significant rise in antibody titer in a number of patients with endocarditis who were followed longitudinally (Table 9–7). Consequently, we have adopted Tuazon's approach in our clinic and have achieved good results, although in a small number of patients.

Streptococcal Infections

The traditional serologic tests employed to diagnose group A streptococcal infections consist of antibody assays directed against enzymes produced by streptococci in the course of the infection. These assays are helpful only retrospectively and are employed in the assessment of poststreptococcal sequelae, such as rheumatic fever and glomerulonephritis. Among these tests, the most useful ones have been antistreptolysin-O (ASO), antihyaluronidase (AH), antistreptokinase (ASK), antideoxyribonuclease-B (anti-DNase-B), and the streptozyme test. The ASO assay is based on the observation that during streptococcal infection, a hemolysin, streptolysin-O, is

TABLE 9–7.—Serial Teichoic
Acid Antibody Titers by CIE in
a Patient With Endocarditis

HOSPITAL DAY	TITER
5	1:1
7	1:8
9	1:8
12	1:8
20	1:16
28	1:32
35	1:32
42	1:16
49	1:8
56	1:8
63	1:8
93	1:8

produced that stimulates development of neutralizing antibodies. When such antibodies interact with streptolysin-O in vitro, an antigen-antibody reaction takes place, streptolysin (added in standard amount) is neutralized, and fewer RBCs are lysed. The degree of hemolysis is measured spectrophotometrically. Depending on the laboratory, the normal ASO levels are taken to be approximately 150 Todd units or 200 IU/ml.

The AH test measures the degree of inhibition of a standard amount of hyaluronidase by antibodies in the patient's serum. The amount of remaining hyaluronidase is determined by its ability to hydrolyze potassium hyaluronate. The titer is the reciprocal of the highest dilution showing a clot formation in vitro. Normal levels are less than 1:500.

In the ASK test, sheep RBCs coated with a mixture of streptokinase and streptodornase are agglutinated by antibody in serially diluted serum. Normal levels are 1:640 or below. The anti-DNase-B assay commences with inactivation of patient's serum to remove native DNase. The serum is then diluted and reacted with a standard amount of DNase antigen, and the reaction mixture is incubated to allow antibody to combine with antigen. When a DNA substrate is added, nonneutralized DNA will form a mucin-like clot. Polymerized DNA is detected with one of several reagents, depending on the system used. Normal titers are approximately 150 units or less.

One of the more recent additions to the streptococcal antibody assay armamentarium is the streptozyme test. The reagents in this test consist of aldehyde-stabilized sheep RBCs sensitized with extracellular products (containing the enzymes that are used in individual tests described above, plus additional enzymes) obtained from broth supernates of group A streptococcal cultures. Sera in various dilutions are mixed with a standard volume of the reagent on a glass slide. Following a 2-minute agitation, the highest dilution giving a definite agglutination is taken as the streptozyme titer. Normal titers are less than 1:100.

The various tests usually reach their peak titers in 2–4 weeks following the infection and may remain elevated for several months. In streptococcal pharyngitis, the ASO test is "positive" (i.e., diagnostically elevated) in 78% of infections; if the ASO is combined with two other assays, such as AH and ASK, the ratio of positivity will become 95%.[91] In skin infections, by contrast, only 25% of patients develop an elevated ASO titer, and one must depend on a test such as anti-DNase-B, which has been reported to be positive in 60% of patients with poststreptococcal glomerulonephritis.[88]

Bisno and Ofek reported that the streptozyme test was positive in titers of 400 or higher in acute sera from virtually all patients with acute rheumatic fever (20/20), acute glomerulonephritis (21/22), convalescent streptococcal pharyngitis (10/11), and pyoderma (21/22). The test was positive in low titer in 25% of patients with a variety of nonstreptococcal illnesses.[92]

Useful as these tests are for detecting streptococcal antibodies, they are helpful only retrospectively in diagnosing streptococcal infections. Attempts have, therefore, been made to develop immunologic assays which could be employed in diagnosing acute streptococcal infections by detection of antigens in clinical specimens obtained by throat swabs or scrapings, either directly or after a short incubation period in vitro. Some of these methods are listed in Table 9–8. In order to be useful, these tests must provide results more rapidly than throat culture on sheep blood agar plate (BAP) coupled with the bacitracin disk inhibition of group A streptococci, which provides results in 48 hours or less. Also, they must have the specificity of the Lancefield method of identifying streptococcal antigens. This method entails a number of steps. A throat swab is plated on a BAP and incubated overnight. Any β-hemolytic streptococci identified morphologically are then inoculated into a Todd-Hewitt (T-H) broth and incubated overnight. The streptococci are harvested and group antigen is extracted from the bacteria, usually by hot hydrochloride treatment. The grouping is then completed by a precipitin reaction with specific rabbit antisera in capillary tubes. The assay takes 24–48 hours.

Some of the larger laboratories employ the FA method. The throat swab is immersed into a broth and incubated for several hours. The broth is centrifuged and the pellet is smeared and stained by a group-specific antibody coupled to a fluorochrome. This method takes 2–5 hours and correlates well with throat culture results. However, it does require an experienced microscopist and a fluorescence microscope.[93] The test is limited to group A and B streptococci, for which antisera are commercially available.

In 1973, Edwards and Larson used a combination of autoclaving and enzyme digestion in the extraction of group-specific antigen and substituted for capillary tube precipitation the more sensitive CIE.[94] They cultured the throat swab in 5 ml of T-H broth for 4 hours and then did the extraction and CIE. They reported a 100% correlation in 25 culture-positive throat swabs. This method takes 5–6 hours, and the least number of bacteria needed for the antigen to be detected is 4×10^8/ml.

A new method has recently been proposed which claims to be able to detect as little as one colony (about 10^6 organisms/ml) and takes less than 1 hour.[95] In this method, instead of using a swab cultured in 5 ml of broth, the authors used a small spatula to scrape the throat and tonsils and put the scraping into 20 μl of solution. A nitrous acid was used that is thought to extract more antigen than HCL. This method detected 28 of the 34 culture-positive throat cultures (82%).

Edwards and associates were able to identify soluble group A antigen directly from throat gargle by an LA test, "Streptex, group A" (Wellcome

TABLE 9–8.—MORE RAPID WAYS OF DIRECT IDENTIFICATION OF GROUP A STREPTOCOCCAL INFECTIONS

METHOD	SPECIMEN	CULTURE	ANTIGEN EXTRACTION	TIME TO COMPLETE	SENSITIVITY	COMMENTS
Fluorescent antibody technique[93]	Throat swab	Broth 2–5 hr	Not necessary	2–5 hr	Few bacteria	Requires fluorescence microscopy
CIE[94]	Throat swab	Broth 4 hr	Autoclave 15 minutes, then digestion by pronase B for 2 hr	6.5 hr	$\geq 4 \times 10^8$ bacteria	100% correlation with culture results in 25 specimens
Direct capillary precipitin[95]	Throat scraping	Not necessary	Throat scraping in 20 µl NaNO$_2$, 3 µl glacial acetic acid	30 min	10^6 bacteria, 82% positive	Throat scraping theoretically recovers more bacteria New method of antigen extraction claimed to increase Ag yield Small final volume theoretically increases concentration of antigen in the extract
Latex agglutination ("Streptex, Group A")[96]	Throat gargle	Not necessary	Not necessary	50 min	84% positive	Gargle must be centrifuged and heated Trypsin required to destroy nonspecific agglutinins

Labs). Fifty specimens were tested by culture and directly: 26 were positive by both procedures, 5 by culture only, 3 by LA only, and 19 were negative by both tests.[96]

Legionellosis

In most cases, laboratory diagnosis of Legionnaires' disease has been achieved only retrospectively, by detection of antibody rise by indirect fluorescence antibody (IFA) microscopy. Diagnosis of acute infection is best done by detection of the organism in a body fluid (pleural, transtracheal aspirate, rarely sputum) by direct FA microscopy, but not all laboratories are equipped to perform this test. The organisms can also be isolated on special media (Isovitalex), but the process may take several days. Thus, there is an urgent need to develop rapid but simple means of diagnosis.

One such approach has been to detect antibodies by a simpler procedure than IFA, such as CIE, for example. Recently, Holliday[97] reported that results of CIE and IFA on 22 sera from patients with Legionnaires' disease and 27 sera from healthy control subjects showed 100% correlation and that studies on 75 paired sera from patients with pneumonia of undetermined etiology showed 96.7% correlation. Titers by CIE tended to be low, 1:1 to 1:16, but could be detected by day 10 of infection. Specimens from control subjects had no detectable antibodies.

A more direct diagnostic approach would be detection of antigens. CIE has been tried for this purpose by Smith et al.,[98] but the method, despite certain modifications, was not sensitive enough. In vitro, only 15.6 μg/ml of antigen by carbohydrate content could be detected, compared with detection of as little as 0.01 μg/ml of pneumococcal polysaccharide antigen by the same method.

Interestingly, the antigen, unlike most other polysaccharide antigens, was found to have cathodal migration. No clinical specimens were tested in this study. RIA[99] and ELISA[57, 58] have been used by different investigators to detect *L. pneumophila* antigen in sputum and urine. Both assays appear to be highly specific and sensitive.

In a study by Kohler et al.,[99] urine of all 9 patients with Legionnaires' disease was clearly differentiated from that of 241 control subjects. Antigen was detected as early as 2 days after initiation of therapy and as late as 10 days. There was only one probable false positive reaction. Antigen in the urine was partially characterized. It was stable at 100 C for 30 minutes and was not degraded by trypsin. Its estimated molecular weight was 10,000.

Other investigators using ELISA on more limited populations were also successful in identifying *Legionella* antigen. Tilton[57] found antigen in the urine of a patient with proved Legionnaires' disease, whereas urines from

TABLE 9–9.—TESTS USED IN IMMUNODIAGNOSIS OF LEGIONELLOSIS FROM
CLINICAL SPECIMENS*

TEST	SPECIMEN TYPE	COLLECTION TIME (Days After Onset)	SUBSTANCE DETECTED
IFA[100]	Serum	<7, 21–42	Antibody (IgG, IgM, IgA)†
CIE[97]	Serum	10–182	Antibody‡
ELISA; MAT[50]	Serum	<7, 21–42	Antibody (IgG, IgM, IgA)‡
ELISA[57]	Urine	<7	Antigen‡
ELISA[58]	Urine	<6–<24	Antigen‡
RIA[99]	Urine	<2–10	Antigen‡

*Table adapted from Wilkinson.[101] IFA, indirect fluorescent antibody; CIE, counter immunoelectrophoresis; ELISA, enzyme-linked immunosorbent assay; MAT, microagglutination; RIA, radioimmunoassay.
†Routine.
‡Experimental.

four other patients with suspected but not proved disease were negative. Berdal and associates[58] found antigen in urine from two of three patients with serologically proved legionellosis. Twenty urine specimens from healthy control subjects were negative; no control specimens from patients with other infections were studied.

RIA and ELISA are generally thought to be of the same order of sensitivity. For reasons discussed above, ELISA is considered a superior procedure.[100] Additional studies, employing perhaps amplified modifications of ELISA that would give it even greater sensitivity, are awaited.

The tests used in the serologic diagnosis of legionellosis are summarized in Table 9–9. The serodiagnosis of legionellosis has recently been extensively reviewed by Wilkinson.[101]

Pseudomembranous Colitis

Antibiotic-associated pseudomembranous colitis (APMC) is now recognized as being caused by a toxin of *C. difficile*. The most widely used method for detecting the toxin is a classic neutralization test, whereby the toxin is rendered harmless to indicator cells in culture by preincubation with a cross-reacting antibody to *C. sordellii*.[102]

More recently, several authors reported detection of the toxin by CIE.[103, 104] In the first report, stool culture at 24 hours was required, and the toxin was detected in culture filtrates. In the second study, 50 fecal specimens were tested by three methods—bacterial isolation, CIE, and tissue culture. Ten specimens (20%) were positive by all three methods. An additional eight specimens were toxin positive only by CIE. All 18 patients whose feces contained the toxin showed evidence of enterocolitis, and 17 were positive for *C. difficile* by bacterial isolation.

A word of caution, however, was sounded recently by West and Wilkins,[105] who found that the antitoxins currently used for detection of *C. difficile* by CIE reacted with other *C. difficile* antigens in addition to the toxins produced by the bacterium. These authors recommend that CIE be used as a presumptive test but that the results be confirmed by the cytotoxicity test, which uses antitoxins that specifically neutralize the currently recognized *C. difficile* toxins A and B. Further, they presented data showing that CIE is not sensitive enough to detect toxin A. It is hoped that a more sensitive assay, such as ELISA, could detect the specific antitoxins. A more rapid method than the cell culture assay is needed in APMC.

CONCLUSIONS

The ever expanding application of immunologic techniques in the diagnosis of bacterial infections is gratifying, particularly to the clinicians who have to deal with the all-too-common situation of fever in a patient with no etiologic diagnosis forthcoming from standard microbiologic methods. It is likely that in the future, detection of antigens in body fluids will provide a rapid and accurate etiologic diagnosis in many infectious diseases. This will enable the clinician to employ more specific, narrow-spectrum antimicrobial agents. The results could well mean better survival rates, particularly in immunocompromised patients, as well as reduction in development of resistant strains of bacteria brought on by exposure of these organisms to broad-spectrum antimicrobial agents.

I have stressed two immunodiagnostic methods in this chapter, CIE and ELISA. CIE is already used in many diagnostic laboratories and probably will remain a permanent member of the diagnostic armamentarium. ELISA is only now coming into its own. It is still primarily used in research and reference laboratories. Commercially available kits for the diagnosis of various infections are being developed in increasing numbers. Few, however, are available as yet for antigen detection. Once the technical problems encountered in their development are surmounted, it is likely that ELISA will replace most of the currently employed tests for detection of both antibodies and antigens.

REFERENCES

1. Cherry W.B., Moss C.W.: The role of gas chromatography in the clinical microbiology laboratory. *J. Infect. Dis.* 119:658, 1969.
2. Mitruka B.M., Kundargi R.S., Jonas A.M.: Gas chromatography for rapid differentiation of bacterial infections in man. *Med. Res. Eng.* 11:7, 1972.
3. Brooks J.B., Kellogg D.S., Alley C.C., et al.: Gas chromatography as a potential means of diagnosing arthritis: I. Differentiation between staphylococcal, streptococcal, gonococcal, and traumatic arthritis. *J. Infect. Dis.* 129:660, 1974.

4. Craven R.B., Brooks J.B., Edman D.C., et al.: Rapid diagnosis of lymphocytic meningitis by frequency-pulsed electron capture gas-liquid chromatography: Differentiation of tuberculous, cryptococcal, and viral meningitis. *J. Clin. Microbiol.* 6:27, 1977.
5. Mitruka B.M., Bonner J.J.: *Methods of Detection and Identification of Bacteria.* Cleveland, CRC Press, Inc., 1976.
6. Kronvall G.: A rapid slide-agglutination method for typing pneumococci by means of specific antibody absorbed to protein A-containing staphylococci. *J. Med. Microbiol.* 6:187, 1973.
7. Edwards E.A., Larson G.L.: New method for grouping beta-hemolytic streptococci directly on sheep blood agar plates by coagglutination of specific sensitized protein A-containing staphylococci. *Appl. Microbiol.* 28:972, 1974.
8. Edwards E.A., Hilderbrand R.L.: Method for identifying *Salmonella* and *Shigella* directly from the primary isolation plate by coagglutination of protein A-containing staphylococci sensitized with specific antibody. *J. Clin. Microbiol.* 3:339, 1976.
9. Suksanong M., Dajani A.S.: Detection of *Haemophilus influenzae* type b antigens in body fluids, using specific antibody-coated staphylococci. *J. Clin. Microbiol.* 5:81, 1977.
10. Thirumoorthi M.D., Dajani A.S.: Comparison of staphylococcal coagglutination, latex agglutination and counterimmunoelectrophoresis for bacterial antigen detection. *J. Clin. Microbiol.* 9:28, 1979.
11. Edwards E.A., Coonrod J.D.: Coagglutination and counterimmunoelectrophoresis for detection of pneumococcal antigens in the sputum of pneumonia patients. *J. Clin. Microbiol.* 11:488, 1980.
12. Sanborn W.R., Lesmann M., Edwards E.A.: Enrichment culture co-agglutination test for rapid, low-cost diagnosis of salmonellosis. *J. Clin. Microbiol.* 12:151, 1980.
13. Smith L.P., Fischer G.W.: Rapid detection of bacterial antigen in false negative blood culture bottles by modified co-agglutination test, in *21st Conference on Antimicrobial Agents and Chemotherapy.* Chicago, American Society for Microbiology, 1981, abstract No. 266.
14. Bloomfield N., Gordon M.A., Elmendorf D.F. Jr.: Detection of *Cryptococcus neoformans* antigen in body fluids by latex particle agglutination. *Proc. Soc. Exp. Biol. Med.* 114:64, 1963.
15. Bennett J.E., Hasenclever H.F., Tynes B.S.: Detection of cryptococcal polysaccharide in serum and spinal fluid: Value in diagnosis and prognosis. *Trans. Assoc. Am. Physicians* 77:145, 1964.
16. Gordon M.A., Vedder D.K.: Serologic tests in diagnosis and prognosis of cryptococcosis. *JAMA* 197:961, 1966.
17. Goodman J.S., Kaufman L., Koenig M.G.: Diagnosis of cryptococcal meningitis: Value of immunologic detection of cryptococcal antigen. *N. Engl. J. Med.* 285:434, 1971.
18. Newman R.B., Stevens R.W., Gaafar H.A.: Latex agglutination test for the diagnosis of *Haemophilus influenzae* meningitis. *J. Lab. Clin. Med.* 76:107, 1970.
19. Severin W.P.J.: Latex agglutination in the diagnosis of meningococcal meningitis. *J. Lab. Clin. Med.* 25:1079, 1972.
20. Coonrod J.D., Drennan D.P.: Pneumococcal pneumonia: Capsular polysaccharide antigenemia and antibody responses. *Ann. Intern. Med.* 84:254, 1976.

21. Coonrod J.D., Rytel M.W.: Determination of aetiology of bacterial meningitis by counterimmunoelectrophoresis. *Lancet* 1:1154, 1972.

22. Finch C.A., Wilkinson H.W.: Practical considerations in using counterimmunoelectrophoresis to identify the principal causative agents of bacterial meningitis. *J. Clin. Microbiol.* 10:519, 1979.

23. Feldman W.E.: Relation of concentrations of bacteria and bacterial antigen in cerebrospinal fluid to prognosis in patients with bacterial meningitis. *N. Engl. J. Med.* 296:433, 1977.

24. Perlino C.A., Shulman J.A.: Detection of pneumococcal polysaccharide in the sputum of patients with pneumococcal pneumonia by counterimmunoelectrophoresis. *J. Lab. Clin. Med.* 87:496, 1976.

25. Miller J.: Diagnosis of pneumococcal pneumonia by antigen detection in sputum. *J. Clin. Microbiol.* 7:459, 1978.

26. Leach R.P., Coonrod J.D.: Detection of pneumococcal antigens in the sputum in pneumococcal pneumonia. *Am. Rev. Respir. Dis.* 116:847, 1977.

27. McCracken G.H. Jr., Sarff L.D., Glode M.P., et al.: Relation between *Escherichia coli* K1 capsular polysaccharide antigen and clinical outcome in neonatal meningitis. *Lancet* 2:246, 1974.

28. Rytel M.W.: Counterimmunoelectrophoresis in diagnosis of infectious diseases. *Hosp. Pract.* 10:75, 1975.

29. Edwards E.A.: Counterimmunoelectrophoresis and double immunodiffusion, in Rytel M.W. (ed.): *Rapid Diagnosis in Infectious Diseases.* Boca Raton, Fla., CRC Press, 1979, pp. 19–37.

30. Tuazon C.U., Sheagren J.N., Choa M.S., et al.: *Staphylococcus aureus* bacteremia: Relationship between formation of antibodies to teichoic acid and development of metastatic abscesses. *J. Infect. Dis.* 137:57, 1978.

31. Schuurs A.H.W.M., Van Weemen B.K.: Enzyme immunoassay. *Clin. Chim. Acta* 81:1, 1977.

32. Beasley W.J., Joseph S.W., Weiss E.: Improved serodiagnosis of *Salmonella* enteric fevers by enzyme-linked immunosorbent assay. *J. Clin. Microbiol.* 13:106, 1981.

33. Lentsch R.H., Batema R.P., Wagner J.E.: Detection of *Salmonella* infections by polyvalent enzyme-linked immunosorbent assay. *J. Clin. Microbiol.* 14:281, 1981.

34. Dahlberg T., Branefors P.: Enzyme-linked immunosorbent assay for titration of *Haemophilus influenzae* capsular and O antigen antibodies. *J. Clin. Microbiol.* 12:185, 1980.

35. Carlsson H.E., Hurvell B., Lindberg A.A.: Enzyme-linked immunosorbent (ELISA) for titration of antibodies against *Brucella abortus* and *Yersinia enterocolitica. Acta Pathol. Microbiol. Scand.* [C] 84:168, 1976.

36. Saunders G.C., Clinard E.H., Bartlett M.L., et al.: Application of the indirect enzyme-labeled antibody microtest to the detection and surveillance of animal diseases. *J. Infect. Dis.* 136(Suppl.):S-258, 1977.

37. Goodman Y.E., Wort A.J., Jackson F.L.: Enzyme-linked immunosorbent assay for detection of pertussis immunoglobulin A in nasopharyngeal secretions as an indicator of recent infection. *J. Clin. Microbiol.* 13:286, 1981.

38. Smith J., Holmgren J., Ahlstedt S., et al.: Local antibody production in experimental pyelonephritis: Amount, avidity, and immunoglobulin class. *Infect. Immun.* 10:411, 1974.

39. Veldkamp J., Visser A.M.: Application of the enzyme-linked immunosorbent

assay (ELISA) in the serodiagnosis of syphilis. *Br. J. Vener. Dis.* 51:227, 1975.

40. Stiffler-Rosenberg G., Fey H.: Messung von Tetanus-Antitoxin mit dem Enzyme Linked Immunosorbent Assay (ELISA). *Schweiz. Med. Wochenschr.* 107:1101, 1977.

41. Nassau E., Parsons E.R., Johnson G.D.: The detection of antibodies to *Mycobacterium tuberculosis* by microplate enzyme-linked immunosorbent assay (ELISA). *Tubercle* 57:67, 1976.

42. Sippel J.E., Mamay H.K., Weiss E., et al.: Outer membrane protein antigens in an enzyme linked immunosorbent assay for *Salmonella* enteric fever and miningococcal meningitis. *J. Clin. Microbiol.* 7:372, 1978.

43. Basta M.T., Russell H., Guirguis N.I., et al.: Enzyme-linked immunosorbent assay for determination of human antibodies to group C meningococcal polysaccharide. *Proc. Soc. Exp. Biol. Med.* 169:7, 1982.

44. Halle S., Dasch G.A., Weiss E.: Sensitive enzyme-linked immunosorbent assay for detection of antibodies against typhus *Rickettsiae*, *Rickettsia prowazekki* and *Rickettsia typhi*. *J. Clin. Microbiol.* 6:101, 1977.

45. Herrmann J.E., Hollingdale M.R., Collins M.F., et al.: Enzyme immunoassay and radioimmunoprecipitation tests for the detection of antibodies to *Rochalimaea* (Rickettsia) *quintana*. *Proc. Soc. Exp. Biol. Med.* 154:285, 1977.

46. Holmgren J., Svennerholm A.M.: ELISA for the study of entertoxic diarrhoel diseases. *Scand. J. Immunol.* 8(suppl. 7):111, 1978.

47. Brodeur B.R., Fraser E.A., Diena B.B.: Enzyme-linked immunosorbent assays for the detection of *Neisseria gonorrhoeae* specific antibodies. *Can. J. Microbiol.* 24:1300, 1978.

48. Lewis V.J., Thacker W.L., Mitchell S.H.: Enzyme-linked immunosorbent assay for chlamydial antibodies. *J. Clin. Microbiol.* 6:507, 1977.

49. Rissing J.P., Buxton T.B., Moore W.L. III, et al.: Enzyme linked immunospecific antibody test for detecting antibody to *Klebsiella*. *J. Clin. Microbiol.* 8:704, 1978.

50. Farshy C.E., Klein G.C., Feeley J.C.: Detection of antibodies to Legionnaires' disease organism by microagglutination and micro enzyme-linked immunosorbent assay tests. *J. Clin. Microbiol.* 7:327, 1978.

51. Russell H., Facklam R.R., Edwards L.R.: Enzyme-linked immunosorbent assay for streptococcal M protein antibodies. *J. Clin. Microbiol.* 3:501, 1976.

52. Svenson S.B., Larsen K.: An ELISA for the determination of diphtheria toxin antibodies. *J. Immunol. Methods* 17:249, 1977.

53. Carlsson H.E., Lindberg A.A., Lindberg G., et al.: Enzyme-linked immunosorbent assay for immunological diagnosis of human tularemia. *J. Clin. Microbiol.* 10:615, 1979.

54. Yolken R.H., Greenberg H.B., Merson M.H., et al.: Enzyme-linked immunosorbent assay for detection of *Escherichia coli* heat-labile enterotoxin. *J. Clin. Microbiol.* 6:439, 1977.

55. Beuvery E.C., Van Rossum F., Lauwers S., et al.: Comparison of counterimmunoelectrophoresis and ELISA for diagnosis of bacterial meningitis. *Lancet* 1:208, 1979.

56. Crosson F.J., Winkelstein J.A., Moxon E.R.: Enzyme linked immunosorbent assay for detection and quantitation of capsular antigen of *Haemophilus influenzae* type b. *Infect. Immun.* 22:617, 1978.

57. Tilton R.C.: Legionnaires' disease antigen detected by enzyme-linked immunosorbent assay. *Ann. Intern. Med.* 90:697, 1979.

58. Berdal B.P., Farshey C.E., Feeley J.C.: Detection of *Legionella pneumophila* antigen in urine by enzyme-linked immunospecific assay. *J. Clin. Microbiol.* 9:575, 1979.

59. Carlsson H.E., Lindberg A.A.: Application of ELISA for the diagnosis of bacterial infections, in Chang T.M.S. (ed.): *Biomedical Application of Immobilized Enzymes and Proteins.* New York, Plenum Press, 1977, vol. 2., p. 97.

60. Saunders G.C., Bartlett M.L.: Double antibody solid phase enzyme immunoassay for the detection of staphylococcal enterotoxin A. *Appl. Environ. Microbiol.* 34:518, 1977.

61. Holmgren J., Svennerholm A.M.: Enzyme-linked immunosorbent assays for cholera serology. *Infect. Immun.* 7:759, 1973.

62. Jones G.L., Herbert G.A., Cherry W.B.: *Fluorescent Antibody Techniques and Bacterial Applications.* Atlanta, Centers for Disease Control, November 1977.

63. Jones G.L., Herbert G.A. (eds.): *"Legionnaires" Disease, the Bacterium and Methodology.* Atlanta, Centers for Disease Control, October 1978.

64. Anhalt J.P.: Fluorescent antibody procedures and counterimmunoelectrophoresis, in Washington J.A. (ed.): *Laboratory Procedures in Clinical Microbiology.* New York, Springer-Verlag, 1981, pp. 249–277.

65. Kawamura A. Jr.: *Fluorescent Antibody Techniques and Their Application,* ed. 2. Baltimore, Md., University Park Press, 1977.

66. Dercon W.E., Lucas J.B., Price E.V.: Fluorescent treponemal antibody absorption (FTA-ABS) test for syphilis. *JAMA* 198:624, 1966.

67. Ling C.M., Overby L.R.: Prevalence of hepatitis B virus antigen as revealed by direct immune assay with ^{125}I-antibody. *J. Immunol.* 109:834, 1972.

68. Overby L.R., Mushahwar I.K.: Radioimmune assays, in Rytel M.W. (ed.): *Rapid Diagnosis in Infectious Disease.* Boca Raton, Fla., CRC Press, 1979, pp. 39–69.

69. Ito M., Tagaya I.: Immune adherence haemagglutination test as a new sensitive method for titration of animal virus antigens and antibodies. *Jpn. J. Med. Sci. Biol.* 19:109, 1966.

70. Mayumi M., Okochi K., Nishioka K.: Detection of Australia antigen by means of immune adherence haemagglutination test. *Vox Sang.* 20:178, 1971.

71. Nelson D.S.: Immune adherence. *Adv. Immunol.* 3:131, 1963.

72. Lennette E.T., Lennette D.A.: Immune adherence hemagglutination: Alternative to complement-fixation serology. *J. Clin. Microbiol.* 7:282, 1978.

73. Weiner M.H., Young W.J.: Mannan antigenemia in the diagnosis of invasive *Candida* infections. *J. Clin. Invest.* 58:1045, 1976.

74. Lew M.A., Siber G.R., Danahue D.M., et al.: Enhanced detection with enzyme-linked immunosorbent assay of *Candida* mannan in antibody-containing serum after heat extraction. *J. Infect. Dis.* 145:45, 1982.

75. Palmer D.F.: Serologic procedures, in Balows A., Hausler W.J. (eds.): *Diagnostic Procedures for Bacterial, Mycotic and Parasitic Infections,* ed. 6. Washington, D.C., American Public Health Association, 1981, pp. 75–88.

76. Gorbach S.L., Khurana C.M.: Toxigenic *Escherichia coli.* *N. Engl. J. Med.* 287:791, 1973.

77. Bartlett J.G., Chang T.W., Gurwith M., et al.: Antibiotic-associated pseudomembranous colitis due to toxin producing clostridia. *N. Engl. J. Med.* 298:531, 1978.

78. Freter R.: Agglutinin titration (Widal) for the diagnosis of enteric fever and

other enterobacterial infections, in Rose N.R., Friedman H. (eds.): *Manual of Clinical Immunology*. Washington, D.C., American Society for Microbiology, 1976, pp. 285–288.

79. Portnoy J., Brewer J.H., Harris A.: Rapid plasma reagin card test for syphilis and other treponematoses. *Public Health Rep.* 77:645, 1962.

80. Portnoy J.: Modification of the rapid plasma reagin card test for syphilis for use in large scale testing. *Am. J. Clin. Pathol.* 40:473, 1963.

81. Logan L.C., Cox P.M.: Evaluation of a quantitative automated microhemagglutination assay for antibodies to *Treponema pallidum. Am. J. Clin. Pathol.* 53:163, 1970.

82. Reed E.L.: Rapid reagin tests in the public health laboratory RPR card test. *J. Conf. Public Health Laboratory Directors* 27:8, 1969.

83. Johnston N.A.: *Treponema pallidum* haemagglutination test for syphilis: Evaluation of a modified micro-method. *Br. J. Vener. Dis.* 48:474, 1972.

84. Lesinski J., Krach J., Kadziewicz E.: Specificity, sensitivity, and diagnostic value of the TPHA test. *Br. J. Vener. Dis.* 50:334, 1974.

85. Jaffe H.W.: The laboratory diagnosis of syphilis. *Ann. Intern. Med.* 83:846, 1975.

86. Crowder J.G., White A.: Teichoic acid antibodies in staphylococcal and non-staphylococcal endocarditis. *Ann. Intern. Med.* 77:87, 1972.

87. Nagel J.G., Tuazon C.U., Cardella T.A., et al.: Teichoic acid serologic diagnosis of staphylococcal endocarditis. *Ann. Intern. Med.* 82:13, 1975.

88. Wheat L.J., White A.C.: Rapid diagnosis of staphylococcal infections, in Rytel M.W. (ed.): *Rapid Diagnosis in Infectious Disease.* Boca Raton, Fla., CRC Press, 1979, pp. 115–130.

89. Jackson L.J., Sotille M.I., Aguilar-Torres F.G., et al.: Correlation of antistaphylococcal antibody titers with severity of staphylococcal disease. *Ann. Intern. Med.* 64:629, 1978.

90. Tuazon C.U., Sheagren J.N.: Teichoic acid antibodies in the diagnosis of serious infections with *Staphylococcus aureus. Ann. Intern. Med.* 84:543, 1976.

91. Stollerman G.H., Lewis A.J., Schultz I., et al.: The relationship of the immune response to group A streptococci to the course of acute, chronic and recurrent rheumatic fever. *Am. J. Med.* 20:163, 1956.

92. Bisno A.L., Ofek I.: Serologic diagnosis of streptococcal infection. *Am. J. Dis. Child.* 127:676, 1974.

93. Moody M.D., Siegel A.C., Pittman B., et al.: Fluorescent antibody identification of group A streptococci from throat swabs. *Am. J. Public Health* 53:1083, 1963.

94. Edwards E.A., Larson G.L.: Serological grouping of hemolytic streptococci by counterimmunoelectrophoresis. *Appl. Microbiol.* 26:899, 1973.

95. El Kholy A., Facklam R., Sabri G., et al.: Serological identification of Group A streptococci from throat scrapings before culture. *J. Clin. Microbiol.* 8:725, 1978.

96. Edwards E.A., Phillips I.A., Suiter W.C.: Diagnosis of Group A streptococcal infections directly from throat gargle. *J. Clin. Microbiol.* 15:481, 1982.

97. Holliday M.G.: The diagnosis of Legionnaires' disease by counterimmunoelectrophoresis. *J. Clin. Pathol.* 33:1174, 1980.

98. Smith R.A., DiGiorgio S., Damer J., et al.: Detection of *Legionella pneumophila* capsular-like envelope antigens by counterimmunoelectrophoresis. *J. Clin. Microbiol.* 13:637, 1981.

99. Kohler R.B., Zimmerman S.E., Wilson E., et al.: Rapid radioimmunoassay diagnosis of Legionnaires' disease. *Ann. Intern. Med.* 94:601, 1981.

100. Wilkinson H.W., Farshy C.E., Fikes B.J., et al: Measure of immunoglobulin G-, M-, and A- specific titers against *Legionella pneumophila* and inhibition of titers against nonspecific gram-negative bacterial antigens in the indirect immunofluorescent test for legionellosis. *J. Clin. Microbiol.* 10:685, 1979.

101. Wilkinson H.W.: Serodiagnosis of legionellosis. *Am. J. Pathol.* 103:454, 1981.

102. Chang T.W., Gorbach S.L., Bartlett J.G.: Neutralization of *Clostridium difficile* toxin by *Clostridium sordellii* antitoxin. *Infect. Immun.* 22:418, 1978.

103. Welch D.F.: Identification of toxigenic *Clostridium difficile* by counterimmunoelectrophoresis. *J. Clin. Microbiol.* 11:470, 1980.

104. Ryan R.W., Kwasnik I., Tilton R.C.: Rapid detection of *Clostridium difficile* toxin in human feces. *J. Clin. Microbiol.* 12:776, 1980.

105. West S.E.H., Wilkins T.D.: Problems associated with counterimmunoelectrophoresis assays for detecting *Clostridium difficile* toxin. *J. Clin. Microbiol.* 15:347, 1982.

10

Interpretation of Immunologic Assays for Mycotic Infections

Michael Lange, M.D.

IN THE LAST THREE DECADES it has been increasingly recognized that fungi are able to cause serious systemic infections, particularly in immunocompromised hosts. Diagnostic verification of these infections is difficult and requires careful consideration of signs and symptoms, knowledge of the immune status of the host, and knowledge of epidemiologic data. Taking these factors into consideration, a presumptive diagnosis of a specific fungal infection may be made and ideally should be confirmed by standard microbiologic and histologic laboratory methods, including specially stained cultures. Clinical signs and symptoms, however, are frequently nonspecific, and specific diagnosis requires isolating the fungal organism. Such isolation is often difficult, despite efforts to culture clinical biopsy specimens promptly. Therefore, immunologic testing frequently gives the first clue as to the existence of a fungal infection.

It must be remembered that many of the antigens used for diagnostic immunologic testing are crude mixtures and that fungi are highly complex substances containing many antigens, some of which are common to fungi of several different species. Furthermore, because many fungal infections occur in severely immunocompromised hosts, immunologic reactions to their antigens may be lacking, owing to the host's inability to produce antibodies to the invading fungal organism. In addition, the widespread distribution of many fungal organisms in the environment may lead to the development of specific fungal antibodies in a large number of normal hosts who do not have clinical disease. This situation not infrequently results in positive serologic evidence of mycotic infection in the context of insignificant colonization or of asymptomatic benign primary infection, and, on the other hand, lack of evidence of antibodies in a patient with widespread systemic dissemination of a fungal organism. Therefore, only a complete knowledge of the patients' clinical history and symptoms taken together with serologic and microbiologic test results will permit accurate diagnosis of systemic fungal infections.

Microbiologically, pathogenic fungi may be classified as true yeasts, true molds, or dimorphic fungi. Yeasts include such organisms as *Cryptococcus neoformans, Candida* sp., and *Torulopsis glabrata.* True molds are represented by *Aspergillus* sp. and *Rhizopus* sp. Dimorphic fungi, which under certain temperatures can grow as a yeast as well as a mold, include what are generally referred to as the geographic fungi, such as *Coccidioides immitis, Blastomyces dermatitidis, Histoplasma capsulatum,* and *Paracoccidioides* sp., as well as *Sporothrix schenckii* (Table 10–1).

Of the major clinical groups of pathogenic fungi, the dermatophytes generally produce only superficial mycoses and keratomycosis, whereas the systemic mycoses produce infections that result in widespread disseminated disease. A subgroup of systemic mycoses are the saprophytic systemic mycoses. Saprophytes are organisms that exist widely throughout the environment and are not usually able to produce disease in a normal host. It is only in immunocompromised hosts, in whom natural immune defenses have broken down, that saprophytic mycoses have the opportunity to instigate widespread systemic infection.

Various immunologic tests have been developed for the detection of my-

TABLE 10–1.—OPPORTUNISTIC FUNGI
(SAPROPHYTES)

True molds
  Aspergillus sp.
    A. flavus
    A. fumigatus
    A. niger
  Zygomyces sp.
True yeasts
  Candida sp.
    C. albicans
    C. guilliermondii
    C. krusei
    C. parapsilosis
    C. stellatoidea
    C. tropicalis
    C. pseudotropicalis
  Cryptococcus neoformans
  Torulopsis glabrata
Dimorphic fungi ("geographic" fungi)
  Blastomyces dermatitidis
  Coccidioides immitis
  Histoplasma capsulatum
  (H. capsulatum var. *duboisii)*
  Paracoccidioides brasiliensis
  Sporothrix schenckii

cotic infections. These include skin tests as well as serologic tests for antibodies, antigens, and, more recently, for metabolic products produced by some fungi. Immunologic tests may yield the first evidence of the existence of mycotic disease. This in turn may lead to more careful search to isolate and identify the etiological fungal agent. Results of these tests are a valuable guide to the prognosis and extent of a mycotic infection as well as to the response of the infection to therapy.

A thorough familarity with an individual mycotic infection and its clinical manifestations will permit the clinician to use the available immunologic testing methods for specific fungal organisms to arrive at an understanding of the nature and extent of such illnesses. This chapter reviews the clinical manifestations of the major pathogenic fungi and discusses available immunodiagnostic methods and their significance and specificity in making a diagnosis and prognosis. The organisms are grouped according to the two major clinical situations in which they produce disease: the saprophytic or opportunistic fungi, which produce disease most often in an immunocompromised host, and the geographic fungi, which may produce disease in normal as well as immunocompromised hosts, but whose clinical manifestations generally occur following exposure in specific geographic settings.

OPPORTUNISTIC FUNGAL INFECTIONS (SAPROPHYTES)

The immunologic tests for saprophytic fungi are listed in Table 10–2. Infections and their diagnoses are discussed in detail below.

Aspergillosis

Aspergillus organisms are ubiquitous in soil and decaying vegetable matter throughout the world. The spores can survive in nature for long periods. Of eight species that are known to cause human disease, *A. fumigatus, A. flavus,* and *A. niger* are the ones most commonly identified. *Aspergillus*

TABLE 10–2.—IMMUNOLOGIC TESTS FOR SAPROPHYTIC FUNGI

ORGANISM	TEST	COMMENT
Aspergillus	Agar gel diffusion	Frequently false negative in severe infections
	Radioimmunoassay for antigen	Experimental
Candida	Agglutination test	Limited usefulness
	Precipitin test	Limited usefulness
	Assays for antigen	Experimental
Cryptococcus	IFA test	Helpful in extrameningeal cryptococcal
	Tube agglutination	infections
	Latex agglutination	Helpful in CNS cryptococcal infections
Zygomycetes	Agar gel diffusion	Experimental

organisms produce three distinct forms of disease in the human host, each with a distinct clinical presentation and vastly different prognosis. These three forms, bronchopulmonary aspergillosis, fungus ball, and systemic aspergillosis, are described below.

Bronchopulmonary aspergillosis.—The clinical entity represents an allergic reaction of the bronchial tree to inhaled *Aspergillus* spores, which germinate to form hyphae within the bronchi without causing invasion. The disease is associated with fluctuating pulmonary infiltrates, eosinophilia, and an increase in the serum IgE level. Clinical manifestations consist primarily of bronchospasm. Symptoms usually respond well to steroid therapy.

Aspergillus fungus ball (mycetoma).—Preexisting pulmonary cavities, such as may be produced by tuberculosis or sarcoidosis, are colonized by *Aspergillus* spores, which, on germinating, form dense mycelial balls. Superficial invasion of the surrounding cavity may lead to hemorrhage. Systemic invasion ordinarily does not occur, and therapeutic intervention in the form of surgical extirpation of the mycetoma is required only if hemorrhage becomes a severe or recurrent problem.

Systemic aspergillosis.—Systemic aspergillosis is the most serious form of *Aspergillus* infection. It usually occurs in granulocytopenic patients, e.g., patients with acute myelogenous leukemia. Classically, the infection manifests after the patient has been treated with broad-spectrum antibiotics for a bacterial infection. *Aspergillus* hyphae can grow across tissue planes and frequently will cut off the blood supply, leading to embolization and infarction. The entry point in most cases is the respiratory tract (lungs and sinuses), but hematogenous metastatic foci may be established in almost any organ system and occur particularly in the bones, kidney, and CNS. Systemic aspergillosis frequently has a fatal outcome unless it is diagnosed early and treated with amphotericin B. Because the isolation of *Aspergillus* organisms, even in progressive pulmonary aspergillosis, is rare and may be missed even when an open lung biopsy is performed, a number of serologic tests have been developed in an effort to obtain an early diagnosis. Two methods, antibody detection and antigen detection, are described below.

Antibody Detection

Agar gel diffusion (Ouchterlony technique) is ordinarily employed to detect antibodies to *Aspergillus*. Two difficulties with serologic testing for *Aspergillus* antibodies are the number and the antigenic variability of strains and species of *Aspergillus*. For example, different strains of *A. fumigatus* have been shown to share 73%–89% of several antigens, whereas species such as *A. flavus*, *A. fumigatus*, and *A. niger* have been shown to share only 19%–35% of their antigens.[1] Since each *Aspergillus* species has more than 50 different antigens, as demonstrated by crossed immunoelectrophoresis, and since it is unknown which of these specific antigens is the most immunogenic in the human, false negative reactions on serologic testing have frequently been reported in patients in whom subsequent biopsy or autopsy demonstrated invasive *Aspergillus* infection (Fig 10–1).[2] Heavy

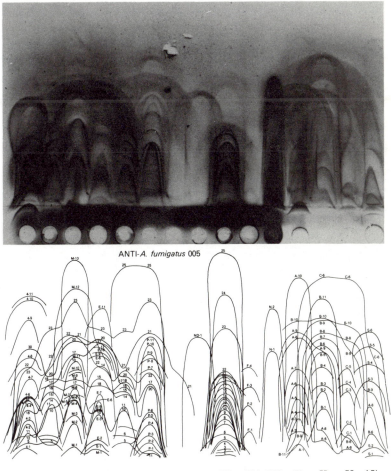

Fig 10–1.—Fused rocket immunoelectrophoresis of extracts of species of *Aspergillus* and fractions of *A. fumigatus* with anti-*A. fumigatus* 005 strain serum. ACT, *A. clavatus; AFE, A. fumigatus* var. *ellipticus; AFV, A. flavus; AND, A. nidulans; ANG, A. niger; APS, A. phialiseptus; ME, 004,* and *005, A. fumigatus* strains; *ASI, FA, FB, FC,* fractions derived from mycelial extract of *A. fumigatus.* (Courtesy of Kim and Chaparas.[1] Reproduced by permission.)

precipitin bands are frequently seen on agar gel diffusion in the nonfatal bronchopulmonary aspergillosis and in *Aspergillus* fungus balls.[3] Unfortunately, in immunocompromised patients, where the development of systemic disseminated aspergillosis poses a life-threating complication, positive serologic results, if present, are usually very weak. It has been suggested that concentrated serum and sequential weekly or biweekly testing of sera from patients at high risk for the development of systemic aspergillosis will give the highest yield of positive reactions.[3, 4] Schaefer et al., using sera that had been concentrated fourfold, demonstrated a conversion from negative to positive immunodiffusion tests that correlated with invasive aspergillosis in 7 of 10 patients proved to have disseminated aspergillosis on biopsy or autopsy.

Antigen Detection

Because of the generally poor antibody response in patients with systemic aspergillosis,[5] attempts have been made to detect circulating antigen in serum and body fluids.[6-8] Shaffer et al.[7] demonstrated circulating *Aspergillus* antigen in a rabbit model of disseminated aspergillosis. More recently, Weiner,[8] using a radioimmunoassay to detect *A. fumigatus* carbohydrate antigen, was able to detect *Aspergillus* antigenemia in sera obtained ante mortem from 4 of 7 patients with systemic aspergillosis, as well as in the pleural fluid from a patient with *Aspergillus* empyema. Sera or pleural fluids from 43 patients not having aspergillosis and from 27 normal donors were negative for antigen. Weiner found that in relation to the clinical onset of disease, antigenemia constituted an early sign of infection. Thus, although it is still considered experimental and is not generally available, this radioimmunoassay permits early specific immunodiagnosis of aspergillosis.

Candidiasis

Although thrush was first described in antiquity, it was not until the antibiotic era that *Candida* infections became a major cause of morbidity and mortality among hospitalized patients. Patients with underlying malignancies, particularly leukemia or lymphoma, and those receiving prolonged courses of broad-spectrum antimicrobial agents are at high risk of developing systemic invasion with *Candida* sp. In addition, an increased incidence of systemic infection with *Candida* sp. has been observed with the use of hyperalimentation fluids,[9] polyethylene catheters,[10] and pressure-monitoring devices.

Candida sp. appears to be mainly confined to mammals, although it has been recovered from soil, hospital environments, and food.[11] The organisms are normal human commensals and are found in sputum, the entire gastrointestinal tract, skin, genital tract (particularly in the female), and in the urine of patients with indwelling Foley catheters. Some 15%–20% of healthy people in a community are colonized with *Candida* sp., most commonly *C. albicans.*[12] The number rapidly rises in hospital populations.[12] Heavy colonization may present as thrush, which can lead to a heavy overgrowth of the mucous membranes of the esophagus and intestines, resulting in dysphagia and esophageal or intestinal candidiasis. Overgrowth of the small intestine leads to persorption: transmission of the yeast across the small bowel into the portal circulation and seeding of the liver, from where, if the phagocytic capacity of the liver cells has been decreased, there may be seeding to various tissues of the body via the hepatic artery.[13]

The clinical manifestations of *Candida* infections have been increasingly well defined during the last 20 years, and several excellent reviews describing the various manifestations have appeared.[14, 15] Clinical manifestations are divided into two major disease forms: mucocutaneous candidiasis, usually manifested by infection of the skin, mucous membranes, nails, and esophagus; and which does not often result in systemic invasion, and disseminated systemic candidiasis, which occurs mostly in granulocytopenic patients and is associated with a high mortality rate.

Although *Candida* infections have become the most common fungal infection in the hospital setting, producing severe and often fatal disease in many patients, the diagnosis of systemic candidiasis is often difficult to make. Definitive therapy is associated with a high degree of toxicity, which prevents the clinician from using antifungal agents on an empirical basis. Because of the lack of pathognomonic signs and symptoms, the lack of positive blood cultures in many patients who have systemic invasion with *Candida* organisms, and the frequency with which peripheral sites are colonized with *Candida* organisms without evidence of systemic disease, acute awareness of predisposing factors and persistent clinical evaluation of the patient at risk are the most important aspects in achieving a diagnosis.[14, 15] Nevertheless, it is has been estimated that a premortem diagnosis in time for appropriate therapy is made in only 15%–40% of patients.[16]

To achieve earlier diagnosis, much attention and effort have been devoted to developing serologic tests for serum antibodies in order to differentiate colonization from invasion and dissemination. Despite more than 75 publications on the topic in the last 10 years, there remains considerable doubt about the value of serologic testing in candidiasis. It has been clearly shown that both false positive and false negative results occur on testing for *Candida* antibodies by either the agglutinin or precipitin tests.[17] Attempts at serodiagnosis in *Candida* infections include studies to measure antibody, antigen, or metabolites. Crossed immunoelectrophoresis has shown the presence of more than 80 different precipitation arcs, indicating a complex antigenic composition.[18] One of the difficulties with antibody and antigen measurements has been the lack of knowledge of which of the more than 80 antigens are most likely to produce antibody or detectable antigen that will correlate well with a confirmed diagnosis of clinically significant candidiasis. Because of the lack of specificity of these tests, biopsy or autopsy demonstrating the organism in tissues is the only valid method of confirming a clinically suspected diagnosis of candidiasis. Nevertheless, some conclusions may be drawn from the available data on serologic testing and will be discussed in the following paragraphs.

Antibody Detection

A negative test for either agglutinin or precipitin antibodies does not rule out the diagnosis of systemic invasive candidiasis.[17] The inability of severely debilitated patients to mount an effective precipitin response and the high rate of false positive agglutinin reactions in healthy individuals have severely limited the usefulness of these serologic methods. Attempts to heighten the sensitivity of detection by counterimmunoelectrophoresis (CIE) or crossed immunoelectrophoresis,[18, 19] as well as efforts to improve the sensitivity of the precipitin test, have been disappointing in regard to specificity.

Antigen Detection

The shortcomings of serologic testing for antibodies to *Candida* antigen have recently led several investigators to attempt detection of antigens or metabolites of the *Candida* organism in blood and other body fluids of infected patients. Assay techniques that have been used include gas-liquid chromatography,[20] radioimmunoassay,[21] CIE,[22] enzyme-linked immunosorbent assay (ELISA),[23, 24] ELISA inhibition,[25] and hemagglutination inhibition (HAI).[26] These studies have shown that fungal products (mannan, arabinitol, etc.) are detectable in at least some infected animals and patients. The sensitivity of these tests, however, has not been determined. A recent report by Lew et al. describing the detection of *Candida* mannan by a solid-phase double antibody technique emphasized that circulating antibodies reduced the sensitivity of this test.[27] The authors demonstrated that *Candida* mannan antigen was detectable at an early stage of systemic infection with a sensitivity of 1 ng/ml in buffer. However, the test was 1,000 times less sensitive in detecting mannan in pooled human serum. It was shown that immune complexes with mannan antigen appeared to be the major blocking factor in serum. By using a rapid heat-extraction method it was possible to recover mannan from antibody-containing serum.[27] In

30 rats with lethal *Candida* infections, Lew et al. detected circulating mannan antigen within 24 hours of infection; the antigenemia subsequently persisted until death. In 8 of 16 patients with documented or suspected candidiasis, mannan antigen levels ranged from 5 to more than 100 ng/ml.

Kiehn et al.[28] reported the detection of D-arabinitol by gas-liquid chromatography in patients with candidiasis. Arabinitol, a metabolic product of the multiplying *Candida* organism, was detected in blood and urine of patients with systemic candidiasis. As the arabinitol was cleared by the kidney, renal dysfunction led to falsely elevated titers (>1.0) suggestive of candidiasis.

Although serologic tests devised to detect antigens and metabolites are considered experimental at this time and are not commercially available, the availability of monoclonal antibodies from hybridomas may lead to further refinement and clinical applicability of these techniques.

Cryptococcosis

Cryptococcus neoformans is a true yeast organism. The organism has been isolated in every part of the world and is always associated with pigeon droppings and pigeon nests. It has been reported to cause disease in every age group, from newborns to adults over 70 years old. Invasion may involve lungs, skin, and other parts of the body, but the organism has a predilection for the brain and meninges. It is thought that the organism most often enters the body by inhalation into the lungs, although it may enter via the nasopharyngeal mucosa or, after swallowing, from the gastrointestinal tract.

Cryptococcal infection has been associated with the disease processes underlying suppressed cell-mediated immunity, such as Hodgkin's disease and other lymphomas, myelogenous, lymphocytic, and monocytic leukemia, sarcoidosis, diabetes, and vasculitis. Immunosuppressive therapy with chemotherapeutic agents and therapy with corticosteroids is frequently a predisposing factor in patients who have cryptococcal infections. Nevertheless, no underlying disease can be identified in approximately 50% of patients.[29]

Microbiology

Cryptococcus neoformans appears in tissue, sputum, or exudate as a thick-walled spherical organism surrounded by a thick, wide capsule. It produces single buds. Because of the thick capsule, cryptococcal infection can be diagnosed with great specificity by detection of cryptococcal antigen.

Diagnosis

The diagnosis of cryptococcosis infection is made by (1) identification of the organism in fluids or tissues, (2) cultural isolation, or (3) detection of cryptococcal antigen in body fluids (serum, urine, and CSF). In identifying the *Cryptococcus* organism in the spinal fluid, the fluid should be centrifuged and the sediment examined directly under the microscope with the help of an India ink preparation. Identification of a single-budding, thick-walled, yeastlike organism 5–20 μm in diameter is highly suggestive of cryptococcosis.

Serologic Testing

Patients who have symptoms suggestive of either pulmonary or CNS infection should be tested for a cryptococcal antigen, antibody, or both. Skin, bone, and visceral lesions due to *C. neoformans* are thought to represent dissemination, usually from a primary focus. Serologic tests for cryptococcosis include an indirect immunofluorescence antibody (IFA) technique for antibody, a charcoal particle agglutination test for antibody, a tube agglutination test for the detection of antibody, and a latex agglutination (LA) test for detection of antigen. Of these tests, the IFA and tube agglutination assays react with 50% of sera from patients with active extrameningeal infection. The specificity of the IFA test is approximately 77%, whereas that of tube agglutination is 89%.[30]

The LA test, used for detection of cryptococcal antigen, has been of greatest value in the diagnosis of CNS cryptococcal infection.[31] Testing for cryptococcal antigen in sera and urine has shown that this test is also valuable in detecting nonmeningeal cryptococcosis at an early stage. The test is considerably more sensitive than the India ink stain. A titer of 1:8 or greater is considered strong evidence for active infection. Titers of 1:4 or less should be considered presumptive evidence of infection until culture results have been obtained. Every possible effort should be made to confirm positive cryptococcal antigen test results with smears and culture. If CSF India ink and Gram stain are negative in a specimen that is positive for cryptococcal antigen, an attempt should be made to obtain a larger (10–20 ml) specimen of CSF. Centrifuging a larger amount of fluid frequently leads to isolation of the organism.[32] False positive serum reactions for cryptococcal antigen are rare and occur most often in patients with a positive rheumatoid factor.[33] For this reason, a control test should be performed to exclude patients with positive rheumatoid factors.

The cryptococcal antigen titer in CSF is a valuable prognostic sign to be followed during treatment.[34] If treatment is successful, it usually should be continued for 4 weeks after antigen has disappeared from the CSF.[32] Failure of the CSF antigen titer to fall indicates inadequate therapy. In a few patients, however, a low titer has remained for months or years following successful therapy with amphotericin B.

In cryptococcal infection outside the CNS, optimal results are obtained by performing tests for antigen and antibody simultaneously.[35] Antibodies may be detected in the early phase of the infection, whereas the antigen will predominate in the later phase, when infection is more widespread. The reemergence of measurable antibody after a serious infection may therefore be a favorable prognostic sign.

Zygomycosis

In the class Zygomycetes, Mucorales and Entomophthorales may lead to human disease. Of these the Mucorales are the most common, and the genera *Absidia*, *Mucor*, and *Rhizopus* account for most cases of human infection.

Mucormycosis results in clinical infections that closely resemble aspergillosis. Like the *Aspergillus* organism, its hyphae can cross tissue planes and invade blood vessels, resulting in hemorrhagic lesions and infarction. The organism most frequently invades the paranasal sinuses, from where it may move directly into contiguous structures of the CNS. It is also known to cause pulmonary and, rarely, gastrointestinal infection. It has been observed to cause serious infection in patients with uncontrolled diabetic ketoacidosis and has also caused invasive disease in patients with prolonged granulocytopenia.

A high degree of suspicion and an aggressive approach to obtaining clinical biopsy specimens for identification is required to make the diagnosis.

Serologic testing has not proved to be helpful in confirming the diagnosis of mucormycosis. An agar gel diffusion test in which one or several precipitin lines may appear has been developed that uses antigens prepared from cultures of several zygomyces species *(M. pusillus, R. arrhizus, R. oryzae,* and *A. corymbifera)*. The test awaits further evaluation before its diagnostic sensitivity and specificity can be assessed. A preliminary series indicated antibody detection in 8 of 11 (73%) proved or suspected cases of zygomycoses.[36]

GEOGRAPHIC MYCOSES

The immunologic tests for geographic fungi are listed in Table 10–3. The infections and their diagnoses are described in detail below.

TABLE 10–3.—IMMUNOLOGIC TESTS FOR GEOGRAPHIC FUNGI*

ORGANISM	TEST	COMMENT
Blastomyces	Skin test	Not reliable
	CF test	High positive titer may be helpful
	ID test	Not clearly useful
Coccidioides	Skin test	May be diagnostically helpful
	TP test	Indicates recent infection
	LA test	More sensitive but less specific than TP test
	CF test	Available as a kit; most valuable serologic test in diagnosis and prognosis; should be done in a reference laboratory
	ID test	Clinically useful; can be done in standard laboratory
Histoplasma	Skin test	Usually not helpful in diagnosis
	Agar gel diffusion ⎫	"H band" in patients with systemic disease
	CIE ⎬	M band less diagnostically helpful
	CF test	Less specific than gel diffusion or CIE
Paracoccidioides	ID test	Specific for diagnosis
	CF test	Useful for monitoring response to therapy
Sporothrix	Skin testing	Not helpful
	LA test	Highly specific
	Tube agglutination	Sensitive but less specific
	CF and ID tests	Not adequately sensitive

*CF, complement fixation; ID, immunodiffusion; TP, tube precipitin; LA, latex agglutination, CIE, counterimmunoelectrophoresis.

Blastomycosis

Of the three geographic mycoses endemic to the United States, infection with *Blastomyces dermatitidis* is the least common. However, when identified, unlike infection with *H. capsulatum* or *C. immitis* it probably results more frequently in clinically serious infection. The spectrum of illness is extremely variable and ranges from an accidentally discovered, self-limited pulmonary infection to a rapidly progressive, fatal illness involving multiple organ systems.[37]

Immunologic testing that has been used in an attempt to diagnose individual acute cases of blastomycosis and to define the epidemiology of this infection has included skin testing (with blastomycin, a crude mycelial phase extract), the complement fixation (CF) test, and the immunodiffusion test. None of these three methods has proved to be very useful, and the prospect for improving any of them is dubious. Blastomycin is not a reliable antigen.[38] It is not at all specific, and positive skin tests frequently occur in histoplasmosis and to a lesser degree in coccidioidomycosis. Diagnostic reliability is further diminished since the areas in which blastomycosis is evident overlap the large geographic areas in which histoplasmosis is endemic. Moreover, skin test reactivity for blastomycin is frequently transient and may disappear rapidly in patients who have acute infection.

Antigen used for the CF test is prepared from either the mycelial or yeast phase. Patients with proved blastomycosis are usually negative by this test; indeed, they are more likely to have a positive result on the CF test for histoplasmin. A negative test is therefore quite meaningless. A high positive titer cannot be used to make a specific diagnosis but should raise clinical suspicion and indicates a careful search for the organism.

Kaufman et al.[38] were able to identify A and B precipitins by immunodiffusion which they felt were specific for blastomycosis. By using control sera and establishing lines of identity between control and patient sera for A and B lines or A lines alone, these investigators demonstrated antibody in 80% of 113 patients. There was little cross reactivity with other fungal antigens. Nevertheless, a positive test result only identified existing or recent infection; a negative test result did not rule out the diagnosis of blastomycosis, nor did a positive test result have prognostic significance, as does the CF test for coccidiodomycosis.

In summary, the diagnostic cornerstone of blastomycosis remains the early identification of the organism in body fluids or in tissues by culture or specific stains. Sputum, pus from skin lesions, and prostatic secretions (particularly following prostatic massage) all provide good specimens from which to isolate the organism. The best method for examining fresh materials is 10% potassium hydroxide digestion and subsequent examination by direct microscopy. This method yields no false positive results and has the added advantage of permitting institution of specific therapy. On microscopy, the organism has a double refractile wall with a broad neck of attachment to the daughter cell, as well as multiple intracellular nuclei.

Coccidioidomycosis

Coccidioides immitis exists in the soil in the mycelial phase. The fungus is endemic in seven Southwestern states and in areas of Mexico and Central and South America. Approximately 100,000 people are infected annually in the United States alone.

Spores released from the maturing soil mycelial phase become airborne and can undergo two cycles: (1) the saprophytic cycle, a new cycle that remains within the soil, and (2) the parasitic cycle, in which spores inhaled by an animal host from soil or dust swell and form a spherule that differentiates internally into endospores (one spherule may form up to 800 endospores). When a spherule ruptures, each endospore can lead to formation of a new spherule. When a spherule is returned to soil, endospores bud into mycelia, thus reestablishing the saprophytic cycle. On the other hand, a spherule that ruptures within an animal host may result in dissemination by the hematogenous or lymphatic route, causing widespread disease outside the initial pulmonary locus.

Clinical Manifestations

Coccidioidomycosis closely resembles tuberculosis in its clinical and pathologic manifestations. Tissue reaction to the organism is predominantly in the form of granuloma around the characteristic spherule. It is estimated that 60% of infected persons are asymptomatic, having at most a mild upper respiratory tract infection. The other 40% develop a lower respiratory tract infection with cough, chest pain, malaise and fever, chills, and night sweats, usually 1–3 weeks following inhalational exposure. Five percent have chronic residual pulmonary disease, and in 0.5% the infection develops into disseminated extrapulmonary disease. Extrapulmonary loci of infection may develop in any organ system, including bone, joint, muscle, and the CNS, where it presents as a chronic, predominantly basal meningitis. The disease may also spread in a rapidly disseminating miliary form that is usually fatal. Dissemination is more common in Orientals, blacks, and Indians, in descending order of incidence.[39]

Serologic Diagnosis

In no other fungal disease are the results of skin testing and serologic tests as accurate and important in correlation with the clinical diagnosis and prognosis. The serologic titers not only help in confirming the diagnosis but also provide an invaluable guide to the course of the disease. The immunologic responses that the normal host mounts against the inhaled organism involve initial phagocytosis and degradation, processing by macrophages, and subsequent sensitization of lymphocytes, which in turn results in the development of delayed-type hypersensitivity and activation of macrophages. B lymphocytes first produce IgM and then IgG antibodies, which are thought to play a role as opsonins. Antigen overload is believed to result in anergy in some patients with disseminated disease and is a poor prognostic sign.[39]

Skin Tests

Coccidioidin, the mycelial antigen, has been the standard skin test agent.[40] It is used in dilutions of 1:10 and 1:100. Recently a parasitic phase antigen material, spherulin, has been found to be more sensitive than and as specific as coccidioidin. Spherulin detects exposure in approximately one third more persons than does coccidioidin.[41] Although use of either agent has not affected serologic testing for coccidioidomycosis, the coccidioidin test has been reported to induce antibody formation that will cross-react with histoplasmin.[42]

Skin test positivity (5 mm induration or greater) usually develops 10–45 days after infection, or 2–21 days after the first clinical symptoms appear. If a patient presents with erythema nodosum, a frequent clinical manifestation of coccidioidomycosis, the customary concentration of coccidioidin causes a severe reaction. Therefore, reagent diluted at 1:100 should be used initially.

It is important to measure reactivity after both 24 and 48 hours, as reactions positive at 24 hours may be negative at 48 hours.

Skin testing with either coccidioidin or spherulin is an important epidemiologic tool. Clinically it is used to assess the cell-mediated immune status of patients with coccidioidal infections. A negative test, however, does not rule out the diagnosis. Indeed, a test will frequently revert from positive to negative in patients who develop disseminated disease, and the return of a positive reaction in these patients is a good prognostic sign, as it indicates restoration of the cell-mediated response.[40] On the other hand, a positive test in itself indicates only that previous exposure occurred at an unknown time and does not indicate active infection. A low incidence of cross reactivity is seen with antigens from *H. capsulatum* and *B. dermatidis*.

Serologic Testing

Tests have been developed to measure serum IgM response to coccidioidin using tube precipitin (TP), LA, CF, and immunodiffusion methods.

Except on rare occasions, a positive TP test indicates recent infection. In patients who develop asymptomatic infection, the TP test result may remain negative, whereas in symptomatic patients the test result is positive in 53% during the first week, 91% during the second and third week, and 86% during the fourth week of illness. Thereafter the incidence of positive titers decreases rapidly.[43] The TP test may again become positive at the time of dissemination. Because the large IgM molecule is unable to penetrate the blood-brain barrier, the CSF is never positive for precipitins, even in meningitis.

The LA test is thought to measure the same IgM antibody as the TP test. The test is more sensitive and is available as a commercial kit. However, it is less specific than the TP test, and false positive results have been reported in 6 of 10 patients with noncoccidioidal infections.[44] It is also possible to have false negative tests, as the level of IgM antibodies may be too low in the early phase of disease. False positive results may occur when the CSF is tested, since the low CSF protein content causes latex particles to become unstable.[45] Nevertheless, the LA test is easy to perform and so is frequently used as an initial screening test. If the result is positive, it should always be confirmed by using other techniques (TP, CF).

The CF test for IgG antibodies is the most valuable serologic test for assessing the diagnosis and prognosis of coccidioidal infection; is also costly and time-consuming to perform. A standardized reference laboratory should be used in performing this test, as only careful attention to methodology will give consistently reliable results. When IgG CF antibody develops in patients, it follows temporally the TP IgM response. The temporal relationship between the coccidioidin skin test and the TP and CF tests is illustrated in Figure 10–2.

When asymptomatic disease follows initial exposure to *C. immitis* spores, the CF test frequently remains negative. Smith et al. reported that only 2 of 27 patients with coccidioidin skin test conversion but without a history of clinical disease had a positive response on CF testing.[46] Nevertheless, it is the prognostic implications of the CF test, as demonstrated by Smith and colleagues during the years 1939–1952, that make the CF test a highly valuable adjunct in assessing the prognosis of coccidioidomycosis.[43, 46] It must be emphasized, however, that Smith's observations should not be used uncritically in patient management, as the CF test was not performed

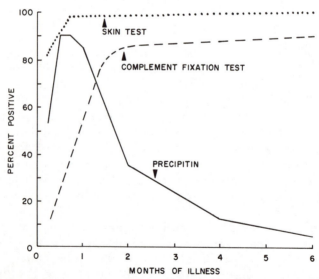

Fig 10–2.—Temporal relationship between coccidioidin skin test reactivity and tube precipitin and complement fixing antibody titer. (Courtesy of Huppert M.: Serology of coccidioidomycosis. *Mycopathol. Mycol. Appl.* 41:107, 1970. Reproduced by permission.)

in precisely the same manner as it is by serologic laboratories today.[39] Following are general guidelines on the relationship of the CF test to the clinical disease:

1. High or rapidly rising CF titers (1:16 or 1:32 or above) are often associated with a poor prognosis, usually reflecting extrapulmonary dissemination of the organism.

2. A significant decrease in the CF titer reflects an improved prognosis. Due to the technical variability of the test, it is essential that sequential specimens of sera be measured simultaneously for CF antibody and that frozen aliquots of serum, CSF, and other body fluids found positive at one time be stored for future use in all patients who are evaluated for coccidioidal disease.

3. Although a "critical serum titer" of 1:16 or 1:32 is suggestive, it is not indicative of dissemination in an individual case; rather, it leads one to become "increasingly apprehensive of dissemination," in Smith's words.

4. A titer below the critical serum titer does not rule out dissemination. Sixty percent of patients with an isolated pulmonary lesion, 30% with meningitis, and 5%–10% with extensive disseminated disease have a CF titer of 1:8 or less.

5. A low-grade CF titer (< 1:8) is common, particularly after recovery from severe disease, and may remain perpetually at this level.

6. CF antibodies may be measured in body fluids other than serum, where they are usually measured at one of two dilutions below that in the serum.

7. A positive CF titer in the CSF is indicative of meningitis, with the rare exception of infection present only in contiguous bone lesions. As demonstrated by Pappagianis, an overnight CF binding assay leads to a positive titer in 95% of patients with coccidioidal meningitis, as opposed to 75% when Smith's technique was used.[39]

Because CF testing using coccidioidin has yielded negative results in 40% of patients with residual pulmonary disease, and because spherulin is more sensitive than coccidioidin in skin testing, spherulin has also been tried in CF testing. However, spherulin cross-reacts with sera from patients with histoplasmosis, candidiasis, cryptococcosis, and actinomycosis much more frequently than does coccidioidin (56% vs. 20%), and so coccidioidin is believed to have a much higher specificity in CF testing.[47]

Immunodiffusion testing using heated sera (heating inactivates the CF coccidioidin antibody) corresponds to the TP test and is called the IDTP.[48] Unheated serum subjected to ultrafiltration used in immunodiffusion corresponds to the CF test and is called the IDCF.[49] The IDCF can be done with a commercial kit and is of particular value in sera that are anticomplementary, which precludes using the CF test.[50] The IDCF test is easily performed in the standard hospital laboratory and yields results very similar to the CF test when done in serial dilutions. Counterimmunoelectrophoresis has been used, but its specificity is less than that of ID, and experience with it limited.[51]

Coccidioidomycosis is diagnosed by isolation of the organism on artificial media or by demonstration of the typical spherules in body fluids or tissue biopsy specimens. Serologic assays and skin testing should be used to make a tentative diagnosis. The major role of serologic testing, however, is in assessing the prognosis of the disease, and it is here that the role of serologic testing in the form of the CF or IDCF test has a unique place among the immunodiagnostic techniques available for assessing the mycotic diseases.

Histoplasmosis

Histoplasmosis, a mycosis produced by the yeast phase of the dimorphic fungus *H. capsulatum*, is the fungal infection with the widest geographic distribution in the United States. The disease is contracted by inhalation of spores from the environment (soil, dust, bird droppings, tree bark, etc.). Isolated cases have been reported from other continents, and a distinct African variety, *H. capsulatum* var. *duboisii*, produces disease that differs from histoplasmosis by the paucity of pulmonary lesions.

Histoplasma capsulatum spores, when inhaled, germinate in the lung tissue, leading to primary infection that closely parallels the initial infection with tuberculosis. Local growth of the organism in lung tissue is followed by lymphatic and hematogenous spread. Metastatic hematogenous foci of infection develop primarily in the liver, spleen, and bone marrow but may rarely occur in other organs. Cases of osteomyelitis, endocarditis, arthritis, meningitis, and adrenal gland involvement have been reported. As hypersensitivity to the organism develops, an intense inflammatory reaction leads to granuloma formation, which may result in caseous necrosis.[52, 53]

The disease has been classified into major syndromes on the basis of clinical manifestations. Benign infection in the normal host includes acute pulmonary histoplasmosis (asymptomatic; symptomatic: influenza-like syndrome with a self-limiting course; and residual foci: mediastinitis, hilar lymphadenopathy, pericarditis, pulmonary histoplasmoma). Opportunistic infections in an immunocompromised host include chronic cavitary pulmonary histoplasmosis (this form of the disease is always thought to be superimposed on pulmonary centrilobular or bullous emphysema); progressive disseminated histoplasmosis (associated with immunodeficiency); and primary cutaneous inoculation.

The diagnosis of histoplasmosis is based on clinical suspicion, a history of exposure, and a compatible incubation period. Because it is difficult to obtain culture or histologic proof of infection, considerable effort has been devoted to developing confirmatory diagnostic tests by skin tesing and serology.

Skin Testing

The histoplasmin skin test has proved to be a useful epidemiologic tool but has not been helpful in making a diagnosis except when used in young children in nonendemic areas. Skin test conversion occurs 2–3 weeks after primary exposure, and in the endemic area more than 90% of the population are positive, precluding any diagnostic significance of the test result.[54, 55] Indeed, because the skin test can result in false conversion of the CF test from negative to positive, many workers believe the skin test has no place in diagnosis and that its use should be strictly confined to epidemiologic survey.[56]

Serology

Various techniques, including CF, immunodiffusion, and CIE, have been used to detect antibodies in histoplasmosis.

Agar Gel Diffusion and CIE

Heiner, using a crude histoplasmin filtrate, demonstrated six distinct precipitin bands,[57] of which only two were seen in all sera tested. These were designated M and H bands. The M band appeared following skin testing in histoplasmin-sensitive normal adults. H bands, on the other hand, were found consistently in sera from patients with histoplasmosis proved by culture. Picardi et al.,[58] using the more rapid CIE technique, were able to show that H precipitins occurred primarily in patients with disseminated disease, chronic pulmonary disease, or mediastinal lymphadenopathy of several months' duration and that this antibody disappeared with resolution of the infection. The H band was uncommon in acute disease. The M band appeared earlier and persisted for months to years following resolution of the infection and was therefore less helpful in making a diagnosis. Positive serum controls to permit designation of H and M bands must be used with both agar gel diffusion and CIE.

The CF test can be used with a mycelial (histoplasmin) as well as with a yeast phase antigen. Its advantage is that it can be quantitated, but it is felt to be less specific than the agar gel diffusion test. False positive results are not rare and have been observed in patients with coccidioidomycosis and blastomycosis.[59] Moreover, false negative results have been reported in 10%–30% of large series of patients with the chronic form of pulmonary histoplasmosis, and the figure is thought to be even higher in the other clinical forms. Higher titers (1:32) are believed to have more diagnostic correlation, but even at this titer level, confirmation by culture was not possible in 36% of positive CF tests when the mycelial antigen was used and in 55% when the yeast phase antigen was used.[60, 61]

Despite extensive work on serologic testing for histoplasmosis, the disease in any of its clinical manifestations cannot be ruled in or out by immunodiagnostic techniques. Serologic data, although helpful in suggesting a diagnosis, must be carefully correlated with clinical data in order to arrive at a presumptive clinical diagnosis. A definitive diagnosis of histoplasmosis can be made only after biopsy or culture.

Paracoccidioidomycosis (South American Blastomycosis)

Paracoccidioidomycosis is produced by *Paracoccidioides brasiliensis*. The only host known for this dimorphic fungus is man. The infection is geographically restricted to areas of Central and South America with a mild humid climate, from Mexico to Argentina.[62, 63] The route of infection remains controversial, although the organism most likely enters by inhalation.

Clinical disease is found predominantly in men over 30 years old and is most common in agricultural workers.[63, 64] The disease is noted for its potential latency, cases having been reported 30 years following a visit to an endemic area. Ulcerations of the oropharyngeal mucosa, nose, vocal cords, and skin are the most common clinical manifestations. The disease may spread from there to lymph nodes, causing sinus tracts and pustules. Involvement of liver, spleen, bone, CNS, gastrointestinal system, and lungs, as well as genitourinary system and adrenal glands, has been reported. If untreated, the disease will run a slowly progressive course ending in death.

At 37 C the fungus grows as a yeast that reproduces by multiple budding, at times producing the characteristic "pilot wheel."[63, 64] At 20–28 C the organism grows as a mold. The classic tissue reaction is granulomatous and is found in the chronic progressive form of the infection. The differential diagnosis includes tuberculosis, other fungal infections, leprosy, leishmaniasis and lues. The diagnosis can be definitely established only by identifying the organism in direct microscopic preparations (10% potassium hydroxide preparation of sputum, pus, etc.) or by culture or in histologic preparations of biopsy material.

Serology

Immunodiagnostic tests are helpful in diagnosis as well as in monitoring the response to therapy.[65] Two tests are available: the agar gel diffusion test (immunodiffusion) and the CF test. Paracoccidioidin antigens used in both tests are prepared from the yeast phase of the organism. The immunodiffusion test, which is specific in this disease, is positive in 95% of cases, and three precipitin bands have been identified. In a study by Kaufman, the presence of precipitin bands 1 and 2, when used with reference sera, established the diagnosis in 95%–98% of cases.[50] The immunodiffusion test remains positive for many years following infection and cannot be used to monitor the activity of the disease. Although it cross-reacts with *Histoplasma* antigens, the CF test is more useful in monitoring the response to therapy, because it is quantifiable. The test is positive in 80%–96% of cases, and the height of the titer, which has ranged from 1:8 to 1:16,384, corresponds to the severity of the infection. A good response to therapy should be accompanied by a decrease in titer level.

Sporotrichosis

Sporothrix schenckii, a dimorphic fungus, has a worldwide distribution. It presents as a chronic infection, usually in the form of a cutaneous nodule or ulcer at the site of implantation with subsequent localized nodular lymphatic spread. Rarely, it may present at an extracutaneous location, resulting in focal or multifocal osteoarticular, pulmonary, ocular, or CNS infection. Because the organism survives in soil as well as in decaying vegetation,- it is most frequently associated with certain occupations and is found in farmers, gardeners, and florists.

Diagnosis of all forms of the disease is made by culturing the organism from tissue or pus specimens. Identification by direct stain of the cigar-shaped yeast organism using silver methenamine or periodic acid Schiff stain is difficult, as features of the organism are not pathognomonic, and differential diagnosis of the tissue granulomas includes tuberculosis, sarcoidosis, and foreign body granuloma. Nocardiosis, blastomycosis, coccidioidomycosis, paracoccidioidomycosis, and leishmaniasis enter the differential diagnosis unless a specific organism is identified in tissue sections.

Immunodiagnosis

Skin testing has not been found to be helpful in making a diagnosis of sporotrichosis. Serologic testing using tube agglutination and LA has been helpful, especially in the diagnosis of extracutaneous or systemic forms of sporotrichosis. The CF test and immunodiffusion test are not adequately sensitive.

Slide LA titers of 1:4 or greater are considered presumptive evidence of sporotrichosis. False positives in the range of 1:4 to 1:8 have been reported. Titers ranging from 1:4 to 1:28 have been reported in patients with localized cutaneous, subcutaneous, and systemic sporotrichosis. A rising or sustained high titer is of help in establishing a diagnosis of pulmonary infection. The LA test is not thought to be of prognostic value, as elevated titers may remain stationary long after convalescence has occurred.[66] The LA test has a sensitivity of 94% and is highly specific. The ability to perform it rapidly (5 minutes) makes it preferable to tube agglutination. The latter assay has the same degree of sensitivity but may exhibit cross reactions at a titer of 1:8 to 1:16 in patients with leishmaniasis.

REFERENCES

1. Kim S.J., Chaparas S.D.: Characterization of antigens from *Aspergillus fumigatus:* III. Comparison of antigenic relationship of clinically important aspergilli. *Am. Rev. Respir. Dis.* 120:1297, 1979.
2. Kim S.J., Chaparas S.C., Buckley H.R.: Characterization of antigen from *Aspergillus fumigatus:* IV. Evaluation of commercial and experimental preparations and fractions in the detection of antibody in aspergillosis. *Am. Rev. Respir. Dis.* 120:1305, 1979.
3. Schaefer J.C., Yu B., Armstrong D.: An *Aspergillus* immunodiffusion test in the early diagnosis of aspergillosis in adult leukemia patients. *Am. Rev. Respir. Dis.* 113:325, 1976.
4. Yu B.H., Armstrong D.: Serological tests for invasive *Aspergillus* and *Candida* infections in patients with neoplastic disease, in *Proceedings of the Sixth Congress of the International Society for Human and Animal Mycology.* Tokyo, University of Tokyo Press, 1977, p. 47.
5. Bardana E.J., Gerber J.D., Craig S., et al.: The general and specific humoral immune response to pulmonary *Aspergillus. Am. Rev. Respir. Dis.* 112:799, 1975.
6. Lehman P.F., Reiss E.: Invasive aspergillosis: Antiserum for circulating antigen produced after immunization with serum from infected rabbits. *Infect. Immunol.* 20:570, 1978.
7. Shaffer P.J., Kobayashi G.S., Medoff G.: Demonstration of antigenemia in patients with invasive aspergillosis by solid phase (protein A-rich *Staphylococcus aureus*) radioimmunoassay. *Am. J. Med.* 67:627, 1979.
8. Weiner M.H.: Antigenemia detected by radioimmunoassay in systemic aspergillosis. *Ann. Intern. Med.* 92:793, 1980.
9. Curry C.R., Quie P.G.: Fungal septicemia in patients receiving parenteral hyperalimentation. *N. Engl. J. Med.* 285:1221, 1971.
10. Bernhardt H.E., Orlando J.C., Benfield J.R., et al.: Disseminated candidiasis in surgical patients. *Surg. Gynecol. Obstet.* 134:819, 1972.
11. Stone H.H., Geheber C.E., Kolb L.D., et al.: Alimentary tract colonization by *Candida albicans. J. Surg. Res.* 14:273, 1973.
12. Stone H.H.: Studies in the pathogenesis, diagnosis and treatment of *Candida* sepsis in children. *J. Pediatr. Surg.* 9:127, 1974.
13. Stone H.H., Kolb L.D., Currie C.A., et al.: *Candida* sepsis: Pathogenesis and principles of treatment. *Ann. Surg.* 179:697, 1974.
14. Louria D.B., Stiff D.P., Bennett B.: Disseminated moniliasis in the adult. *Medicine* 141:307, 1962.
15. Edward J.E. (moderator): Severe candidal infections: Clinical perspective, immune defense mechanisms and current concepts of therapy. *Ann. Intern. Med.* 89:91, 1978.

16. Gaines J.D., Remington J.S.: Diagnosis of deep infection with *Candida:* A study of *Candida* precipitins. *Arch. Intern. Med.* 132:699, 1973.
17. Filice G., Yu B., Armstrong D.: Immunodiffusion and agglutination tests for *Candida* in patients with neoplastic disease: Inconsistent correlation of results with invasive infections. *J. Infect. Dis.* 135:349, 1977.
18. Glew R.H., Buckley H.R., Rosen H.M., et al.: Serologic tests in the diagnosis of systemic candidiasis: Enhanced diagnostic accuracy with crossed immuno-electrophoresis. *Am. J. Med.* 64:586, 1978.
19. Marier R., Andriole V.T.: Usefulness of serial antibody determinations in diagnosis of candidiasis as measured by discontinuous counter immunoelectrophoresis using HS antigen. *J. Clin. Microbiol.* 8:15, 1978.
20. Miller G.G., Witwer M.W., Braude A.I., et al.: Rapid identification of *Candida albicans* septicemia in man by gas-liquid chromatography. *J. Clin. Invest.* 54:1235, 1974.
21. Weiner M.H., Coats-Stephen M.: Immunodiagnosis of systemic candidiasis: Mannan antigenemia detected by radioimmunoassay in experimental and human infections. *J. Infect. Dis.* 140:989, 1979.
22. Kerkering T.M., Espinez-Ingroff A., Shadow S.: Detection of *Candida* antigenemia by counter immunoelectrophoresis in patients with invasive candidiasis. *J. Infect. Dis.* 140:659, 1979.
23. Warren R.C., Richardson M.D., White, L.O.: Enzyme-linked immunosorbent assay of antigens. *Mycopathologia* 66:179, 1979.
24. Scheld W.M., Brown R.S. Jr., Harding S.A., et al.: Detection of circulating antigen in experimental *Candida albicans* endocarditis by an enzyme-linked immunosorbent assay. *J. Clin. Microbiol.* 12:679, 1980.
25. Segal E., Berg R.A., Pizzo P.A., et al.: Detection of *Candida* antigen in sera of patient with candidiasis by an enzyme-linked immunosorbent assay-inhibition technique. *J. Clin. Microbiol.* 10:116, 1979.
26. Weiner M.H., Yount W.J.: Mannan antigenemia in the diagnosis of invasive *Candida* infections. *J. Clin. Invest.* 58:1045, 1976.
27. Lew M.A., Siber G.R., Donahue D.M., et al.: Enhanced detection with an enzyme-linked immunosorbent assay of *Candida* mannan in antibody-containing serum after heat extraction. *J. Infect. Dis.* 145:45, 1982.
28. Kiehn T.E., Bernard E.M., Gold J.W.M., et al.: Candidiasis: Detection by gas-liquid chromatography of D-arabinitol, a fungal metabolite in human serum. *Science* 206:577, 1979.
29. Diamond R.D., Bennett J.E.: Prognostic factors in cryptococcal meningitis: A study of 111 cases. *Ann. Intern. Med.* 80:176, 1974.
30. Kaufman L., Blumer S.: Cryptococcosis: The awakening giant, in *Proceedings of the Fourth International Symposium on Mycoses.* Washington, D.C., Pan American Health Organization Scientific Publication No. 356, 1977, p. 176.
31. Bloomfield N., Gordon M.A., Elmendorf D.F. Jr.: Detection of *Cryptococcus neoformans* antigen in body fluids by latex particle agglutination. *Proc. Soc. Exp. Biol. Med.* 114:64, 1963.
32. Ellner J.J., Bennett J.E.: Chronic meningitis. *Medicine* 53:341, 1976.
33. Bennett J.E., Bailey J.W.: Control for rheumatoid factor in the latex test for cryptococcosis. *Am. J. Clin. Pathol.* 56:360, 1971.
34. Chernik N.L., Armstrong D., Posner J.B.: Central nervous system infections in patients with cancer: Changing patterns. *Cancer* 40:268, 1977.
35. Bindschadler D.D., Bennett J.E.: Serology of human cryptococcosis. *Ann. Intern. Med.* 69:45, 1968.

36. Jones K.W., Kaufman L.: Development and evaluation of an immunodiffusion test for diagnosis of systemic zygomycosis (mucormycosis): Preliminary report. *J. Clin. Microbiol.* 7:97, 1978.

37. Sarosi G.A., Davies S.F.: Blastomycosis: State of the art. *Am. Rev. Respir. Dis.* 120:911, 1979.

38. Kaufman L., McLaughlin D.W., Clark M.J., et al.: Specific immunodiffusion test for blastomycosis. *Appl. Microbiol.* 26:244, 1973.

39. Drutz D.J., Catanzaro A.: Coccidioidomycosis: State of the art. *Am. Rev. Respir. Dis.* 117:727, 1978.

40. Smith C.E., Whiting E.G., Baker E.E., et al.: The use of coccidioidin. *Am. Rev. Tubercul.* 57:330, 1948.

41. Levine H.B., Cobb J.B., Scalarone G.M.: Spherule coccidioidin in delayed dermal sensitivity reactions of experimental animals. *Sabouraudia* 7:20, 1969.

42. Deresinski S.C., Levine H.B., Kelly P.C., et al.: Spherulin skin testing and histoplasmal and coccidioidal serology: Lack of effect. *Am. Rev. Respir. Dis.* 116:1116, 1977.

43. Smith C.E., Saito M.T., Simons S.A.: Pattern of 39,500 serologic tests in coccidioidomycosis. *JAMA* 160:546, 1968.

44. Huppert M., Peterson E.T., Sun S.H., et al.: Evaluation of a latex particle agglutination test for coccidioidomycosis. *Am. J. Clin. Pathol.* 49:96, 1968.

45. Pappagianis D., Kragnow R.I., Beall S.: False-positive reactions of cerebrospinal fluid and diluted sera with the coccidioidal latex-agglutination test. *Am. J. Clin. Pathol.* 66, 916, 1976.

46. Smith C.E., Saito M.T., Beart R.R., et al.: Serologic tests in the diagnosis and prognosis of coccidioidomycosis. *Am. J. Hygiene* 52:1, 1950.

47. Huppert M., Krasnow I., Vukovich K.R., et al.: Comparison of coccidioidin and spherulin in complement fixation tests for coccidioidomycosis. *J. Clin. Microbiol.* 6:33, 1977.

48. Huppert M., Bailey J.W.: The use of immunodiffusion tests in coccidioidomycosis: II. An immunodiffusion test as a substitute for the tube precipitin test. *Am. J. Clin. Pathol.* 44:369, 1965.

49. Huppert M., Bailey J.W.: Immunodiffusion as screening test for coccidioidomycosis serology. *Sabouraudia* 2:284, 1963.

50. Kaufman L.: Current status of immunology for diagnosis and prognostic evaluation of blastomycosis, coccidioidomycosis, in *Proceedings of the Third International Conference on the Mycoses*. Washington, D.C., Pan American Health Organization Scientific Publication No. 304, 1975, p. 137.

51. Avilar-Torres F.G., Jackson L.J., Ferstenfeld J.E., et al.: Counter-immunoelectrophoresis in the detection of antibodies against *Coccidioides immitis*. *Ann. Intern. Med.* 85:740, 1976.

52. Goodwin R.A. Jr., Des Prez R.M.: Histoplasmosis: State of the art. *Am. Rev. Respir. Dis.* 117:929, 1978.

53. Goodwin R.A. Jr., Lloyd J.E., Des Prez R.M.: Histoplasmosis in normal hosts. *Medicine* 60:231, 1981.

54. Furclow M.L.: Airborne histoplasmosis. *Bacteriol. Rev.* 25:301, 1961.

55. Buechuer A.A., Seabury J.H., Campbell C.C., et al.: The current status of serologic, immunologic and skin tests in the diagnosis of pulmonary mycoses: Report of the committee of fungus diseases and subcommittee on criteria for clinical diagnosis. *Chest* 63:259, 1973.

56. Campbell C.C., Hill G.B.: Further studies on the development of complement

fixing antibodies and precipitins in healthy histoplasmin-sensitive persons following a single histoplasmin skin test. *Am. Rev. Respir. Dis.* 90:927, 1964.

57. Heiner E.D.: Diagnosis of histoplasmosis using precipitin reactions in agar gel. *Pediatrics* 22:616, 1958.

58. Picardi J.L., Kaufman C.A., Schwartz J., et al.: Pericarditis caused by *Histoplasma capsulatum. Am. J. Cardiol* 37:82, 1976.

59. Newberry W.M., Tosh F.E., Doto I.L., et al.: The complement fixation antibody test in the diagnosis of chronic pulmonary histoplasmosis and blastomycosis. *J. Chron. Dis.* 20:203, 1967.

60. Lowell J.R., Shuford E.H.: The value of the skin test and complement fixation test in the diagnosis of chronic pulmonary histoplasmosis. *Am. Rev. Respir. Dis.* 114:1069, 1976.

61. Furcolow M., Schubert J., Tosh F.E., et al.: Serologic evidence of histoplasmosis in sanatoriums in the U.S. *JAMA* 180:109, 1962.

62. Restrepo A., Geer D.L., Vasconcellos M.: Paracoccidioidomycosis: A review. *Rev. Med. Vet. Mycol.* 8:97, 1973.

63. Greer D.L., Restrepo A.: The epidemiology of paracoccidioidomycosis, in Al-Doory (ed.): *The Epidemiology of Human Mycotic Diseases.* Springfield, Ill., Charles C Thomas, Publisher, 1975, p. 117.

64. Angulo-Ortega A., Pollak L.: Paracoccidioidomycosis, in Baker R.D. (ed.): *The Pathologic Anatomy of the Mycoses: Human Infections With Fungi, Actinomycetes and Algae.* Berlin, Springer-Verlag, 1971, p. 507.

65. Fava-Netto C.: Immunologia da paracoccidioidomicose. *Rev. Inst. Med. Trop. (Sao Paulo)* 18:42, 1976.

66. Palmer D.F., Kaufman L., Kaplan W., et al.: *Serodiagnosis of Mycotic Diseases.* Springfield, Ill., Charles C Thomas, Publisher, 1977.

11

Infectious Diseases: Viral, Chlamydial, Mycoplasmal, and Rickettsial Immunology

Peter A. Gross, M.D.

"IT'S A VIRAL ILLNESS" no longer has to be a statement of diagnostic default. Techniques for growing viruses to determine the presence of antibody have been available for several decades. Widespread adoption of these techniques has languished because results are achieved too slowly (or so it is thought) to benefit patient care. Many viruses, however, can be identified in 1–3 days, which is comparable to the time required for isolation of bacteria. Other viruses still take 1–2 weeks to identify. The advent of rapid diagnostic methods in virology will increase the demand for viral diagnostic tests. Identifying an illness as viral will obviate further diagnostic evaluation, antibacterial therapy, and extended hospitalization. If an antiviral drug is available, its use may prolong the patient's life; though this situation is infrequent today, it may not be so in the future.

The isolation of viruses in cell cultures is still the starting point in most diagnostic virus laboratories. The proper timing of attempted virus isolation is important in minimizing false negative results. In most viral illnesses, the duration of virus shedding is short. It begins early and peaks near the onset of clinical illness; then the titer drops off rapidly (Fig 11–1). Serum antibody, in contrast, is usually absent at the beginning of the clinical illness, accumulates toward the end of the illness, and peaks when the patient is well. Some types of antibody, such as neutralizing and hemagglutination inhibition (HI) antibodies, last longer than others, such as complement fixing (CF) antibodies. The relationship of virus titer and antibody level to disease course determines the optimal time to obtain specimens for viral isolation and to demonstrate an increase in serum antibody levels. Tests for cell-mediated immunity are not discussed because they are not readily available and their place in clinical evaluation is just becom-

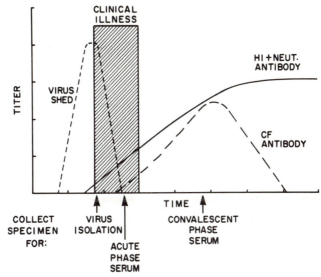

Fig 11–1.—Temporal relationship between clinical illness and virus shedding or development of serum antibody Virus is most likely to be detected very early in the clinical illness. By contrast, levels of antibody do not rise significantly until late in the illness. The time serum is obtained and the interval between the two serum specimens determines the likelihood of demonstrating a fourfold rise in antibody titer. Different types of antibody (complement fixation *(CF)*, hemagglutination inhibition *(HI)*, neutralization *(Neut)*) have different time courses of appearance and disappearance. These generalizations, with a few exceptions, apply to most types of primary viral infections.

ing clear. The same guidelines apply to most other classes of microorganisms discussed in this chapter.

There are several fine comprehensive reference texts.[1–4]

CLASSIFICATION

The viruses, chlamydiae, mycoplasmata, and rickettsiae that infect man are listed in Tables 11–1 through 11–4.

METHODS

Collection of Specimens

Proper collection of specimens is as important as the analysis of the test subsequently performed. Most specimens for virus isolation are collected onto a calcium alginate swab with a plastic applicator stick, because the oil in cotton on a wood stick may be toxic to the cell culture. The virus is then

TABLE 11–1.—VIRUSES OF MAN

I. RNA VIRUSES

FAMILY	GENUS	COMMON SPECIES (NUMBER OF IMMUNOTYPES)
Picornaviridae	Enterovirus	Polioviruses (3)
		Coxsackieviruses (types A & B) (23)
		Echoviruses (31)
		Enteroviruses 68–71 (4)
		Possible member: hepatitis A virus
	Rhinovirus	Virus types 1A-114 (> 115)
Caliciviridae	Calicivirus	Possible member: human calicivirus
Reoviridae	Reovirus	Types 1–3
	Orbivirus	Seventeen subgroups, including Colorado tick fever and Kemerovo viruses (> 80)
	Rotavirus	Human rotavirus (4)
Togaviridae	Alphavirus (arbovirus group A)	Sindbis virus and many other mosquito-borne viruses, including the viruses of eastern equine, Venezuelan, and western equine encephalitis, and Semliki Forest virus (22)
	Flavivirus (arbovirus group B)	Yellow fever virus, and other mosquito-borne viruses, including the viruses of dengue, Japanese, Murray Valley, and St. Louis encephalitis, and West Nile fever (25)
		Tick-borne viruses, including the viruses of Kyasanur Forest disease, Omsk hemorrhagic fever, European and Far Eastern tick-borne encephalitis (11)
		Viruses whose vectors are unknown (17)
	Rubivirus	Rubella virus
Orthomyxoviridae	Influenzavirus	Influenza virus type A (many)
		Influenza virus type B (several)
		Influenza virus type C (1)
Retroviridae	Not designated	Human T cell leukemia virus (HTLV)
Paramyxoviridae	Paramyxovirus	Parainfluenza virus (4)
		Mumps virus
	Morbillivirus	Measles virus
	Pneumovirus	Respiratory syncytial virus
Rhabdoviridae	Vesiculovirus	Vesicular stomatitis virus of horses, cattle, swine, with some human infections
	Lyssavirus	Rabies virus
Arenaviridae	Arenavirus	Lymphocytic choriomeningitis virus
		Lassa fever virus
		Tacaribe complex viruses, including Junin and Machupo viruses of South American hemorrhagic fevers (8)

TABLE 11–1.—Continued

I. RNA VIRUSES

FAMILY	GENUS	COMMON SPECIES (NUMBER OF IMMUNOTYPES)
Coronaviridae	Coronavirus	Human coronavirus
Bunyaviridae	Bunyavirus	Bunyamwera virus
		California encephalitis viruses (>11)
		Twelve other groups of antigenically related viruses plus ungrouped agents (> 102)
	(Ungrouped genus or genera)	Eleven other serological groupings plus ungrouped agents; included are viruses of the Uukuniemi group and well-known human pathogens such as the Crimean hemorrhagic fever-Congo group, phlebotomus fever group, Rift Valley fever virus, as well as other agents (> 95)

II. DNA VIRUSES

Parvoviridae	Parvovirus	Possible member: Norwalk gastroenteritis virus (2)
	Adeno-associated virus group	AAV (adeno-satellite virus) (4)
Papovaviridae	Papovavirus A	Wart virus (several)
		Papilloma viruses (several)
	Papovavirus B	BK and JC viruses
Adenoviridae	Mastadenovirus	Virus types 1–34
Herpesviridae		
Alphaherpesvirinae		Herpes simplex virus (2)
		Varicella-zoster virus
Betaherpesvirinae		Cytomegalovirus
Gammaherpesvirinae		Epstein-Barr virus
Poxviridae		
Chordopoxvirinae	Orthopoxvirus	Smallpox virus (variola)
		Vaccine virus
	Parapoxvirus	Virus of milker's node

eluted into the transport medium, usually Hank's balanced salt solution or veal infusion broth. Gelatin or albumin is added to stabilize the virus. Antibiotics are usually incorporated into the medium to suppress bacterial growth.

The type of swab used is similar for most classes of microorganisms. For mycoplasmata, trypticase soy broth is preferred as the transport medium. The antibiotics used are penicillin and fungicides; tetracycline, macrolides, and aminoglycosides inhibit or kill mycoplasmata. For chlamydiae, any nutrient broth will suffice, but the antibiotics should be aminoglycosides and fungicides and not tetracycline, penicillin, or macrolides, as these inhibit or kill the organism. For rickettsiae, the safest approach is not to isolate the organism.

TABLE 11–2.—Chlamydiaceae

MICROORGANISM	CLINICAL SYNDROME
Chlamydia psittaci	Pneumonia
C. trachomatis	
Serotypes A, B, Ba, C	Trachoma
	Inclusion conjunctivitis
Serotypes D–K	Nongonococcal urethritis
	Pneumonia
Serotypes L₁, L₂, L₃	Lymphogranuloma venereum

TABLE 11–3.—Mycoplasmatales

MICROORGANISM	CLINICAL SYNDROME
Mycoplasma pneumoniae	Pneumonia
M. hominis	Opportunist
Ureaplasma urealyticum	Nongonococcal urethritis
(T strain mycoplasma)	
M. salivarium	Normal oral flora
M. orale	Normal oral flora
M. buccale	Normal oral flora
M. faucium	Normal oral flora
M. fermentans	Rarely, in genitourinary tract flora
Acholeplasma laidlawii	Rarely, in oral flora and burn
(M. laidlawii)	wound flora

TABLE 11–4.—Rickettsial Diseases of Humans

DISEASE	ETIOLOGIC AGENT
Spotted fever group	
Rocky Mountain spotted fever	Rickettsia rickettsii
Boutonneuse fever	R. conorii
Rickettsialpox	R. akari
Siberian tick typhus	R. siberica
Queensland tick typhus	R. australis
Typhus group	
Epidemic typhus	R. prowazekii
Murine typhus	R. typhi (mooseri)
Brill-Zinsser disease	R. prowazekii
Q fever	Coxiella burnetii
Trench fever	Rochalimaea quintana
Scrub typhus	R. tsutsugamushi

Storage

Ideally, all specimens should be inoculated into the appropriate host system as soon as possible after collection to maximize yield. If that is not possible, most viruses, chlamydiae, and mycoplasmata are stable for 24 hours when refrigerated at 4 C. Beyond that period, specimens should be stored at − 70 C. The titer or quantity of the organism will diminish with one or more cycles of freezing and thawing, and the degree of reduction is variable for organisms within each class.

Detection of Antibody

The principles of the numerous serologic tests available are outlined below (see also Chap. 2).

COMPLEMENT FIXATION.—The CF test is a widely used procedure that is based on the ability of complement to fix or bind to antigen-antibody complexes. When either antigen or antibody is absent, no binding occurs and complement is free to react with the indicator system. This test requires special care in processing the complement.

HEMAGGLUTINATION INHIBITION.—Many viruses and other microorganisms agglutinate red blood cells (RBCs) from various animal species. When virus-specific antibody is added to the system, it will combine with the virus and inhibit the virus from agglutinating the RBCs. The titer of antibody is the dilution of serum at which hemagglutination ceases to be inhibited. This is a simple test to perform.

NEUTRALIZATION.—Many viruses cause cytopathic effect (CPE) in cell culture. In the presence of virus-specific antibody, live virus is neutralized and cannot cause CPE. The neutralization test is tedious to perform.

IMMUNOFLUORESCENCE (IF).—Virus and virus-specific antibody interaction can also be identified by reaction with a fluorescent dye in the IF test, by radioactive label in radioimmunoassay (RIA), or by an enzymatic reaction in the immunoperoxidase test and in the enzyme-linked immunosorbent assay (ELISA). With all of the systems the indicator can usually be linked with either the antigen or the antibody.

Detection of Antigen

Viruses can be grown in cell culture, embryonated hen eggs, or laboratory animals such as suckling mice or monkeys; co-cultivated with cell cultures and cells from diseased tissue; and grown in organ culture such as tracheal rings. Direct demonstration of antigen can be made by electron microscopy, often with the addition of virus-specific antibody (immuno-electron microscopy), by counterimmunoelectrophoresis (CIE), and by IF, immunoperoxidase, RIA, or ELISA. Most of these systems are also used for the detection of mycoplasma, chlamydiae, and rickettsiae.

Cell culture is still the most commonly used method for detection of virus. In cell culture, animal tissues are broken up with proteolytic enzymes (e.g., trypsin) and chelating agents (e.g., EDTA) to form a suspension of cells. These are placed in glass tubes, and a monolayer of cells forms. The cells are covered with an antibiotic-containing nutrient solution. Three types of cell cultures, primary, semicontinuous, and continuous cultures, are regularly used. Primary cultures are composed of epithelial and fibroblastic cells taken directly from animal tissues, for example from monkey kidney tissue (rhesus, cynomologous, or African green) or from primary human embryonic kidney. Semicontinuous cell cultures are derived by subculturing primary cultures repeatedly for a finite number of passages. Only fibroblastic cells survive passage, for example, those of WI-38 (human embryonic lung) or human foreskin. Continuous cell cultures are most often malignant epithelial cells. They are heteroploid, in contrast to the primary and semicontinuous types of cell cultures, which are diploid. Cells in continuous cell cultures grow rapidly and usually overgrow one another because of lack of contact inhibition. They can be passed indefinitely. Examples are Hep-2 (human epidermoid laryngeal carcinoma) and HeLa (human cervical carcinoma).

Virus is identified in cultures by one of three methods. First, virus infection alters cell morphology, resulting in a CPE. Cells round up and may cluster or form syncytiae. The time of development and appearance of the cellular alteration is characteristic for many viruses. Second, some viruses alter the surface of cells they infect and permit RBCs to adhere. This process is called hemadsorption. Finally, virus infection may induce neither CPE nor hemadsorption, but infected cells can be detected because they are resistant to superinfection with a virus known to cause CPE in those cells. For example, rubella virus infects African green monkey kidney cells without causing CPE. If the cells are later infected with echovirus type 2 or several other types of virus that induce CPE, typical CPE does not appear because the rubella virus interferes.

IMMUNODIAGNOSIS BASED ON CLINICAL SYNDROMES

In the following discussion, viral, chlamydial, mycoplasmal, and rickettsial infections are considered by clinical syndrome rather than by microorganism. The clinician, in attempting to ferret out the cause of a clinical syndrome, is better prepared to request the appropriate test if he knows the most likely organisms.

Respiratory Tract Infections

A list of syndromes and common causes of respiratory tract infections is given in Table 11–5. The appropriate specimens from the respiratory tract include nasal or throat washings, if the patient can cooperate, or combined nasal and throat swabs or sputum. If the etiology is unclear in a severe pneumonia, transtracheal aspirate, bronchial brushing or washing, or lung

TABLE 11–5.—Respiratory Tract Infections: Syndromes and Causes

SYNDROME	COMMON CAUSES	LESS COMMON CAUSES
Upper respiratory tract infection: cold, pharyngitis, etc.	Rhinoviruses Coronaviruses Parainfluenza viruses Influenza A and B viruses Herpes simplex virus (HSV) Adenoviruses Echoviruses Coxsackieviruses Respiratory syncytial virus Epstein-Barr virus	Influenza C virus Many other agents
Croup and bronchiolitis	Influenza A and B Respiratory syncytial virus Parainfluenza viruses	Adenoviruses
Pneumonia (adults)*	Influenza A *Mycoplasma pneumoniae*	*Coxiella burnetii* Adenoviruses *Chlamydia trachomatis*
Pneumonia (children)	Respiratory syncytial virus *Mycoplasma pneumoniae* Parainfluenza viruses Influenza A *Chlamydia trachomatis*	*Mycoplasma* sp. Adenoviruses Varicella-zoster virus (VZV)

*In the compromised host, herpesviruses (HSV, VZV, and cytomegalovirus [CMV]) are less common causes of pneumonia.

biopsy may be warranted. In contrast to bacterial pneumonia, upper respiratory secretions are valuable for detecting viral pneumonia. Herpes simplex virus (HSV) is the only virus that might be considered normal flora of the upper respiratory tract throughout the year.

Upper Respiratory Tract

Hundreds of different viruses are responsible for the common cold syndrome.[5-8] The rhinoviruses (115+ types) cause about 25%–30% of cases. Coronaviruses account for at least 10%. Influenza types A and B (rarely C), parainfluenza viruses (4 types, but mostly types 1, 2, and 3), respiratory syncytial virus, and adenoviruses (34 types) together are responsible for 10%–15% of common colds; most of these agents can also cause epidemic disease. Several of the respiratory viruses can cause reinfection in the presence of high titers of serum antibody (e.g., parainfluenza and respiratory syncytial viruses). Many other viruses associated with predominantly nonrespiratory clinical syndromes, such as measles, rubella, varicella, enteroviruses, and hepatitis viruses, are also associated with the common cold syndrome; perhaps 5% of colds are accounted for by these latter agents.

This leaves 50% or more of infections with no detectable etiologic agent. Although a small number may be caused by group A streptococci, most are probably due to unrecognized viruses.

The expected incidence in various age groups is important epidemiologic information. Pre-school-aged children have about 12 colds a year. The incidence decreases in older children to 6–8 colds per year and declines further in adults to 2–4 colds per year. Adults with children at home are likely to have more colds than those without.

Because of the innumerable causes, the self-limited nature of the disease, the minimum morbidity, and lack of effective treatment, the search for an etiologic agent is not cost effective and is rarely pursued except in research studies. The occasional complication of otitis media or sinusitis is usually due to bacterial superinfection.

DETECTION OF ANTIBODIES.—Detection of coronaviruses is usually done serologically, as isolation of viruses ordinarily requires obtaining organ specimens for culture. Strains 229E, OC-38, and OC-43 can be detected by CF.[9] Detection of antibodies to the other common agents will be discussed later.

DETECTION OF ANTIGEN.—Rhinoviruses are usually isolated in WI-38 and HeLa-M cell cultures, but a temperature of 33 C and a roller drum should be used.[10] Serologic methods are not routinely used for the identification of rhinoviruses because of the multiplicity of specific serotypes and lack of a group antigen.[10] Techniques for isolating other common viruses will be discussed later.

Lower Respiratory Tract

Viral infections cause most cases of pneumonia and tracheobronchitis in adults and bronchiolitis and croup in young children. Most lower respiratory tract infections occur in midwinter and early spring. In children, respiratory syncytial virus, parainfluenza viruses, and influenza A and B, and in adults, influenza A and B are the major viral agents.[11-14] Among military recruits adenovirus types 4 and 7 are also important. Many other viral agents are found less frequently in infections of the lower respiratory tract. For example, other serotypes of adenovirus and enteroviruses, such as coxsackieviruses and echoviruses, are found in adults and children. Rhinoviruses are responsible for some acute exacerbations in patients with chronic bronchitis. Measles is infrequently responsible since the advent of widespread immunization. The herpesviruses—varicella-zoster virus (VZV), cytomegalovirus (CMV), and HSV—are more often present in the immunosuppressed host, and prolonged shedding of respiratory syncytial virus may occur in this host setting.

Mycoplasma pneumoniae causes pneumonia throughout the year but the incidence tends to peak in late summer and fall.[15, 16] Older children and young adults are most often affected in epidemic and interepidemic periods.

Chlamydia psittaci is a well-recognized cause of pneumonia following exposure to many types of birds.

Chlamydia trachomatis is a newly recognized cause of pneumonia. It was first recognized as a slowly developing pneumonia in infants younger than 6 months and recently it has been proposed as a not uncommon cause of community-acquired pneumonia in adults.[17, 18] It also may cause an acute pharyngitis that resembles streptococcal pharyngitis.[19]

Rickettsiae are unusual causes of pneumonia. *Coxiella burnetii* is the agent responsible for the illness referred to as Q (query or Queensland) fever. The unique epidemiologic condition of exposure to infected products of cattle, sheep, or goats is required for transmission to occur.[20]

DETECTION OF ANTIBODIES.—One of the more common applications of diagnostic virology in a clinical setting is the ordering of a battery of serologic tests to determine the cause of a suspected viral lower respiratory tract infection. Influenza A and B virus, parainfluenza viruses, adenoviruses, and respiratory syncytial virus are usually included.

As with most serologic tests, an acute-phase serum should be obtained at or within a few days of the onset of illness and a convalescent phase serum obtained 10–14 or more days after onset (Table 11–6). A fourfold or greater increase in the antibody titer is considered significant (an acute phase titer of 1:8 and a convalescent phase titer of 1:32 represents a fourfold increase). A twofold increase is not considered significant, as it is within the limits of error of the test (e.g., 1:8 vs. 1:16, a twofold difference). Exceptions to this rule are rare. Dilutions, incidentally, are serial twofold dilutions (undilute, 1:2, 1:4, 1:8, 1:16, etc.). Dilutions may also be expressed as the reciprocal of the dilution, hence 0, 2, 4, 8, 16, etc. Serum in an initial test may be undilute or in low dilution—1:8. For example, in tests for orthomyxoviruses and paramyxoviruses, the serum is treated with receptor-destroying enzyme to inactivate nonspecific inhibitors of hemagglutination. This results in an initial serum dilution of 1:8 or 1:10, depending on laboratory method.

TABLE 11–6.—INTERPRETATION OF SEROLOGIC TESTS: GENERAL GUIDELINES

1. Fourfold or greater rise in titer between acute and convalescent specimen is usually diagnostic of infection.
2. A single high titer in convalescent specimen is usually only suggestive of recent infection.
3. Range of error of tests is a twofold dilution.
4. Cross-reactions with closely related agents should be considered.

In general, isolation of virus and the finding of a fourfold rise in serum antibody to that virus permits the clinician to relate the patient's illness to that virus. But it should be understood that these findings are not strict proof of causation.

Influenza.—Influenza is perhaps the most clinically significant of the respiratory viruses. It is responsible for greatest mortality.[21] Because of this clinical reality, much has been learned of the immunology of influenza virus infection. The most common serologic test, the HI test, requires a fourfold rise in titer to be compatible with acute infection. The test is sensitive, specific, and inexpensive. Serum antibody titers of 1:40 or greater are associated with protection from reinfection,[22, 23] titers of 1:20 and 1:10 are associated with lesser degrees of protection. A titer less than 1:10 is considered negative and indicates the need for vaccination. In addition to antibody to the hemagglutinin (H) protein already described, the human host develops antibody to the neuraminidase (N) protein. These appear to be the viral proteins of major immunologic significance. Antihemagglutinin antibody is thought to protect against infection, while antineuraminidase (or neuraminidase inhibition) antibody protects against clinical illness if infection occurs; this dichotomy has recently been disputed.[24, 25]

There are several different types of H and N proteins (Table 11-7).[26-27] These viruses, are named by the type (A, B, or C), the country or city where they were isolated, the number of the isolate in that locale that year, the year the strain was first isolated, and the H and N subtype. The B strains have no subtype designation. The influenza strains used in the recent vaccines are influenza A/Brazil/11/78 (H1N1), A/Bangkok/1/79 (H3N2), and B/Singapore/222/79.

When the prevalent strain in a community changes from a virus with one hemagglutinin subtype to another, the phenomenon is called antigen

TABLE 11-7.—ARCHAEOLOGY OF INFLUENZA A VIRUSES

VIRAL SURFACE ANTIGENS		APPROXIMATE YEAR OF INTRODUCTION	ERA	EARLY AND RECENT REPRESENTATIVE STRAINS
Hemagglutinin	Neuraminidase			
HSW*	N1	1918		A/Swine/1976/37
				A/New Jersey/8/76
HO*	N1	1929	Swine	A/Puerto Rico/8/34
H1*	N1	1946		A/Fort Meade/1/47
				A/Brazil/11/78
H2	N2	1957		A/Singapore/1/57
			Asian	
H3	N2	1968		A/Hong Kong/1/68
				A/Bangkok/1/79

*These three H subtypes are antigenically related. They are now grouped together as the H1 subtype.

shift [e.g., from A/Taiwan/64 (H2N2) to A/HongKong/68 (H3N2)]; this represents a shift from one subtype (H2N2) to another subtype (H3N2). When the prevalent strain maintains the same hemagglutinin but the antigenic composition of the hemagglutinin changes slightly, it is referred to as antigenic drift [e.g., from A/USSR/77 (H1N1) to A/Brazil/77 (H1N1)]; this represents a drift within the same H1N1 subtype. Antigen drift occurs within types A and B influenza virus, but shift occurs with type A only.

The probable public health significance of a shift in virus strain is self-evident—a new strain has a reasonable chance of causing a worldwide pandemic. The importance of drift is less evident. The degree of drift determines the need for changing the vaccine strain of the same subtype. Slight antigenic drift may not require a change in vaccine composition, but a drift that takes place over 2–3 years usually does.

Neutralization tests are more sensitive in detecting low levels of antibody than HI tests but are more costly and time-consuming.[28] CF tests are used less often than HI tests because they are not specific for the hemagglutinin but detect antibody to the ribonucleoprotein. They are, therefore, type-specific (Type A or B) but not subtype-specific, as is the HI test. Nevertheless, CF is occasionally used to define acute infections when an acute specimen is not available for the HI test. CF antibodies are predominately of the IgM class, so they last for a shorter period than HI, neutralization, and neuraminidase inhibition antibody. Rapid disappearance of CF antibody in the context of a persistently elevated HI antibody titer is compatible with acute infection.

Antibody elaborated by mucosal surfaces is known as secretory antibody. Each antibody molecule is composed of two IgA molecules plus two additional moieties, secretory piece and J chain, to prevent degradation of IgA molecules. Secretory antibody levels in the nasal mucosa are important in parainfluenza virus infection but less so in influenza.[29, 30]

Other respiratory viruses.—Most of the other respiratory viruses also require demonstration of a fourfold or greater rise in antibody from the acute to the convalescent phase. For parainfluenza viruses, HI, CF, and neutralization testing can be done. However, heterotypic antibody responses, especially with repeated infection, are the rule, so it is often difficult to be certain which one of the four types has caused infection. Some mild infections in primed adults do not result in a rise in antibody titer.[31]

For adenoviruses, the same three serologic tests can be used. The CF test is more commonly used as it is group-specific and can detect infection with most types. The HI and neutralization tests are type-specific and so are used when the type number of the infecting strain is known. Heterotypic antibody responses occur to a lesser extent in adenoviruses than in parainfluenza.[32]

Respiratory syncytial virus commonly occurs in infants in the first 6 months of life, yet an antibody response may not be elicited during this period. This is also a problem in the elderly. The CF test is most commonly used for serodiagnosis, but neutralization, plaque reduction neutralization, and ELISA are more sensitive techniques. In respiratory syncytial virus as in parainfluenza virus infections, the level of serum antibody correlates poorly with protection from reinfection. Local IgA antibody production in the nasal mucosa is more important.[33, 34]

Mycoplasmata.—CF is the standard test for detection of *M. pneumoniae.* However, it will miss 20% or more of cases. More sensitive tests are growth inhibition and mycoplasmacidal methods,[35] but these are not ordinarily available.

Ureaplasma urealyticum may also be an agent of respiratory infection. Additional confirmatory studies are necessary.

Chlamydiae.—There are 15 immunotypes of *C. trachomatis.* Endemic trachoma is usually caused by types A–C. Genital infections, including neonatal infection acquired from the cervix, and adult ocular infections in developed countries are most often due to types D–K. Lymphogranuloma venereum is caused by type L.

With the microimmunofluorescence (micro-IF) method, a fourfold rise in IgG or IgM *Chlamydia*-specific antibody is diagnostic of acute infection. IgM titers of 1:64 or greater in a single specimen is suggestive of recent infection in adults and infants.[17, 18] The CF test is not used as it detects a group-specific antigen and is not immuno-type-specific, as is micro-IF. Micro-IF can also be used to detect tear antibody and so is useful in the diagnosis of ocular infections.

For *C. psittaci,* the CF test is most often used. A fourfold rise in titer should be sought between acute and convalescent specimens. A single titer of 1:16 in the proper host setting is suggestive of psittacosis. Appropriate antibiotics may delay the appearance of serum antibody in the convalescent period.[36]

Rickettsiae.—Of the *Rickettsia* associated with pneumonia, *Coxiella burnetii* is most often diagnosed by CF. Again, a fourfold rise in titer is sought to establish the association with an acute illness.

The antigens used in the CF test and other serologic tests (microagglutination, IF, and radioimmune precipitation) can employ either suspensions of phase II *Rickettsia,* which react with antibody from an acute infection or past exposure, or phase I *Rickettsia,* which react only with antibody from past exposure or current chronic infection (such as endocarditis).[37]

The Weil-Felix test is negative in Q fever.

DETECTION OF ANTIGEN.—Influenza viruses can be isolated in tissue culture such as primary monkey kidney (rhesus or cynomologous) or a continuous cell line (Madin-Darby canine kidney). Embryonated hen eggs can also be used. Virus growth is then detected in several days by hemadsorption of cell cultures or by hemagglutination of amniotic or allantoic fluid, or both. With influenza viruses, as with most respiratory viruses, nasal, and throat swabs, nasal washings, throat gargles, or sputum can be used. The last three give the highest yield.

If virus is not detected in several (3–5) days, an aliquot of culture fluid can be passed to another culture ("blind passage") to attempt to increase the yield.[38] This is done with all respiratory and most other viruses.

Parainfluenza viruses are detected in primary monkey kidney or human embryonic kidney cell cultures by hemadsorption (Fig 11–2). Type 2

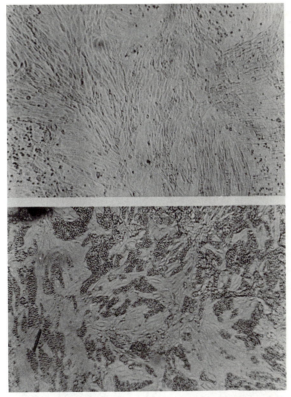

Fig 11–2.—Hemadsorption of a myxovirus-infected RhMK culture (10 ×). *Top,* uninoculated RhMK culture. *Bottom,* RhMK culture infected with parainfluenza virus type 1, showing hemadsorption of guinea pig erythrocytes. (From Hsiung G.D.: *Diagnostic Virology,* rev. ed. New Haven, Yale University Press, 1973, p. 87. Reproduced by permission.)

strains may product CPE in the initial culture passage.[39] The four virus types are distinguished by HI methods.

Adenoviruses are rapidly grown in various human epithelial cell lines, where they show a typical CPE of grapelike clusters of cells and long strands between infected clusters (Fig 11–3). The individual type is determined by serologic methods after being grouped by hemagglutination characteristics.[32]

Respiratory syncytial virus also grows in human epithelial cell lines and produces characteristic syncytium as its CPE (Fig 11–4). An IF technique has been successful in the rapid diagnosis of infection when sputum or upper respiratory tract cells from washings are used. IF techniques may be available in the near future for the rapid diagnosis of most common respiratory viruses.[1, 2]

Mycoplasma pneumoniae can be grown on diphasic media in a few days but may take 2–3 weeks. Detection should be done in a facility separate

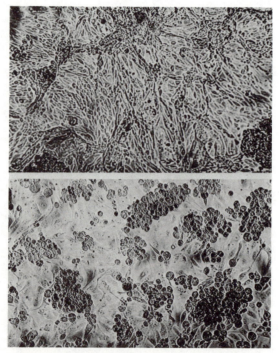

Fig 11–3.—Cytopathic effect (CPE) induced by an adenovirus in HEK cell culture (10×). *Top,* uninfected HEK cultures. *Bottom,* CPE induced by adenovirus type 3. (From Hsiung G.D.: *Diagnostic Virology,* rev. ed. New Haven, Yale University Press, 1973, p. 120. Reproduced by permission.)

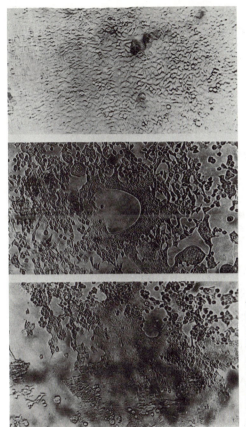

Fig 11–4.—Syncytial cell formation induced by RS virus in Hep-2 cell cultures (10×). *Top,* uninoculated cell control. *Middle,* RS virus-infected cells at 3 days. *Bottom,* RS virus-infected cells at 5 days. (From Hsiung G.D.: *Diagnostic Virology,* rev. ed. New Haven, Yale University Press, 1973, p. 101. Reproduced by permission.)

from the virology laboratory to avoid persistent contamination of viral cell cultures with mycoplasma.

Chlamydia trachomatis is grown in monkey cells that are either X-irradiated or treated with nucleic acid or protein synthesis inhibitors to decrease cell reproduction and permit chlamydiae to successfully compete for cell nutrients. Growth is detected by staining for intracytoplasmic inclusions.

Attempts to isolate *C. psittaci* are too hazardous for laboratory personnel. *Coxiella burnetii* can be grown in the yolk sac of eggs, as can most rickettsiae. These methods are not without hazard. Serologic methods of diagnosis are preferred.

Rapid diagnostic techniques using primarily IF methods are gradually being instituted in virus laboratories.[40, 41] Broader application will follow when reliable reagents are commercially available.

Detection of metabolites.—The diagnostic value of cold agglutinins (actually cold hemagglutinins) are often confused with the more specific serologic procedures used in the diagnosis of *M. pneumoniae* infections discussed above. High titers of cold agglutinins are present in infections due to not only *M. pneumoniae* but also adenovirus and influenza virus infections. A positive cold agglutinin test is suggestive of *M. pneumoniae* most often when the titer is 1:64 or greater for the bedside test on 1:128 or greater for the conventional test.[42]

Gastrointestinal Infections

Many diarrheas are referred to as viral when the etiology is not apparent. Some are bacterial and require special growth media (e.g., *Campylobacter fetus*), some are truly viral, and many are of unknown etiology. The viruses that are now recognized as causing diarrhea are rotaviruses, a reovirida, and Norwalk-like agents, which are parvoviruses.[43–54] Adenoviruses, astroviruses, caliciviruses, coronaviruses, and enteroviruses have been suggested as causes of gastroenteritis,[43] but Koch's and River's postulates for causation have not been regularly satisfied.

Detection of Antibodies

For rotaviruses, multiple serologic techniques are available—immunoelectron microscopy, CF, IF, immune adherence hemagglutination, and ELISA.[44, 45] ELISA offers the advantage of distinguishing IgM from IgG immune responses. In addition, the immune responses appear to be serotype-specific.

For the parvovirus-like agents, there are several antigenically distinct agents—Norwalk, Hawaii, Montgomery County (MC), W, Ditchling, and Cockle. Immunity lasts for 6 weeks to 2 years and is agent-specific.[46, 47] Local secretory IgA antibody in the gastrointestinal tract may be more important than serum IgG antibody in protection from reinfection.[48] Immune adherence assays and RIAs can document the presence of infection, as serum antibody rises within 2 weeks after infection, but the assays are not agent-specific.

None of these serologic tests is currently commercially available for either virus group, so the more common method of detection is to look for antigen.

Detection of Antigen

Rotavirus can be easily detected by a commercially available ELISA that rapidly (within hours) detects virus in stool samples. The original technique for detection—immunoelectron microscopy—although efficient, is too cumbersome for the average laboratory. Other methods such as IF, CIE, and RIA are more expensive or more elaborate than ELISA. Cell culture techniques are not used, as the virus does not grow readily.[45, 49, 51]

The parvovirus-like agents are optimally detected by immunoelectron microscopy.[50, 51] Immune serum must still be used, in contrast to rotavirus detection, where it is not necessary. Virus shedding is readily detectable within 1–2 days of onset of illness. Thereafter it is unusual to find virus in the stool with most Norwalk-like agents.[53] An RIA has recently been developed that may simplify detection.[54]

Hepatitis

Most cases of viral hepatitis are caused by hepatitis A virus (HAV), hepatitis B virus (HBV), and one or more non-A, non-B hepatitis viruses. There are, however, several other common viruses that can present as acute hepatitis. These agents include Epstein-Barr virus (EBV), CMV, rubella, rubeola, mumps, adenoviruses and coxsackie B viruses; other clinical signs, however, should distinguish them. In immunosuppressed hosts, HSV, VZV, and CMV can present with hepatitis as part of a disseminated infection. Outside the United States, yellow fever virus is a rare cause of hepatitis.[55]

Detection of Antibodies

Detection of HAV antibody has recently become possible. On a single serum specimen, IgM and IgG antibody to HAV (anti-HAV) is determined. During the early stage of illness IgM anti-HAV is present in high titer and indicates acute infection. This antibody first appears about 4 weeks after exposure and at the onset of jaundice, and persists for 6–8 weeks more (Fig 11–5). IgG anti-HAV appears later and is predominant in the convalescent phase of illness; it appears about 6 weeks after exposure and persists for years. The presence of IgG anti-HAV alone is not compatible with an acute illness but is more consistent with infection at an indeterminant time in the past. A micro-solid-phase RIA blocking test (SPRIA-blocking) is commonly used to test for the presence of the two antibodies. Immunoelectron microscopy is also effective. Other tests used in the immunodiagnosis for anti-HAV are an ELISA blocking test, immuno-adherence hemagglutination, and CF.[56–58]

False positive tests are common unless a highly purified antigen preparation is used. Serum antibodies to non-HAV antigens in crude stool extracts account for the false positive results.[56]

In the presence of IgG anti-HAV, protection against reinfection should

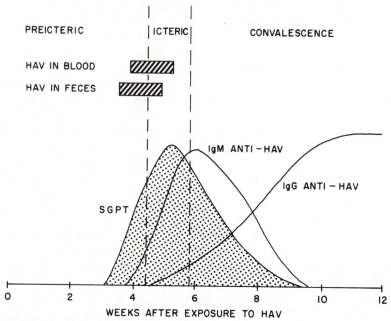

Fig 11–5.—Schematic diagram indicating the appearance and disappearance of seroimmunologic markers of hepatitis A infection (antibodies to hepatitis A, *anti-HAV*) during the course of typical disease and their relationship to SGPT elevation. The period of viremia and fecal excretion of hepatitis A virus *(HAV)* is shown at the top. (Adapted from Koff R.S.: *Viral Hepatitis.* New York, John Wiley & Sons, Inc., 1978, p. 136. Reproduced by permission.)

be lifelong. In the detection of HBV infection, HBV antibodies and HBV antigens are both sought. HBV is composed of several clinically detectable components. A central core, the Dane particle, has on its surface a core antigen (HBcAg) and within it the viral DNA and DNA polymerase. The e antigen (HBeAg) may also be associated with this particle. The Dane particle is in turn surrounded by surface antigen (HBsAg).

In the typical patient (70% of cases), early in the course of an HBV infection, HBsAg is the first viral marker to appear (Fig 11–6). HBeAg, Dane particles and DNA polymerase activity subsequently appear. All of these markers are present before the onset of clinically apparent hepatitis. Antibody to HBcAg (anti-HBc) develops at the onset of clinical disease, and antibody to HBsAg (anti-HBs) appears later during the convalescent phase. Anti-HBe develops also during the convalescent period.[59]

The diagnosis of HBV infection is usually based on determination of three of the seven described markers: HbsAg, anti-HBc, and anti-HBs. If

HBsAg and anti-HBc are present or if anti-HBc alone is present, the patient is in the acute phase of illness, and the disease is communicable. When anti-HBs with or without anti-HBc is present the patient is either in the convalescent phase of illness or has had HBV infection at some time in the past; in this phase the illness is not contagious. The presence of anti-HBs provides immunity from reinfection. If HBsAg remains in the blood for 20 or more weeks, the patient is considered to be a chronic HBsAg carrier and may remain infectious for as long as 20 years. High titers of IgM anti-HBc might help distinguish patients with acute hepatitis.[60]

About 25% of patients have self-limited HBV infections without the detection of HBsAg. In this group of patients, anti-HBs appears before the onset of clinical disease. Anti-HBc also appears earlier and is present in lower titers than in the first type of patient described.

The remaining 5% of patients become chronic carriers. Tests for HBeAg

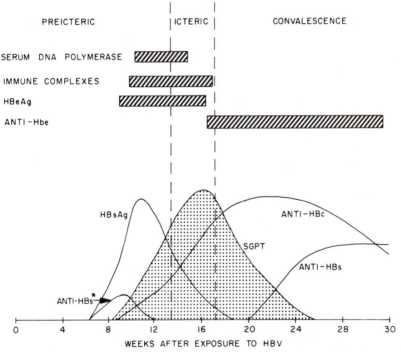

Fig 11–6.—Schematic diagram indicating typical seroimmunologic alterations in relation to SGPT elevations during the course of acute hepatitis B. The presence of serum DNA polymerase activity, immune complexes, and HBeAg is shown at the *top left. Asterisk* indicates that anti-HBs is present but not detectable as free antibody. (Adapted from Koff R.S.: *Viral Hepatitis.* New York, John Wiley & Sons, Inc., 1978, p. 137. Reproduced by permission.)

and anti-HBe are now commercially available. These two new tests should be ordered when HBsAg is detectable. The subtle interrelationships of all the serologic markers are outlined in Table 11–8.[61] Most tests used for detection of HBV markers have gone through several stages of development. First-generation tests, agarose gel diffusion, are the least sensitive. Second-generation tests, CIE, rheophoresis, and CF, improved detection 10- to 100-fold. The currently used third-generation tests, RIA, hemagglutination, ELISA, immune adherence, and latex agglutination; are up to 10,000-fold more sensitive than the first-generation tests.

For epidemiologic studies, advantage is taken of the point that there are at least five antigenic specificites on the HBsAg particles: A group determinant, a, and two pairs of subtype determinants, d and y (for Darmouth and Yale) and w and r (for Walter and Reed). Strains adw, adr, ayw, ayr can then be identified to serve as epidemiologic markers. Antigenic heterogenicity was recently described for the w determinant, and additional determinants q, g, or x may exist.[59]

Also recently described is the delta antigen associated with HBsAg. Its presence usually correlates with a subgroup of HbsAg chronic carriers who have chronic active and progressive hepatitis. Anti-delta antibody can be identified by RIA or ELISA.[62]

TABLE 11–8.—PATTERNS OF HEPATITIS B VIRUS (HBV) SEROLOGIC MARKERS

| INTERPRETATION | SEROLOGIC MARKERS | | | | | |
	HBsAg	HBeAg	IgM Anti-HBc	Total Anti-HBc	Anti-HBe	Anti-HB
Acute infection						
Incubation period	+ *	+ *	−	−	−	−
Acute phase	+	+	+	+	−	−
Early convalescent phase	+	−	+	+	+	−
Convalescent phase	−	−	+	+	+	−
Late convalescent phase	−	−	− †	+	+	+
Long past infection	−	−	−	+ ‡	+ or −	+ ‡
Chronic infection						
Chronic active hepatitis	+ §	+ or −	+ or −	+ §	+ or −	− §
Chronic persistent hepatitis	+ ¶	+ or −	+ or −	+	+ or −	−
Chronic HBV carrier state	+ ¶	+ or −	+ or −	+	+ or −	−
HBsAg immunization	−	−	−	−	−	+

Table courtesy of Swenson and Escobar.[61] Reproduced by permission.
*HBsAg and HBeAg are occasionally undetectable in acute HBV infection.
†IgM anti-HBc may persist for over a year after acute infection when very sensitive assays are employed.
‡Total anti-HBc and anti-HBs may be detected together or separately long after acute infection.
§HBsAg-negative chronic active hepatitis may occur where total anti-HBc and anti-HBs may be detected together, separately, or not at all.
¶HBsAg-negative chronic persistent hepatitis and chronic HBV carriers have been observed.

Detection of Antigen

Although HAV is tentatively classified as an enterovirus in the picorna-virus family, it does not grow readily in tissue culture. Detection of virus requires demonstration of virus particles in the stool by immunoelectron microscopy, RIA, or ELISA. However, virus appears early in the incuba-tion period and is usually gone by the time the patient comes to the atten-tion of a physician because of jaundice. IF detection of HAV in liver biopsy tissue after the onset of jaundice is currently being investigated.[56] Liver biopsy, however, is not a procedure that is indicated in the average patient with HAV infection. Because of all of these limitations, the diagnosis of HAV infection is invariably made by searching for IgM and IgG anti-HAV antibodies.[56]

The detection of HBV antigens was discussed previously.

A diagnosis of non-A, non-B hepatitis is currently made by excluding HAV, HBV, and other known causes of hepatitis. As in HAV, the disease is relatively mild in the acute stage, but chronic hepatitis can occur. The infection usually follows blood transfusions; in fact, it is the most common cause of posttransfusion hepatitis. The disease has an incubation period of 5–10 weeks, which is between that for HAV and HBV.[63]

Mononucleosis Syndrome

The syndrome of infectious mononucleosis is most often caused by EBV and most of these cases exhibit heterophile antibody. In heterophile-nega-tive mononucleosis EBV is still the most common cause, followed by CMV, toxoplasmosis, HAV and HBV, rubella, roseola, mumps, and drug reac-tions.[64, 65] The syndrome can also be confused with streptococcal sore throat and infectious lymphocytosis of childhood.

Detection of Antigen

EBV is found in throat washings and in circulating lymphocytes during the acute phase of disease as well as many years afterward. The presence of virus, then, is not diagnostic of acute disease. In addition, the virus is difficult to detect; isolation is usually attempted only in research laborato-ries. EBV is known to infect B lymphocytes and to stimulate a proliferation of T cells cytotoxic for the B cells.

CMV can be grown in tissue culture; however, the appearance of CPE usually takes 1–4 weeks. The laboratory must therefore be notified that CMV infection is suspected, so that the culture can be held for the appro-priate time. WI-38 cell cultures, a cell strain used in most virus laboratories, can support the growth of CMV. The best specimens for culture are urine, throat swab, buffy coat, and cervical swab.

Detection of Antibody

Heterophile antibodies are found in 80%–90% of cases of EBV-associated mononucleosis. The viral component that stimulates their production is unknown. In the Paul-Bunnell test, sheep RBCs are agglutinated by heterophile antibodies as well as by Forssman antibodies and antibodies found with serum sickness. To distinguish these three antibodies, the Paul-Bunnell-Davidsohn differential absorption test was devised. The patient's serum is absorbed with guinea pig kidney cells and beef RBCs and then tested again for the persistence of sheep RBC agglutinins (Table 11–9). If the titer of sheep cell agglutinins after guinea pig kidney absorption is only twofold to fourfold less than before absorption (i.e., 128 or 256 vs. 512), and markedly reduced by beef RBCs, the result is compatible with infectious mononucleosis. If guinea pig kidney cells and beef RBCs completely remove the sheep cell agglutinins, serum sickness is more likely. Forssman antibodies found in normal serum are present in low titers and are removed by guinea pig but not beef cells.

The Lee-Davidsohn test uses horse instead of sheep RBCs to increase the sensitivity of the test. Hence, it is the preferred test when evidence for low levels of antibody is sought.

Heterophile antibodies may not appear until late in the illness; therefore, the test should be repeated weekly for the first few weeks if it is negative initially. Prolonged convalescence is associated with delay in their appearance.[66]

The commercial tests currently preferred do not use the classic tube method of Paul-Bunnell-Davidsohn. These new rapid spot and slide tests are at least as sensitive as the classic ones. Lymphoma, malaria, rubella, adenovirus, CMV, mumps, and hepatitis rarely give a false positive result.[67, 68] False negative results may occur in children; the clinical syndrome is also atypical in this age group.

TABLE 11–9.—INTERPRETATION OF HETEROPHILE ANTIBODIES TEST: SAMPLE TITERS

SOURCE OF ANTIBODY	SHEEP RBC AGGLUTININS WITHOUT ABSORPTION	SHEEP RBC AGGLUTININS AFTER ABSORPTION WITH	
		Guinea Pig	Beef RBCs
Infectious mononucleosis	1,024	512	0
Serum sickness	256	0	0
Normal serum: Forssman antibody	32	0	32

A positive spot test should be confirmed by a tube test (e.g., Lee-Davidsohn) only if the blood smears are not compatible with infectious mononucleosis. Conversely, when the blood smears are suggestive and the spot test is negative, a tube test should be done to maximize the chance of detecting heterophile antibodies.

Heterophile antibodies are no longer detectable in most sera 1 year after infection by the Paul-Bunnell-Davidsohn test but they are detectable at that time by the Lee-Davidsohn test.[69]

Specific anti-EBV antibodies can be sought in the unusual case when EBV infection is suspected but heterophile antibodies are repeatedly absent (Fig 11–7). IgM and IgG antibodies to the viral capsid antigen (VCA) are detectable early in the illness. IgM VCA antibodies clear by 4 months in most cases, while IgG VCA remain for life and protect against reinfection.[69] Other early-appearing viral specific antibodies such as antibody to the anti-D and anti-R types of early antigen are not consistently present. The late-appearing antibodies are Epstein-Barr nuclear antigen and soluble complement-fixing antigen. Neutralizing antibodies also appear late but are difficult to measure.

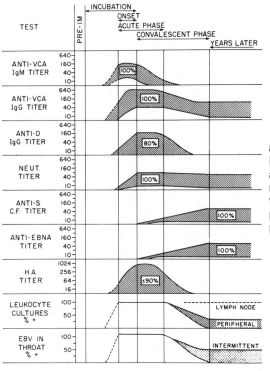

Fig 11–7.—Scheme of antibody responses to Epstein-Barr virus-related antigens in infectious mononucleosis. (Adapted from Lennette and Schmidt, p. 450[1] Reproduced by permission.)

The absence of IgG VCA antibody in an initial serum sample followed shortly by its appearance in a second serum sample is compatible with recent infection.

There are several other causes of heterophile-negative mononucleosis; CMV is the most common. CF is most often used to identify CMV under such circumstances. As with most CF tests it is specific but not optimally sensitive. The less readily available IF tests, indirect fluorescent antibody (IFA) and anticomplementary IF tests, are more sensitive and detect antibody earlier in the course of illness.[70, 71] ELISA assays for IgG and IgM antibodies to CMV are becoming commercially available and should prove to be extremely useful.

Evaluation for the other less common causes of heterophile-negative mononucleosis described at the beginning of this section are discussed elsewhere. CMV is thought to be responsible for almost half of heterophile-negative cases and for about 18% of all cases of the mononucleosis syndrome.

Exanthematous Infections

In general skin lesions are not cultured in exanthematous infections except for vesicular lesions. Throat and rectal swabs are helpful to isolate the putative agents and combine such information with the serologic response and clinical syndrome. IF and electron microscopy may demonstrate the organism in skin biopsy specimens. In the case of vesicular lesions, vesicular fluid should be aspirated; bacterial cultures and Gram stains should not be omitted. Virus may be isolated from whole blood in the hemorrhagic rashes.

The etiologic agents in exanthematous infections can be distinguished from one another when an outbreak occurs, but in an individual patient such distinction may be difficult. A century ago, the common maculopapular rashes were divided into six diseases: measles, scarlet fever, rubella, Duke's disease (probably a rubella variant), erythema infectiosum, and roseola (exanthem subitum).[72] The causes of the first three of these diseases are now known and the diseases are readily evaluable, whereas the causes of the last two are unknown and the diseases are not evaluable in the laboratory. Rubella virus, incidentally, has recently been classified as a togavirus. Some causes of exanthematous infections and the appearance of the associated rash are listed in Table 11–10.

Maculopapular rashes can also be caused by enteroviruses and *M. pneumoniae* (see section on respiratory infection). Vesiculopustular rashes are commonly caused by VZV and HSV, and uncommonly by molluscum contagiosum, orf, and papilloma virus. Because smallpox has been eradicated,

TABLE 11–10.—EXANTHEMATOUS INFECTIONS

APPEARANCE OF RASH	COMMON CAUSES	LESS COMMON CAUSES
Maculopapular	Echoviruses	Epstein-Barr virus
	Coxsackieviruses	*Mycoplasma pneumoniae*
	Measles	Adenoviruses
	Rubella	Cytomegalovirus
Vesiculopustular	Herpes simplex virus	*Rickettsia akari*
	Varicella-zoster virus	Vaccinia
	Coxsackieviruses	
	Echoviruses	
	Enterovirus 71	
Hemorrhagic	Alphaviruses	*Rickettsia typhi*
	Bunyaviruses	Atypical measles
	Flaviviruses	
	Rickettsia rickettsii	
Localized	Herpes simplex virus	Cowpox
	Papilloma virus	Milker's nodule
	Molluscum contagiosum	Orf

vaccination is no longer administered; rashes due to vaccinia or smallpox would therefore be expected only after a laboratory accident while working with these agents.

The agents of hemorrhagic fever are unusual in this country though common in tropical areas of the world; they are arenaviruses, Marburg and Ebola, and the various togaviruses.

Rickettsial diseases, in particular Rocky Mountain spotted fever, are more commonly seen now with the changing life-styles and increased exposure to ticks while camping.

Detection of Antigen

Following widespread immunization, the incidence of measles (rubeola) has been markedly reduced. Though reinfection can occur, there is no associated clinical disease (except for atypical measles) in persons initially vaccinated with killed measles vaccine. Virus isolation is difficult technically and the diagnosis is best established by serologic tests or, if urgent, by direct IF.[73]

The procedure for rubella isolation is tedious, usually requiring demonstration in African green monkey kidney cells of interference-CPE in Vero and RK-13 cell lines.[74] The virus is very labile. Serologic confirmation of infection is preferred, but if it is not possible, isolation can be attempted.

VZV causes chickenpox and herpes zoster or shingles. Differentiation from HSV may be necessary, but distinguishing VZV from smallpox virus is no longer required, as smallpox has been eradicated and should only be a problem in isolated laboratory accidents. In the past, smallpox virus could be rapidly detected by electron microscopy or by searching for Guarnieri bodies with light microscopy. Distinguishing vaccinia (cowpox) from variola (smallpox) virus required observing growth characteristics on the chorioallantoic membrane.[75]

Examination of vesicle scrapings with Giemsa stain (Tzanck smear) or a cervicovaginal Papanicolaou stain will show multinucleated giant cells and intranuclear inclusions with the herpes viruses VZV and HSV, but not with smallpox virus. The test, however, is not specific for the type of herpes virus.

If culture for VZV is planned, special collection techiques are required.[76] The specimen should be collected from fresh vesicles in the first few days for chickenpox and in the first week for zoster (or longer in immunosuppressed subjects). Immunodiffusion and fluorescence antibody techniques provide a more rapid and specific way of distinguishing VZV and HSV.

Growth in tissue culture is difficult and slow for VZV. In contrast, HSV grows quickly in many different tissue culture systems, including ones available in most diagnostic virology laboratories. CPE may develop overnight with HSV if the inoculum is high,[77] whether or not the virus is of type 1 or 2. HSV can be determined by IF or microneutralization.

To make a diagnosis of an enterovirus exanthematous illness, virus isolation must be attempted. The viruses are relatively simple to isolate in standard cell cultures. Multiple sites, including throat, stool, and other symptomatic sites (i.e., spinal or pericardial fluid), should be sampled. If a group A coxsackievirus is suspected in a patient with herpangina, suckling mice should be inoculated. These animals are not available in most virus laboratories. The not infrequent exanthem, hand, foot and mouth disease, is usually due to Coxsackie A-16 and also A-5, 9 or 10.

If an enterovirus is isolated, the exact immunotype can be identified at a central reference laboratory. Neutralization tests are done with multiple antiserum pools, each of which contains antibody to several immunotypes.[78] The results are displayed in a checkerboard format and the isolate is identified by examining the intersecting pools of antiserum.

Warts are caused by papillomavirus in the Papovaviridae family. The virus, however, has not been easy to grow in eggs or tissue culture. Antibody is detectable in many cases by CF or fluorescence antibody methods, but the diagnosis is basically a clinical one today.

Rocky Mountain spotted fever is the most common of the rickettsial infections in the United States. Most cases occur east of the Rockies. Attempts at isolating the organisms are to be avoided because the procedures are complicated and the chance of laboratory-acquired infection is not insignificant.[79] IF of infected tissue is being investigated as a rapid diagnostic method.[80] Diagnosis is preferably made by serologic methods.

Detection of Antibody

Serologic confirmation of a diagnosis of measles is rarely requested. However, suspected acute measles in a vaccinated person, atypical measles, and subacute sclerosing panencephalitis (SSPE) will require serologic confirmation. The presence of acute measles and atypical measles can be shown by demonstrating the standard fourfold or greater rise in antibody titer. The HI method is preferred but neutralization and CF tests are available. For SSPE, the presence of high HI antibody titers in the cerebrospinal fluid (CSF) and serum will help establish the diagnosis.[73]

Determination of rubella antibodies is frequently requested and correct interpretation of the results can have a significant clinical impact. The HI test is most commonly used. Titers of 1:64 or less in those vaccinated with rubella vaccine may not protect against reinfection. Nevertheless, if reinfection occurs it is usually asymptomatic, and viremia is a rare, poorly documented event.[81]

Rubella antibody titers are most frequently requested to determine the immune status in a woman. Here a single specimen is submitted to the laboratory. A passive hemagglutination test is usually done; any positive result (1+ to 4+) is considered evidence of immunity from past infection. An HI test result of 1:8 or greater is also compatible with past infection. If either test is positive, vaccination is not required. The passive hemagglutination test is not used to detect recent infection. ELISA has recently been reported to be as sensitive and specific as the HI test[82] but less time-consuming to perform.

When a pregnant woman is exposed to rubella a serum specimen should be obtained within 7 days of exposure (although up to 21 days is acceptable); if no antibody is found by the HI test, a second specimen should be drawn 3 weeks later. If a fourfold or greater rise in HI antibody is noted, acute rubella infection has occurred; proper guidance and genetic counseling would then be appropriate. If the rise in titer is twofold or less, acute infection is unlikely. The two serum specimens, of course, should be tested simultaneously to avoid the day-to-day variation that is commonplace with laboratory results.

If a single specimen only is available from the convalescent phase of the illness, determination of the presence of acute infection is difficult. An HI titer of 1:16 or less would be unusual in acute rubella infection, as convalescent titers are often very high. Even years after infection, HI titers of 1:512 or 1:1,024 are not uncommon. The presence of rubella IgM antibody may be determined in the convalescent specimen. If IgM antibody is found, it would be compatible with recent infection; however, IgM antibodies may disappear 4–6 weeks after infection. Their absence does not eliminate the possibility of recent infection.[82]

An acute chickenpox infection can usually be confirmed by a fourfold rise in CF antibody between an initial specimen drawn within 1 week of onset of illness and a convalescent specimen drawn 2–4 weeks later. Because CF antibody is transitory, a titer of 1:32 or more is compatible with recent infection.

If a patient, such as an immunocompromised child, has been exposed to chicken pox or shingles, his immune status is better determined by the fluorescent antibody to membrane antigen test or the immune adherence hemagglutination test, as CF antibody is not long-lasting.[76]

Evidence of enteroviral infection is not often obtained by serologic means unless a virus has been isolated from the patient. There are at least 67 immunotypes, and without a viral isolate, it is not economically feasible to screen for this number of possibilities. Some laboratories, however, may do serologic screening for the six coxsackie B viruses in a case of suspected viral myocarditis or pericarditis.[78]

Most common serologic methods have been applied to diagnosing HSV infections. Again, a fourfold rise in titer is indicative of primary infection. Reinfection is another matter. Reinfection can occur in the presence of high titers of serum antibody. Whether local IgA antibody or cell-mediated immunity is important for preventing reinfection is not clear. Distinguishing HSV-1 and HSV-2 antibodies is difficult because of the cross-reactivity of two antibodies. Kinetic neutralization and other methods have been used.[77]

Rickettsia rickettsii, the cause of Rocky Mountain spotted fever is best diagnosed by serologic methods. The Weil-Felix reaction takes advantage of the ability of *Proteus* organisms, OX-19, OX-2, and OX-K, to agglutinate the serum of patients with Rocky Mountain spotted fever. The test is not positive until at least 1 week after illness begins and may be delayed further by antibiotic usage. As in any serologic test, a fourfold rise in titer must be demonstrated between an acute and a convalescent specimen. The test therefore cannot be used to make a diagnosis when the patient is seen early in the illness. Furthermore, cross reactions from infection or vaccination with other gram-negative rods occurs. A single titer must be high (1:80 or more) to be suggestive of recent infection. Consequently, the Weil-Felix test is of no help during the acute illness; the test should be abandoned by clinical laboratories.

If Rocky Mountain spotted fever is suspected, acute and convalescent sera are better studied by the CF for the Spotted Fever group of rickettsiae. The test is more specific and more sensitive than the Weil-Felix reaction.[80]

Hemorrhagic fevers are unusual in the United States. Dengue virus, a flavivirus or group B togavirus, may cause hemorrhagic rash in visitors to Puerto Rico and other parts of the Caribbean. The diagnosis is usually confirmed by the CF test on acute and convalescent sera. There are many other viruses that cause hemorrhagic fever such as Lassa, Marburg, and Ebola viruses, but these usually occur outside the continental United States and will not be considered further.[83]

CNS Infections

Specimens of CSF, throat, and rectal swabs may all be helpful in diagnosing CNS infections. Urine should be collected for mumps and genital lesions cultured for HSV. Whole blood is useful in encephalitis due to alphaviruses and flaviviruses. Brain is considered the specimen of choice for suspected HSV.

The nonbacterial organisms that cause meningitis usually cause encephalitis also. It is the causes of the latter diagnosis which we will consider in detail (Table 11–11).

The encephalitides can be classified by two methods.[84] By groups of organisms, the major categories are arboviral (Western Equine, Eastern Equine, St. Louis, and California encephalitis viruses) and enteroviral forms; the types associated with childhood infections (mumps, measles, rubella, chickenpox), with respiratory tract infections (adenoviruses, influenza A, reovirus) and with immunizations; a general category (HSV, VZV CMV, EBV, Rocky Mountain spotted fever, etc.) and indeterminate. Another

TABLE 11–11.—CNS INFECTIONS

SYNDROME	COMMON CAUSES	LESS COMMON
Aseptic meningitis	Mumps	Herpes simplex virus
	Coxsackievirus	Lymphocytic choriomeningitis
	Echoviruses	Varicella-zoster
		Many other viruses
Paralysis	Polioviruses	Coxsackieviruses
		Echoviruses
Encephalitis	Alphaviruses	Rubella
	Flaviviruses	Varicella-zoster
	Bunyaviruses	Herpes B virus
	Herpes simplex virus	Coxsackieviruses
	Mumps	Echoviruses
		Many other viruses
		Rickettsiae
		Mycoplasma pneumoniae

classification, which we will use here, is by pathogenesis. The first category is viral encephalitis, where viruses cause inflammation and have been isolated from the CNS (e.g., HSV, arboviruses, and enteroviruses). The second group is the postinfectious and postvaccinial encephalomyelitides, which are probably immunologically mediated processes (e.g., naturally occuring measles, mumps, varicella, and rubella and vaccines against smallpox and rabies). The third category is parainfectious inflammatory encephalitis. This group resembles the viral encephalitides clinically but virus or other infectious agents have never been cultured from the CNS (e.g., mycoplasmosis, EBV, and influenza). Pathologically these infections are not associated with the demyelination, gliosis, and perivascular cuffing seen with the second category. Guillain-Barré syndrome, transverse myelitis, and cranial nerve neuropathies also fall into this third group and are pathologically distinct from the second category. The fourth and last category is made up of the parainfectious, noninflammatory encephalopathies, which are characterized by brain swelling without inflammation and gliosis (e.g., Reye's syndrome and various toxic encephalopathies). Increased intracranial pressure with few or no cells in the spinal fluid is characteristic.

Viral Encephalitides

ARBOVIRUSES (ARTHROPOD-BORNE VIRUSES).—There are 388 arboviruses. These organisms were originally grouped because of their mode of transmission via hematophagous arthropods. More recently they have been recognized as a heterogeneous group and so have been reclassified according to their membership in the virus families.[85] The most common of these agents in North America are shown in Table 11–12.

The state health department laboratories will usually provide tests for the arboviruses common in their geographic area. Interpretation of the serologic tests must account for the serologic relatedness of various viruses within each genus or group (i.e., members of flaviviruses may cross-react).[3] In descending order of likelihood, cross reactions may occur with HI, CF, or neutralization tests.[86]

Virus isolation can be attempted in tissue culture or by mouse inoculation but both should be done in reference laboratories or laboratories with appropriate containment facilities. Blood, throat, and spinal fluid can be tested. Serologic confirmation, however, is more productive than attempts at viral isolation. For fatal cases, isolation from brain and spinal fluid should be attempted for epidemiologic purposes.

OTHER VIRUS GROUPS.—Encephalitis may be caused by the arenaviruses (e.g., lymphocytic choriomeningitis and Lassa fever viruses). Lassa is a very hazardous virus to deal with in the laboratory; maximum containment

TABLE 11-12.—COMMON ARBOVIRUSES IN
NORTH AMERICA

VIRUS	INFECTION
Togaviridae	
Alphaviruses	Eastern equine encephalitis
	Western equine encephalitis
	Venezuelan equine encephalitis
Flaviviruses	St. Louis encephalitis
	Yellow fever virus
	Dengue (types 1–4)
	Powassan
Bunyaviridae	
Bunyaviruses	California equine encephalitis
Reoviridae	
Orbiviruses	Colorado tick fever
Rhabdoviridae	
Lyssavirus	Rabies

facilities should be used, and they are available in only a few locations.[87] Enteroviruses were discussed in the section on exanthematous illnesses; spinal fluid cultures provide a high yield in CNS infections. Cross-reacting antibody can be a major confounding factor. For example, some echoviruses may elicit serum antibody against group B coxsackieviruses and polioviruses. Consequently, diagnosing disease on the basis of a clinical isolate or a serum antibody rise in a single case may not be justified. Should this occur in a large number of cases, an etiologic association is stronger.[78]

RABIES VIRUS.—Identification of problems related to the vaccine strain are as important as the wild virus. Diagnostic tests have several specific applications but are most often used in preventive programs rather than in postbite cases.[88] The state department of health rabies control officer should be consulted for all questions relating to a possible rabies exposure.

If a rabid animal is captured, the brain should be studied for Negri bodies (pathognomonic cytoplasmic inclusions) and for viral antigen by IF. The latter test is more specific and sensitive. Virus isolation can also be attempted from animals or humans. Salivary specimens for culture or corneal epithelial cells or skin from the neck at the hairline (in man) can be examined for viral antigen using direct FA.

Serologic studies such as the indirect fluorescence antibody test are done to determine the immune response to vaccination, particularly those given vaccine for prophylaxis such as veterinarians. A rapid fluorescence focus-inhibition test and mouse or plaque reduction neutralization tests are used.

POLIO.—In the United States, a diagnosis of polio is most often entertained following vaccination, and in the contact of a vaccinee more often than in the vaccinee. Both situations, however, are rare: 1 case per 11.5

million vaccine recipients and 1 household contact per 3.9 million persons vaccinated.[89] The immunosuppressed child is at high risk for this complication and should not be vaccinated with the live virus vaccine but rather with the inactivated (Salk) vaccine.

The virus is readily isolated in primary monkey kidney cells from stool specimens for several weeks. Unlike other enteroviruses, poliovirus is not often found in cell cultures of spinal fluid. The isolation of virus from the stool in a vaccinee with asymmetrical paralysis is not, however, diagnostic of the illness poliomyelitis, as one normally expects to find virus in the stool of a vaccinee. The same concern applies to the interpretation of a significant rise in antibody by serologic studies. Ideally, the virus should be isolated from the brain or spinal cord to establish the etiology definitively. This is rarely done, so a "compatible" case of vaccine-associated polio must meet these criteria: (1) onset of illness between 4 and 30 days following feeding of the vaccine type in question and onset of paralysis not sooner than 6 days after the feeding; (2) significant residual lower motor neuron paralysis; (3) laboratory data not inconsistent with respect to multiplication of the vaccine virus feed (i.e., virus can be isolated in stool or there is a rise in serum antibody); and (4) no evidence of upper motor neuron disease, definite sensory loss, or progression or recurrences of paralytic illness 1 month or more after onset.[90] If fever, spinal fluid pleocytosis, and a preceding systemic illness also occur, the association with vaccine is considered even more probable.

Vaccine strains of virus are distinguished from wild strains by antigenic and temperature markers as well as by a monkey neurovirulence test.[91] These tests are done at the Centers for Disease Control, Atlanta, Georgia. Recently, highly strain-specific absorbed sera and oligonucleotide mapping procedures have been added to fingerprint the virus strain.[92]

HSV.—With the advent of effective antiviral drugs, establishing HSV as the cause of encephalitis is more than a formal exercise. Unfortunately, it is unusual to isolate HSV from the spinal fluid in adults. A brain biopsy is required to demonstrate the presence of virus by cell culture electron microscopy or IF staining.[93]

Several avenues are being pursued to obviate brain biopsy. RIA and ELISA techniques are being explored because of the manyfold increase in sensitivity of detection these tests afford. After the disease has been present for 1–3 weeks, a rise in spinal fluid antibody by the CF or other tests (PHA and IAHA) may be demonstrable. A rise in spinal fluid antibody level will not aid in early diagnosis unless IgM antibody is sought in CSF, in which case a positive result is compatible with acute infection.[94] Serum antibody determinations are not helpful, because a rise in titer may merely represent reactivation of HSV by any febrile illness.

Postinfectious and Postvaccinal Encephalomyelitides

This form of CNS disease is thought to resemble Waksman's experimental allergic encephalomyelitis model, which is an inflammatory demyelinating disease of animals produced by immunization with myelin basic protein.[95] Central myelin is thought to be the reactogenic component here. In contrast, in the third category, peripheral myelin is thought to be the reactive component (i.e., in Guillain-Barré-related illnesses).[96] History, clinical presentation, and serologic studies may confirm that one of the viral exanthems (measles, varicella, rubella), mumps, smallpox, or rabies vaccines was associated with this CNS syndrome. These serologic studies were discussed earlier in this chapter.

Other infectious agents encountered in the group are influenza, EBV, and *M. pneumoniae.*

Parainfectious Inflammatory Encephalitides

Guillain-Barré syndrome and various peripheral neuropathies are the syndromes in this category that frequently pose a diagnostic dilemma. Guillain-Barré syndrome has been reported in association with respiratory and gastrointestinal viruses, CMV, live virus vaccines (e.g., mumps, rubella, measles), killed virus vaccines (e.g., influenza and rabies), chronic diseases (e.g., Hodgkin's disease, other malignancies, systemic lupus erythematosus), surgical procedures and other forms of trauma, drugs (such as organophosphates), and metabolic insults.[97-104] Guillain-Barré syndrome following swine influenza vaccine may have been unique to that strain since recent influenza vaccines present no increased risk of the disease.[104]

Parainfectious Noninflammatory Encephalopathies

Reye's syndrome is a typical parainfectious noninflammatory encephalopathy. Types B and A influenza viruses and VZV have been frequently linked epidemiologically. The viruses probably act as co-factors with yet unidentified environmental toxins. Many other viruses and several noninfectious agents have also been associated.[105, 106] Serologic and isolation methods of diagnosis for the infectious agents have been discussed previously.

Slow Viruses

These infectious agents are being treated as a separate category because of the unique nature of the infecting agents and the long incubation period. SSPE is caused by a measles-like virus latent in brain cells. Antibody in serum and CSF is present in high titers in most patients. The presence of antibody in CSF is virtually diagnostic of SSPE; lower titers have been reported in patients with multiple sclerosis.[107] Special co-cultivation methods are necessary to grow the virus in tissue culture.[108]

Chronic rubella CNS disorders are seen in the newborn (progressive congenital rubella encephalomyelitis) and in infants (chronic progressive rubella panencephalitis).[109] Congenital cytomegalic inclusion disease due to CMV is also a chronic CNS disorder. The isolation or serologic methods already described will help in establishing the diagnosis.

Progressive multifocal leukoencephalopathy (PML) appears to be caused by several polyomaviruses (in the Papoviridae family) known as JC and SV40-PML viruses. Relatively few patients have been studied, and viral isolation techniques are difficult.[110] The diagnostic serologic method of choice is the HI test. Serum neutralization, CF, metabolic inhibition, and fluorescent antibody tests have also been used.

Cruetzfeldt-Jakob disease and Kuru are transmitted man-to-man by corneal transplants in the first instance and by cannibalism in New Guinea in the second. Transmissible agents have been identified though not yet characterized; this diagnosis is based on clinical findings and pathologic demonstration of a spongioform encephalopathy.[111, 112]

Sexually Transmitted Diseases

The list of sexually transmitted illnesses grows longer each year. Whereas bacteria were the first known sexually transmitted diseases, several viruses, *Chlamydia,* and *Mycoplasma* organisms have recently become established as causes of sexually transmitted diseases. Enteric bacteria and parasites are the latest additions.

Perhaps the most prevalent of the nonbacterial agents is *C. trachomatis.*[113, 114] It is the most common cause (30%–50% of cases) of nongonococcal urethritis and is now two to four times as frequent a cause of urethritis as is *Neisseria gonorrhoeae.* Often *C. trachomatis* is found with *N. gonorrhoeae* in urethral infections; both organisms are also found in asymptomatic males.

Nongonococcal urethritis with *Chlamydia* is detected by isolation, as described previously in the section on lower respiratory infections. Serologic techniques for nongonococcal urethritis are less sensitive and may not be able to distinguish recent from past infection. *Chlamydia trachomatis* has recently been associated as well with the anterior urethral syndrome.[114]

In women, *C. trachomatis* is also the most common cause of genital tract infections. In addition to cervicitis, salpingitis, peritonitis, endometritis, and perihepatitis have recently been shown to be caused by *C. trachomatis.*[113]

Lymphogranuloma venereum is best detected by demonstrating a four-fold rise in antibody titer by CF or by the more sensitive micro-IF test. Micro-IF can distinguish the three immunotypes (L_1, L_2, L_3). The Frei test is not used anymore as it is too insensitive and nonspecific.[114]

Ureaplasma urealyticum (T strain mycoplasma) is a frequent (20%–30% of cases) but less common cause of nongonococcal urethritis than *C. trachomatis*. It can be isolated in urea broth medium. Growth occurs in 1–2 days. Because there are 11 serotypes and antisera are not generally available, serologic testing is not regularly used. Serodiagnosis is also unsatisfactory because the organisms are not sufficiently invasive to elicit an antibody response in most infected patients.[115]

Mycoplasma hominis, though not found in nongonococcal urethritis, may occasionally cause pelvic inflammatory disease. Growth on solid agar gives the typical "fried egg" appearance, which distinguishes it from *M. pneumoniae*. Serum antibody is more frequently elicited then with *U. urealyticum*. The serologic tests for *M. pneumoniae* described earlier in the chapter are applicable here.[115]

HSV causes genital infection in men and women. Type 1 HSV is less common then type 2 HSV. HSV-1 is also less likely to recur. Recurrences with HSV-2 are more likely in persons with high levels of serum neutralizing antibody. Therefore, the serum antibody level is not an indicator of protection but rather a predictor of recurrence.[116] The virus is readily isolated in cell culture in a short time. The CF and neutralization serologic methods were described in the section on exanthematous illnesses.

CMV causes cervicitis. *Neisseria gonorrhoeae* is found more often when CMV infection is present. As with HSV, the frequency of infection varies with age, sexual promiscuity, socioeconomic class, and parity. Isolation and serologic methods were discussed in the section on the mononucleosis syndrome. IF is more sensitive than CF in cervical infections.

Other Classes of Infections

Serologic methods and agent isolation techniques described previously apply to most of the clinical entities discussed below, except mumps.

Parotitis

Acute parotitis is invariably caused by mumps virus. Rarely, parainfluenza type 3, coxsackieviruses, and influenza type A viruses may be responsible for "recurrences." Pancreatitis and orchitis have also been associated with both mumps and the coxsackieviruses. Viral culture and serology will help distinguish these causes. Mumps virus can be isolated from the saliva for 4–5 days after onset of parotitis and from urine for 2 weeks after onset.

The virus is readily grown in cell cultures available in routine diagnostic laboratories (i.e., primary monkey kidney and HeLa cells). It also can be grown in eggs.

Serologic evidence of infection is by standard HI, CF, or neutralization tests; however, cross-reacting antibody often develops to parainfluenza viruses because both viruses are members of the paramyxovirus group. The frequency of these heterotypic antibodies increases with age. Clinical history, viral isolation, and serologic tests considered together usually resolve this dilemma. CF can be used to distinguish the time of infection, as S-antibody is present early and disappears in a few months. V-antibody appears later and lasts for years.[117]

Torch Syndrome

The diagnosis of rubella, CMV, and HSV in the newborn will be considered here. Toxoplasmosis is reviewed in Chapter 12. Some prefer the term STORCH, which includes syphilis. "O" refers to other congenital infections, such as EBV.

The principle in documenting the presence of one of these congenital infections is to demonstrate high levels of total IgM and virus-specific IgM antibody in the neonate's or cord serum. IgM antibody produced by the mother from recent infection will not cross the placental barrier. IgG antibodies to rubella, CMV, and HSV are likely to be present in the maternal serum and will readily cross the placenta and appear in the newborn's serum. Such passively acquired maternal IgG will decline gradually over 6 months, whereas actively acquired IgG antibody, induced by neonatal infection, will rise and remain at a high level during the same period. This antibody obviously does not favorably alter the course of congenital infection. A defective cell-mediated immune response may be more important.

For rubella, virus isolation is possible from most body sites—pharynx, urine, spinal fluid—and most organs. The frequency of virus isolation declines gradually; even at 1 year after birth 7% of infants will still be shedding virus. Between birth and 3 months of age, demonstration of virus-specific IgM antibody in a single specimen is diagnostic. Separation of IgM and IgG by ultracentrifugation on sucrose gradients, then testing of gradient fractions for HI activity, is the method of choice.[118, 119]

Congenital CMV infections can be documented by demonstrating viruria within 48 hours of birth. Viral isolation is more sensitive than attempting to demonstrate virus-specific IgM antibody. Rheumatoid factor (IgM antibody to maternal IgG) results in false positive reactions in the indirect fluorescence test for IgM antibody. Demonstration of a rising or persistent total IgG antibody in serial samples from the newborn is helpful.[120]

HSV-2 infection in the newborn period is usually acquired at the time of delivery rather than transplacentally. CMV also can be acquired perinatally by the same route. Disseminated disease occurs with virus shedding and antibody production a few weeks after birth.[77] Disseminated disease in the newborn has also been associated with type B coxsackieviruses, echoviruses, hepatitis B, and adenoviruses.

Teratogenic effects may be unique to rubella and perhaps the CMV. Other viruses have been implicated, but repeated documentation is not available. Many viruses and other infectious agents, in contrast, are responsible for stillbirths and premature labor.

Compromised Host

The immunosuppressed patient has an increased risk of herpesvirus infections—HSV, VZV, and CMV. This group of viruses causes latent infection, and infections recur following iatrogenic suppression of cell-mediated immunity in treating malignancies or after major organ transplantation, pregnancy, or aging. These patients are also more susceptible to serious complications when these viruses cause primary infection.

Accurate virologic diagnosis is important since moderately effective antiviral chemotherapy is available for VZV and HSV. Pneumonia, hepatitis, and disseminated infections should be evaluated by viral culture with properly collected specimens from sputum, lung biopsy, skin vesicles (for VZV and HSV), white blood cells, and urine (for CMV). Search for serologic evidence of infection may be hampered by the immunosuppressive dampening of the humoral immune response, particularly in patients with overwhelming infection.

Screening for VZV antibody is done prior to administration of zoster immune globulins (ZIG). If an immunosuppressed child younger than age 15 has been appropriately exposed to chickenpox within the past 4 days and has a negative past history of chickenpox, he may be a candidate for ZIG.[121] It is helpful to screen the sera for VZV antibody by the standard methods already described.[76]

Eye Infections

Conjunctivitis, pharyngoconjunctival fever, and epidemic keratoconjunctivitis all have been attributed to various types of adenovirus. *Chlamydia trachomatis* causes trachoma and inclusion conjunctivitis. HSV, VZV, measles, enteroviruses, vaccinia, and dengue have all been causally related to the conjunctivitis syndrome.

Epidemics of acute hemorrhagic conjunctivitis are usually due to enteroviruses or adenoviruses such as enterovirus 70, adenovirus 11, 8, and 7, or coxsackievirus A-24. Neurologic complications such as radiculomyelitis with flaccid paralysis (polio-like) may be associated.[122] Methods for identifying these organisms have already been described.

Arthritis

Arthritis has been described in association with rubella, viral hepatitis (hepatitis B), mumps, lymphocytic choriomeningitis, adenovirus, echovirus, EBV, and varicella. Erythema infectiosum and Lyme arthritis are associated with synovitis, but the etiology of the former disease is unknown and a spirochete is suspected in the latter illness.

Cardiovascular Infections

Myocarditis and pericarditis are typically associated with group B coxsackieviruses. Serologic diagnosis is possible as there are only six immunotypes. Since these two entities, particularly pericarditis, can also be caused by group A (and B) coxsackieviruses and echoviruses, every attempt should be made to isolate virus from stool and throat swab specimens early in the illness. Without an isolate, a serologic search for 1 of over 100 immunotypes is not feasible. Other etiologic agents include *Chlamydia*, *Coxiella burnetii*, and *M. pneumoniae*. Even rarer causes among the viruses are adenoviruses, CMV, VZV, EBV, HAV, polioviruses, HSV-1 and 2, influenza type A and B viruses, lymphocytic choriomeningitis virus, mumps, rubella, and vaccinia viruses, and among the rickettsia are *R. rickettsii* and *R. typhi (mooseri)*. Even with a careful search, more than 50% of cases still remain without an identifiable etiologic agent.

Endocarditis has been attributed to *C. burnetii*. Here a chronic form presents as "culture-negative" endocarditis. With use of phase 1 antigen, the diagnosis can be attributed to Q fever.[123] *Chlamydia psittaci* has also been associated with culture-negative endocarditis. Serologic methods should point to this etiology.[124]

Myositis

Generalized inflammation of the skeletal muscles has been reported with the togaviruses, influenza B virus, and coxsackieviruses.

Urinary Tract Infections

Hemorrhagic cystitis has been attributed to adenoviruses (types 11, 2, and 21). Viral isolation from the urine and perhaps a single high titer (1:32) will confirm the diagnosis.[125] Hepatitis B may cause glomerulonephritis.

Diseases with Suspected Viral or Rickettsial Cause

The etiology of roseola, erythema infectiosum, cat scratch disease, and Kawasaki's disease may someday be better defined.

REFERENCES

1. Lennette E.H., Schmidt N.J. (eds.): *Diagnostic Procedures for Viral, Rickettsial and Chlamydial Infections*, ed. 5. Washington, D.C., American Public Health Association, 1979.
2. Lennette E.H., Ballows A., Hansler W.J. Jr., et al.: *Manual of Clinical Microbiology*, ed. 3. Washington, D.C., American Society for Microbiology, 1980.
3. Mandell G.L., Douglas R.G., Jr., Bennett J.E. (eds.): *Principles and Practice of Infectious Diseases*. New York, John Wiley & Sons, 1979, vol. 1.
4. Mandell G.L., Douglas R.G., Jr., Bennett J.E. (eds.): *Principles and Practice of Infectious Diseases*. New York, John Wiley & Sons, 1979, vol. 2.
5. Stuart-Harris C.H., Andrews C., Andrews B.E., et al.: A collaborative study of the aetiology of acute respiratory infection in Britain 1961–4: A report of the Medical Research Council working party on acute respiratory virus infections. *Br. Med. J.* 2:319, 1965.
6. Hamre D., Connelly A.P. Jr., Procknow J.J.: Virologic studies of acute respiratory disease in young adults: IV. Virus isolations during four years of surveillance. *Am. J. Epidemiol.* 83:238, 1966.
7. Monto A.S., Ullman B.M.: Acute respiratory illness in an American community; The Tecumseh study. *JAMA* 227:164, 1974.
8. Dingle J.H., Badger G.F., Jordan W.S. Jr.: Illness in the home: Study of 25,000 illnesses in a group of Cleveland families. Cleveland, The Press of Western Reserve University, 1964, p. 1.
9. Schieble J.H., et al.: Coronaviruses, in Lennette E.H., Schmidt N.J. (eds.): *Diagnostic Procedures for Viral, Rickettsial and Chlamydial Infections*, ed. 5. Washington, D.C., American Public Health Association, Inc., 1979, p. 709.
10. Hamparian V.V.: Rhinoviruses, in Lennette E.H., Schmidt N.J. (eds.): *Diagnostic Procedures for Viral, Rickettsial and Chlamydial Infections*, ed. 5. Washington, D.C., American Public Health Association, Inc., 1979, p. 535.
11. Dorff G.J., Rytel M.W., Farmer S.G., et al.: Etiologies and characteristic features of pneumonias in a municipal hospital. *Am. J. Med. Sci.* 266:349, 1973.
12. Fekety F.R., Caldwell J., Gump D., et al.: Bacteria, viruses, and mycoplasmas in acute pneumonia in adults. *Am. Rev. Respir. Dis.* 104:499, 1971.
13. Sullivan R.J., Dowdle W.R., Marine W.M., et al.: Adult pneumonia in a general hospital: Etiology and host risk factors. *Arch. Intern. Med.* 129:935, 1972.
14. Lepow M.L., Balassanian N., Emmerich J., et al.: Interrelationships of viral, mycoplasmal and bacterial agents in uncomplicated pneumonia. *Am. Rev. Respir. Dis.* 97:533, 1968.
15. Grayston J.T., Alexander E.R., Kenney G.E., et al.: *Mycoplasma pneumoniae* infections: Clinical and epidemiological studies. *JAMA* 191:97, 1965.

16. Foy H.M., et al.: *Mycoplasma pneumoniae* pneumonia in an urban area. JAMA 214:1666, 1970.

17. Harrison H.R., English M.G., Lee C.K., et al.: *Chlamydia trachomatis* infant pneumonitis: Comparison with matched controls and other infant pneumonitis. *N. Engl. J. Med.* 298:702, 1978.

18. Komaroff A.L., Aronson M.D., Schacter J.: *Chlamydia trachomatis* infection in adults with community-acquired pneumonia. JAMA 245:1319, 1981.

19. Pantell R.H.: Pharyngitis: Diagnosis and management. *Pediatr. Rev.* 3:35, 1981.

20. Warren J.W., Hornick R.B.: *Coxiella burnetii* (Q fever), in Mandell G.L., Douglas R.G. Jr., Bennett J.E. (eds.): *Principles and Practice of Infectious Diseases.* New York, John Wiley & Sons, 1979, vol. 2, p. 1516.

21. Surgeon General's Meeting: Summary report on influenza, February 12, 1979. U.S. Department of Health, Education and Welfare, Feb. 23, 1979.

22. Couch R.B., Douglas R.G Jr., Rossen R., et al.: Role of secretory antibody in influenza, in Dayton D.H Jr., et al. (eds.): *The Secretory Immunologic System.* Washington, D.C., U.S. Government Printing Office, 1969, pp. 93–112.

23. Kilbourne E.D., Butler W.T., Rossen R.D.: Specific immunity in influenza: Summary of influenza workshop III. *J. Infect. Dis.* 127:220, 1973.

24. Schulman J.L., Khakpour M., Kilbourne E.D.: Protective effects of hemagglutinin and neuraminidase antigens of influenza virus: Distinctiveness of hemagglutinin antigen of Hong Kong-68 virus. *J. Virol.* 2:778, 1968.

25. Douglas R.G., Markoff L.J., Murphy B.R., et al.: Live Victoria/75-ts-1(E) influenza A virus vaccines in adult volunteers: Role of hemagglutinin immunity in protection against illness and infection caused by influenza A virus. *Infect. Immun.* 26:274, 1979.

26. Palese P., Young J.F.: Variation of influenza A, B and C viruses: Genetic and antigenic changes in the virus are determining factors of the epidemiology of influenza. *Science* to be published.

27. World Health Organization: A revision of the system of nomenclature for influenza viruses: A WHO memorandum. *Bull. WHO* 58:585, 1980.

28. Gross P.A., Davis A.E. : Neutralization test in influenza: Use in individuals without hemagglutination inhibition antibody. *J. Clin. Microbiol.* 10:382, 1979.

29. Foy H.M., Cooney M.K., McMahan R., et al.: Single-dose monovalent A₂/Hong Kong influenza vaccine: Efficacy 14 months after immunization. *JAMA* 217:1067, 1971.

30. Mann J.J., Waldeman R.H., Toga R., et al.: Antibody response in respiratory secretions of volunteers given live and dead influenza virus. *J. Immunol.* 100:725, 1968.

31. Chanock R.M., Parrott R.H., Johnson K.M., et al.: Myxoviruses: Parainfluenza. *Ann. Rev. Respir. Dis.* 88:153, 1963.

32. Baum S.G.: Adenoviridae, in Mandell G.L., Douglas R.G., Jr., Bennett J.E. (eds.): *Principles and Practices of Infectious Diseases.* New York, John Wiley & Sons, 1979, vol. 2, p. 1353.

33. Hall C.B.: Respiratory syncytial virus, in Mandell G.L., Douglas R.G. Jr., Benett J.E. (eds.): *Principles and Practices of Infectious Diseases.* New York, John Wiley & Sons, 1979, vol. 2, p. 1186.

34. Welliver R.C., Kaul T.N., Putnam T.I., et al.: The antibody response to pri-

mary and secondary infection with respiratory syncytial virus: Kinetics of class-specific responses. *J. Pediatrics* 96:808, 1980.

35. Brunner H., Horswood R.L., Chanock R.M.: More sensitive methods for detection of antibody to *Mycoplasma pneumoniae. J. Infect. Dis* 127(suppl):S52, 1973.

36. Schaffner W.: Psittacosis, in Mandell G.L., Douglas R.G. Jr., Bennett J.E. (eds.): *Principles and Practices of Infectious Diseases.* New York, John Wiley & Sons, 1979, vol. 2. p. 1476.

37. Elisberg B.L., Bozeman F.M.: The *Rickettsiae,* in Lennette E.H., Schmidt N.J. (eds.): *Diagnostic Procedures for Viral, Rickettsial and Chlamydial Infections,* ed. 5. Washington, D.C., American Public Health Association, 1979, p. 1061.

38. Douglas R.G. Jr., Betts R.F.: Influenza virus, in Mandell G.L., Douglas R.G. Jr., Bennett J.E. (eds.): *Principles and Practices of Infectious Diseases.* New York, John Wiley & Sons, 1979, vol. 2, p. 1135.

39. Hendley J.O.: Parainfluenza virus, in Mandell G.L., Douglas R.G. Jr., Bennett J.E. (eds.): *Principles and Practices of Infectious Diseases.* New York, John Wiley & Sons, 1979, vol. 2, p. 1170.

40. Fulton R.E., Middleton P.J.: Comparison of immunofluorescence and isolation techniques in the diagnosis of respiratory viral infections of children. *Infect. Immun.* 10:92, 1974.

41. Gardner P.S.: Rapid diagnostic techniques in clinical virology, in Health R.B., Waterson A.P. (eds.): *Modern Trends in Medical Virology.* New York, Appleton-Century-Crofts, 1970, vol. 2, p. 15.

42. Griffin J.P.: Rapid screening for cold agglutinins in pneumonia. *Ann. Intern. Med.* 70:701, 1969.

43. Steinhoff M.C.: Viruses and diarrhea: A review. *Am. J. Dis. Child.* 132:302, 1978.

44. Yolken R.H., Wyatt R.G., Kim H.W., et al.: Immunological response to infection with human reovirus-like agent: Measurement of anti-human reovirus-like agent immunoglobulin G and M levels by the methods of enzyme-linked immunosorbent assay. *Infect. Immun.* 19:540, 1978.

45. Yolken R.H., Wyatt R.C., Zissis G.P., et al.: Epidemiology of human rotavirus types 1 & 2 as studied by enzyme-linked immunosorbent assay. *N. Engl. J. Med.* 299:1156, 1978.

46. Wyatt R.G., Dolin R., Blacklow N.R., et al.: Comparison of three agents of acute infectious nonbacterial gastroenteritis by virus challenge in volunteers. *J. Infect. Dis.* 129:709, 1974.

47. Parrino T.A., Schreiber D.S., Trier J.S., et al.: Clinical immunity in acute gastroenteritis caused by Norwalk agent. *N. Engl. J. Med.* 291:86, 1977.

48. Agus S.E., Falchuk Z.M., Sessoms C.S., et al.: Increased jejunal IgA synthesis in vitro during acute infectious nonbacterial gastroenteritis. *Am. J. Dig. Dis.* 19:127, 1974.

49. Kapikian A.Z., Kim H.W., Wyatt R.G., et al.: Reovirus-like agent in stools: Association with infantile diarrhea and development of serologic tests. *Science* 185:1049, 1974.

50. Kapikian A.Z., Wyatt R.G., Dolin R., et al.: Visualization by immune electron microscopy of a 27 nm particle associated with acute infectious non-bacterial gastroenteritis. *J. Virology* 10:1075, 1972.

51. Kapikian A.Z., Yolken R.H., Greenberg H., et al.: Gastroenteritis viruses, in Lennette E.H., Schmidt N.J. (eds.): *Diagnostic Procedures for Viral, Rickettsial and Chlamydial Infections*, ed. 5. Washington, D.C., American Public Health Association, Inc., 1979 p. 927.

52. Ghose L.H., Schnagl R.D., Holmes I.H.: Comparison of an enzyme linked immunosorbent assay for quantitation of rotavirus antibodies with complement fixation in an epidemiological survey. *J. Clin. Microbiol.* 8:268, 1978.

53. Thornhill T.S., Kalica A.R., Wyatt R.G., et al.: Pattern of shedding of the Norwalk particle in stools during experimentally induced gastroenteritis in volunteers as determined by immune electron microscopy. *J. Infect. Dis.* 132:28, 1975.

54. Greenberg H.B., Wyatt R.G., Valdesuso J. et al.: Solid phase microtiter radioimmunoassay for detection of the Norwalk strain of acute non-bacterial epidemic gastroenteritis virus and its antibodies. *J. Med. Virol.* 2:97, 1978.

55. Hoffnagle J.H.: Hepatitis, in Mandell G.L., Douglas R.G. Jr., Bennett J.E. (eds.): *Principles and Practices of Infectious Diseases*. New York, John Wiley & Sons, 1979, vol. 2, p. 1043.

56. Hollinger F.B., Dienstag J.L.: Hepatitis viruses, in *Manual of Clinical Microbiology*, ed. 3. Washington, D.C., American Society for Microbiology, 1980, p. 899.

57. Mathiesen L.R., Feinstone S.M., Purcell R.H., et al.: Detection of hepatitis A antigen by immunofluorescence. *Infect. Immun.* 18:524, 1977.

58. Robinson W.S.: Hepatitis A virus, in Mandell G.L., Douglas R.G. Jr., Bennett J.E. (eds.): *Principles and Practices of Infectious Diseases*. New York, John Wiley & Sons, 1979, vol. 2, p. 1370.

59. Robinson W.S.: Hepatitis B virus, in Mandell G.L., Douglas R.G. Jr., Bennett J.E. (eds.): *Principles and Practices of Infectious Diseases*. New York, John Wiley & Sons, 1979, vol. 2, p. 1388.

60. Lemon S.M., Gates N.L., Simms T.E., et al.: IgM antibody hepatitis B core antigen as a diagnostic parameter of acute infection with hepatitis virus. *J. Infect. Dis.* 143:803, 1981.

61. Swenson P.D., Escobar M.R.: Serologic markers in the diagnosis of viral hepatitis. *Clin. Immunol. Newsletter* 3:7–9, 1982.

62. Crivelli O., Rizzetto M., Lavarini C., et al.: Enzyme-linked immunosorbent assay for detection of antibody to the hepatitis B surface antigen-delta antigen. *J. Clin. Microbiol.* 14:173, 1981.

63. Robinson W.S.: Non-A, Non-B hepatitis, in Mandell G.L., Douglas R.G. Jr., Bennett J.E. (eds.): *Principles and Practices of Infectious Diseases*. New York, John Wiley & Sons, 1979, vol. 2, p. 1424.

64. Wood T.A., Frenkel E.P.: The atypical lymphocyte. *Am. J. Med.* 42:923, 1967.

65. Chin T.D.Y.: Diagnosis of infectious mononucleosis. *South Med. J.* 69:654, 1976.

66. Chretien J.H., Eswein J.G., Holland W.G., et al.: Predictors of the duration of infectious mononucleosis. *South Med. J.* 70:437, 1977.

67. Seitanidis B.: A comparison of the Monospot with the Paul-Bunnell test in infectious mononucleosis and other diseases. *J. Clin. Pathol.* 22:321, 1969.

68. Wolf P., Dorfman R., McClenahan J., et al.: False positive infectious mononucleosis spot test in lymphoma. *Cancer* 25:626, 1970.

69. Evans A.S., Niederman J.C., Cenabre L.C., et al.: A prospective evaluation

of heterophile and Epstein-Barr virus specific IgM antibody tests in clinical subclinical infectious mononucleosis: Specificity and sensitivity of the tests and persistence of antibody. *J. Infect. Dis.* 132:546, 1975.

70. Rao N., Waruszewski D.T., Ho M., et al.: Evaluation of the anticomplement immunofluorescence test in cytomegalovirus infection. *J. Clin. Microbiol.* 6:633, 1977.

71. Reynolds D.W., Stagno S., Alford C.A.: Laboratory diagnosis of cytomegalovirus infections, in Lennette E.H., Schmidt N.J. (eds.): *Diagnostic Procedures for Viral, Rickettsial and Chlamydial Infections*, ed. 5. Washington, D.C., American Public Health Association, 1979, p. 399.

72. Shapiro L.: The numbered diseases: First through sixth. *JAMA* 194:680, 1965.

73. Gershon A.A., Krugman S.: Measles virus, in Lennette E.H., Schmidt N.J. (eds.): *Diagnostic Procedures for Viral, Rickettsial and Chlamydial Infections*, ed. 5. Washington, D.C., American Public Health Association, 1979, p. 665.

74. Hermann K.L.: Rubella virus, in Lennette E.H., Schmidt N.J. (eds.): *Diagnostic Procedures for Viral, Rickettsial and Chlamydial Infections*, ed. 5. Washington, D.C., American Public Health Association, 1979, p. 725.

75. World Health Organization: *Guide to the Laboratory Diagnosis of Smallpox for Smallpox Eradication Programs.* Geneva, WHO, 1979.

76. Weller T.H.: Varicella and herpes zoster, in Lennette E.H., Schmidt N.J. (eds.): *Diagnostic Procedures for Viral, Rickettsial and Chlamydial Infections*, ed. 5. Washington, D.C, American Public Health Association, 1979, p. 375.

77. Rawls W.E.: Herpes simplex virus types 1 and 2 and herpesvirus simiae, in Lennette E.H., Schmidt N.J. (eds.): *Diagnostic Procedures for Viral, Rickettsial and Chlamydial Infections*, ed. 5. Washington, D.C., American Public Health Association, 1979, p. 309.

78. Melnick J.L., Wenner H.A., Phillips C.A.: Enteroviruses, in Lennette E.H., Schmidt N.J. (eds.): *Diagnostic Procedures for Viral, Rickettsial and Chlamydial Infections*, ed. 5. Washington, D.C., American Public Health Association, 1979, p. 471.

79. Johnson J.E., Kadull P.J.: Rocky Mountain spotted fever acquired in a laboratory. *N. Engl. J. Med.* 227:842, 1967.

80. Woodward W.E., Hornick R.B.: *Rickettsia rickettsii* (Rocky Mountain Spotted Fever), in Mandell G.L., Douglas R.G. Jr., Bennett J.E. (eds.): *Principles and Practices of Infectious Diseases.* New York, John Wiley & Sons, 1979, vol. 2, p. 1508.

81. Gershon A.A.: Rubella virus (German measles), in Mandell G.L., Douglas R.G. Jr., Bennett J.E. (eds.): *Principles and Practices of Infectious Diseases.* New York, John Wiley & Sons, 1979, vol. 2, p. 1258.

82. Shekarchi I.C., Sever J.L., Tzan N., et al.: Comparison of hemagglutination inhibition test and enzyme-linked immunosorbent assay for determining antibody to rubella virus. *J. Clin. Microbiol.* 13:850, 1981.

83. Fraser D.W.: Lymphocytic choriomeningitis virus, Lassa virus, and the Tacaribe group of viruses, in Mandell G.L., Douglas R.G. Jr., Bennett J.E. (eds.): *Principles and Practice of Infectious Diseases.* New York, John Wiley & Sons, 1979, p. 1231.

84. Case Records of the Massachusetts General Hospital: Case 35–1981. *N. Engl. J. Med.* 305:507, 1981.

85. Shope R.E., Sather G.E.: Arboviruses, in Lennette E.H., Schmidt N.J. (eds.): *Diagnostic Procedures for Viral, Rickettsial and Chlamydial Infections*,

ed. 5. Washington, D.C., American Public Health Association, 1979, p. 767.

86. Theiler M., Casals J.: The serological reactions in yellow fever. *Am. J. Trop. Med. Hyg.* 7:585, 1958.

87. Casals J.: Arenaviruses, in Lennette E.H., Schmidt N.J. (eds.): *Diagnostic Procedures for Viral, Rickettsial and Chlamydial Infections*, ed. 5. Washington, D.C., American Public Health Association, 1979, p. 815.

88. Plotkin S.A., Clark H.F.: Rabies, in Fergin R., Cherry J.D. (eds.): *Textbook of Pediatric Infectious Disease.* Philadelphia, W.B. Saunders Co. 1981, p. 1267.

89. Nightingale E.O.: Recommendations for a national policy on poliomyelitis vaccination. *N. Eng. J. Med.* 297:249, 1977.

90. Henderson D.A., Witte J.J., Morris L., et al.: Paralytic disease associated with oral polio vaccines. *JAMA* 190:153, 1964.

91. Centers for Disease Control: *Poliomyelitis Surveillance.: Summary 1979.* Atlanta, CDC, April 1981.

92. Nomenclature of strains of poliovirus. *Morbid. Mortal. Weekly Rep.* 30:450, 1981.

93. Shope T.C., Klein-Robbenhaar J., Miller G.: Fatal encephalitis due to herpesvirus hominis: Use of intact brain cells for isolation of virus. *J. Infect. Dis.* 125:542, 1972.

94. Levine D.P., Lauter C.B., Lerner M.: Simultaneous serum and CSF antibodies in herpes simplex virus encephalitis. *JAMA* 240:356, 1978.

95. Waksman B.H.: Experimental allergic encephalomyelitis and the "auto-allergic" disease. *Int. Arch. Allergy Appl. Immunol.* 14(suppl):1, 1959.

96. Griffin D.E., Johnson R.T.: Encephalitis, myelitis, and neuritis, in Mandell G.L., Douglas R.G. Jr., Bennett J.E. (eds.): *Principles and Practice of Infectious Diseases.* New York, John Wiley & Sons, 1979, vol. 1, p. 679.

97. Leneman F.: The Guillain-Barré syndrome. *Arch. Intern. Med.* 118:139–144, 1966.

98. Schonberger L.B., Bregman D.J., Sullivan-Bolyai J.Z., et al.: Guillain-Barré syndrome following vaccination in the national influenza immunization program, United States, 1976–1977. *Am. J. Epidemiol.* 110:105, 1979.

99. Centers for Disease Control: *Guillain-Barré Syndrome Surveillance Report: Summary Jan., 1978–March 1979.* Atlanta, CDC, October 1980.

100. Froelich C.J., Searles R.P., Davis L.E., et al.: A case of Guillain-Barré syndrome with immunologic abnormalities. *Ann. Intern. Med.* 93:563, 1980.

101. Kennedy R.H., Danielson M.A., Mulder D.W., et al.: Guillain-Barré syndrome: A 42-year epidemiologic and clinical study. *Mayo Clin. Proc.* 53:93, 1978.

102. Fisher J.R.: Guillain-Barré syndrome following organophosphate poisoning. *JAMA* 238:1950, 1977.

103. Dowling P., Menonna J., Cook S.: Cytomegalovirus complement fixation antibody in Guillain-Barré syndrome. *Neurology* 27:1153, 1977.

104. Hurwitz E.S., Schonberger L.B., Nelson D.B., et al.: Guillain-Barré syndrome and the 1978–1979 influenza vaccine. *N. Engl. J. Med.* 304:1557, 1981.

105. Linnemann C.C. Jr., Shea L, Partin J.C., et al.: Reye's syndrome: Epidemiologic and viral studies, 1963–1974. *Am. J. Epidemiol.* 101:517, 1975.

106. LaMontagne J.R.: Summary of a Workshop on Influenza B Viruses and Reye's Syndrome: From the National Institute of Allergy and Infectious Diseases. *J. Infect. Dis.* 142:452, 1980.

107. Salmi A.A., Norby E., Panelius M.: Identification of different measles virus-

specific antibodies in the serum and cerebrospinal fluid from patients with subacute sclerosing panencephalitis and multiple sclerosis. *Infect. Immun.* 6:248, 1972.

108. Horta-Barbosa L., Hamilton R., Wittig B. et al.: Subacute sclerosing panencephalitis: Isolation of suppressed measles virus from lymph node biopsies. *Science* 173:840, 1971.

109. Townsend J.J., Baringer J.R., Wolinsky J.S., et al.: Progressive rubella panencephalitis: Late onset after congenital rubella. *N. Engl. J. Med.* 292:990, 1975.

110. Lehrich J.R.: Polyomavirus (progressive multifocal leukoencephalopathy), in Mandell G.L., Douglas R.G. Jr., Bennett J.E. (eds.): *Principles and Practice of Infectious Diseases.* New York, John Wiley & Sons, 1979, vol. 2, p. 1436.

111. Gajdusek D.C.: Unconventional viruses and the origin and disappearance of kuru. *Science* 197:943, 1977.

112. Gajdusek D.C., Gibbs C.J., Asher D.M., et al.: Precautions in medical care of, and in handling materials from, patients with transmissible virus dementia (Creuzfeldt-Jakob disease). *N. Engl. J. Med.* 297:1253, 1977.

113. Gump D.W., Dickstein S., Gibson M.: Endometritis related to *Chlamydia trachomatis* infection. *Ann. Intern. Med.* 95:61, 1981.

114. Bowie W.: *Chlamydia trachomatis* (trachoma, inclusion conjunctivitis, lymphogranuloma venereum), in Mandell G.L., Douglas R.G. Jr., Bennett J.E. (eds.): *Principles and Practice of Infectious Diseases.* New York, John Wiley & Sons, 1979, vol. 2, p. 1464.

115. Couch R.B.: *Ureaplasma urealyticum* (T. strain mycoplasma) and *Mycoplasma hominis*, in Mandell G.L., Douglas R.G. Jr., Bennett J.E. (eds.): *Principles and Practice of Infectious Diseases.* New York, John Wiley & Sons, 1979, vol. 2, p. 1498.

116. Reeves W.C., Corey L., Adams H.G., et al.: Risk of recurrence after first episodes of genital herpes: Relation to HSV type and antibody response. *N. Engl. J. Med.* 305:315, 1981.

117. Hopps H.E., Parkman P.D.: Mumps virus, in Lennette E.H., Schmidt N.J. (eds.): *Diagnostic Procedures for Viral, Rickettsial and Chlamydial Infections,* ed. 5. Washington, D.C., American Public Health Association, 1979, p. 633.

118. Leoin M.J., Oxman M.N., Moore M.G., et al.: Diagnosis of congenital rubella in utero. *N. Engl. J. Med.* 290:1187 1974.

119. Vesikari T., Vahieri A.: Rubella: A method for rapid diagnosis of a recent infection by demonstration of the IgM antibodies. *Br. Med. J.* 1:221, 1968.

120. Reynolds D.W., Stagno S., Alford C.A.: Laboratory diagnosis of cytomegalovirus infections, in Lennette E.H., Schmidt N.J. (eds.): *Diagnostic Procedures for Viral, Rickettsial and Chlamydial Infections,* ed. 5. Washington, D.C., American Public Health Association, 1979, p. 399.

121. Varicella-Zoster Immune Globulin—United States. *Morbid. Mortal. Weekly Rep.* 30:15–23, 1981.

122. Centers for Disease Control: Acute hemorrhagic conjunctivitis. *Morbid. Mortal. Weekly Rep.* 30:463, 1981.

123. Wilson H.G., Neilson G.H., Galea E.G., et al.: Q fever endocarditis in Queensland. *Circulation* 53:680, 1976.

124. Dick D.C., McGregor C.G.A., Mitchell K.G., et al.: Endocarditis as a manifestation of *Chlamydia* B infection (psittacosis). *Br. Heart J.* 39:914, 1977.

125. Mufson M.A., Belshe R.B.: A review of adenoviruses in the etiology of acute hemorrhagic cystitis. *J. Urol.* 115:191, 1976.

12

The Interpretation of Serologic Tests for Parasitic Infections

Dickson D. Despommier, Ph.D.

THIS CHAPTER emphasizes the clinical interpretation of serologic tests for parasitic infections that are difficult to diagnose by other laboratory methods, such as stool examination or stained blood smear. The availability of improved protein separation techniques, including affinity chromatography using monoclonal antibodies and isoelectric focusing coupled with sensitive detection systems for antibody-antigen interactions (e.g. enzyme-linked immunosorbent assay [ELISA])[1] has led to the development of a number of reliable serologic tests for detecting a variety of parasitic organisms, including *Toxoplasma gondii, Entamoeba histolytica, Trichinella spiralis,* and *Toxocara canis.*

The elicitation of antibodies by both protozoan and helminthic infections in infected patient populations has been well established by numerous studies, but positive serologic tests are often difficult to interpret. This discussion reviews guidelines for interpreting these tests in relation to the clinical status of the patient and to offer a modicum of speculation wherever factual information is lacking.

The kinds of serologic tests that have been used for the detection of various species of protozoan and metazoan parasites have been reviewed by Houba[2] and Kagan.[3] Although many tests are available, only a few are considered useful for the clinical diagnosis of active infections caused by the parasite in question. Many tests simply indicate whether or not an individual has ever been infected, and a positive test result therefore must be carefully interpreted in light of the patient's clinical and laboratory data before it can be concluded that the individual currently has a parasitic infection. The limitation of experimentation on human subjects dictates that many such tests most likely will never be correlated with the presence of the organism. Nevertheless, much progress has been made in the serodiagnosis of some parasitic infections, primarily because ancillary diagnostic techniques have also improved. Infection with *Giardia lamblia* is a case in point.[4, 5]

Precise correlation of the serum antibody titer with the course of infection has been achieved for only one parasitic infection, *Toxoplasma gondii* infection.[6] The reasons for this are several. Usually the day of onset of infection is not known for most parasitic infections. Furthermore, the course of the infection prior to the onset of clinical symptoms is unique for each helminth and protozoan. For instance, some helminths migrate throughout the body, seeking their final niche, without multiplying within the host. Various lymphoid tissues are differentially stimulated by such migratory behavior, as has been shown, for example, in experimental infections with *Ascaris* larvae.[7, 8] Hence, the presence of specific antibodies depends on which lymphoid tissues have received antigenic stimulation and can also deliver antibodies to the general circulation. In addition, some of the most serious human helminthic infections have aberrant life cycles and occupy immunologically silent regions of the body, such as *Angiostrongylus cantonensis* infection in the meninges of the brain. In this case, serologic tests should focus on the detection of soluble worm antigens or other parasite products of metabolism that are unique to that pathogen.

In contrast to most helminth parasites, all protozoan pathogens multiply within their host, which increases the antigenic stimulation to the host's defense systems as the infection progresses. In this respect, protozoal infections resemble viral, bacterial, and fungal infections, and correlation of antibody titer with the number of organisms present is theoretically possible. Although this correlation has been made only for *T. gondii*, positive serologic tests and clinical symptoms consistent for any given protozoan parasite have been established for many of these pathogens. The parasitic infections to be discussed in detail in this chapter are ones which are both prevalent and cause serious illness throughout most of the world.

PROTOZOAN INFECTIONS

Toxoplasma gondii

With the possible exception of the influenza virus, no other parasitic organism is as prevalent and as widely distributed throughout the world as *Toxoplasma gondii*. In the United States, approximately 80 million people have serologic evidence of infection with *T. gondii*. Transmission of this infection to humans occurs primarily through the ingestion of raw or undercooked infected meats.[9] Exposure to infected cat feces can also lead to infection,[10, 11] but infection occurs more rarely by this mode. Despite the large numbers of seropositive individuals, the incidence of disease from *T. gondii* infection is low. Hence, the epidemiologic pattern of infection and disease with this protozoan closely resembles that seen in the United States with poliovirus prior to the development of vaccines.

Toxoplasma gondii induces two general disease states, one involving adult patients and one involving the fetus. In both cases, the immune system is stimulated to produce antibodies of the IgM and IgG classes. This antibody production occurs in sequence, with IgM antibody production reflecting the early phase of infection. A positive IgG test for *T. gondii* indicates either a later phase of the infection or convalescence. In addition, the complement fixation (CF) test, which detects mostly IgG class antibodies, parallels the disease more closely than a test that measures only IgM or IgG.

Typically, adult-acquired infection with *T. gondii* elicits IgM antibodies at the onset of exposure. The IgM titer, which is commonly measured by the indirect fluorescent antibody (IFA) test[12] or ELISA,[13] rises during the first few weeks, then declines below detectable levels during the fifth and sixth weeks of infection by IFA and somewhat more slowly by ELISA.[14] Prior to the decline of the IgM titer, the IgG antibody titer rises for as long as 2 months.

The IgG antibody titer usually remains somewhat elevated for years, although the clinical symptoms disappear. Therefore, the clinician must determine the change in IgM and IgG antibody titers over several months in order to fully evaluate the health status of the patient. The CF test is a better indication of clinical disease than tests that measure only IgG class antibodies. However, this test is more difficult to perform and is more time-consuming than IFA-IgG, IFA-IgM, or ELISA. The IFA-IgG test has been shown to be as effective at detecting positive individuals as the indirect hemagglutination test (IHA).[15] IgM antibody titers may subside before clinical signs and symptoms (e.g., lymphadenopathy and fever) become noticeable. Therefore, the IFA-IgM may not be particularly helpful in diagnosing adult-acquired toxoplasmosis. However, IgM-ELISA is a more specific and more sensitive assay than IFA-IgM and should prove to be more useful once commercial reagents are available.[13] Furthermore, the titer point that indicates a positive infection varies for different laboratories. Hence, the cutoff point for positivity must be independently determined by each laboratory.

Immunosuppression, either naturally or iatrogenically induced, can lead to serious, even fatal consequences with *T. gondii* infection.[16] Because the immune system is impaired, serologic tests may be of limited value in diagnosing the infection. Other approaches, such as lymph node biopsy or infection of *Toxoplasma*-free laboratory rodents with biopsy material, may be valuable in ruling in this infection in the immunosuppressed patient. The peroxidase-antiperoxidase (PAP) method to detect *Toxoplasma* antigen in tissue is a recent development in immunopathology that permits detection of this etiologic agent as causally related to encephalitis in immunosuppressed subjects unable to respond serologically.[17]

The detection of antibodies in the newborn against *T. gondii* is an important laboratory approach to the diagnosis of congenital infection. In the United States, approximately 20% of all newly pregnant women already have IgG antibodies to *T. gondii*, and so have acquired their infection sometime before becoming pregnant. The percentage varies from country to country. In France, it has been calculated to be as high as 85%.[18] These women do not risk transmitting the infection to the fetus, even if they are reexposed to the organism. It has been demonstrated that the most serious pathology from infection with *T. gondii* in the fetus occurs during the first 3 months of development, but some damage can result from infection during the last trimester in utero.[19] Detection of *T. gondii*-specific IgM antibodies in the newborn is proof of fetal infection.[12] The IgM antibody titer should be periodically evaluated for several weeks to several months (depending on how long it persists) to gain some insight as to when the fetus might have become infected. In contrast, the presence of IgG antibodies in fetal circulation may indicate infection or may simply reflect maternally transferred antibodies. In this case, both mother and child should be serologically followed for several months after birth. If the mother's titer remains stable and the infant's titer declines, it is very likely that the child was not infected. In contrast, if the titers of both mother and child remain stable for several weeks or months, then it is probable that the fetus was infected. If the mother's titer rises and the child's titer continues to rise, it is highly likely that infection was acquired by both individuals during the third trimester.

The reliability of the IFA-IgM or ELISA-IgM test is variable, due to the lack of consistently high-quality, commercially available reagents that detect IgM antibodies. On the other hand, tests that measure IgG antibodies are highly specific and sensitive, primarily because of the ease with which anti-human IgG conjugate can be produced. The use of hybridomas for detecting class-specific antibodies will most likely eliminate troublesome laboratory difficulties related to specificity and sensitivity. The cost of each test should also decline as hybridoma-produced monoclonal antibodies increase in the marketplace.

Entamoeba histolytica

The causative agent of amebic dysentery, *Entamoeba histolytica,* is ubiquitously distributed throughout the world and is endemic in human populations, infecting all age groups and both sexes. In addition, *E. histolytica* can invade tissues other than the large intestine, often resulting in death. An extra-intestinal infection must be differentiated from abscesses of bacterial, fungal, or larval tapeworm origin. This is largely accomplished by serology, since stool examinations are generally negative for *E. histolytica* when extra-intestinal disease is involved.[20] Various tests have been developed for this purpose, including IHA,[21] ELISA,[1] and counterimmunoelectrophoresis (CIE).[22, 23] Each of these tests is reliable for the detection of antibodies against the trophozoite of *E. histolytica*.

The IHA test has been evaluated in many clinical laboratories around the world, with uniformly good results.[21] In a study by Yap et al., 81 of 91 (89.1%) patients already diagnosed as having *E. histolytica* infection were positive by IHA.[22] In another series, 90% of patients suffering from only extra-intestinal amebiasis were positive by IHA; more than 95% of those same patients were positive by CIE as well. Other investigators have confirmed these findings, and in addition have shown that the IHA test is more sensitive in detecting extra-intestinal than intestinal amebiasis.[21, 23–25] A single titer point of a given patient's serum cannot be correlated with the severity of the disease or with the onset of therapeutic cure. The same is true for CIE and ELISA.[23, 26, 27] Furthermore, a patient who has been treated for and has recovered from extra-intestinal amebiasis will continue to have positive serologic findings for several months. Hence, the physician must correlate positive serologic findings with the patient's medical history if the diagnosis of *E. histolytica* is to be made.

There are reliable commercial sources of *E. histolytica* antigens as well as commercially produced kits for the CIE and ELISA tests.

Newly diagnostic approaches have been directed toward detection of *E. histolytica*-specific antigens in abscess fluid and feces.[28, 29] These tests have employed ELISA using rabbit anti-*E. histolytica* antibodies but require further improvement, since many false positive and false negative reactions have been reported.

Other Protozoan Infections

In addition to the protozoan infections described above, several others of major health importance deserve mention.

GIARDIA LAMBLIA.—*Giardia lamblia* is a flagellate protozoan that lives on the surface of the columnar cells of the villi in the small intestine. It clings tenaciously to the host cell and rarely ventures out into the lumen. For this reason, a stool examination is often negative in an infected individual. Furthermore, the physician may not always be able to use duodenal aspiration or the string test[30] for the diagnosis of this malabsorption-inducing pathogen. An IFA test has been developed that takes advantage of the facts that *G. lamblia* can now be obtained in pure culture and that most infected individuals have some antibody response to the organism.[31] The IFA test is now performed on a limited basis. As with *E. histolytica*, a positive titer indicates only that the patient has been exposed at some time to *G. lamblia*. No studies on the correlation between disease and changes in titer have yet been reported.

TRYPANOSOMA CRUZI.—A number of reliable methods, including CF and IFA tests,[32] are available for serologic testing for American trypanosomiasis, an infection caused by *T. cruzi*. These tests are useful diagnostic tools since it is very difficult to find the trypanomastigote stage of this parasite in peripheral blood. It has been estimated through seroepidemiologic surveys employing the IFA test that more than 10 million people throughout South America may be infected with this parasite (Camargo, personal communication). Since infection with *T. cruzi* lasts many years in the untreated patient, a positive serologic test is a good index of infection. The IFA test has almost no false positivity or false negativity associated with it.

PNEUMOCYSTIS CARINII.—There are no reliable serologic tests for *P. carinii* infections, although one is much needed.[33–35] This lung infection has been responsible for an increasing number of deaths in recent years due to the introduction of combined immunosuppressive therapy for various cancers. In addition, patients with acquired immune deficiency syndrome have been succumbing to *P. carinii* infection for reasons poorly understood.[36] All tests so far have not employed purified antigens, and this is probably the single most important reason why a successful test has not been forthcoming.

A summary of serologic tests for protozoan infections is given in Table 12–1.

HELMINTH INFECTIONS

Trichinella spiralis

Trichinella spiralis, a nematode, causes infection throughout the world. The worms occupy an intracellular niche in altered striated muscle tissue as larvae[38] and an intramulticellular niche in the gut as adults,[37] which makes the laboratory diagnosis of this infection an arduous task. Indeed, the only definitive way of demonstrating the parasite in the infected patient is by muscle biopsy, a procedure preferably avoided. Therefore, serology is a useful diagnostic alternative to biopsy.

Several serologic tests have been developed that offer a high degree of reliability, sensitivity, and specificity: CIE,[39] ELISA,[40] and the bentonite flocculation (BF) test.[41] These methods for the diagnosis of *Trichinella* in-

TABLE 12–1.—SEROLOGIC TESTS FOR PROTOZOAN INFECTIONS

ORGANISM	TEST*	COMMENT
Toxoplasma gondii	IFA-IgG	May detect late phase of infection or convalescence; highly specific and sensitive; commercially available
	IFA-IgM; ELISA-IgM	Positive early in infection; useful in detecting fetal infection; not very useful in adult-acquired disease; commercially available reagents of variable quality and reliability
	CF	Tends to parallel the disease process; not commercially available
Entamoeba histolytica	IHA	Most valuable for diagnosis; not commercially available
	CIE	Similar results to IHA but not as sensitive; commercially available
	ELISA	Commercially available
Giardia lamblia	IFA	Performed on a limited basis; does not indicate active disease; not commercially available
Trypanosoma cruzi	CF; IFA	Both are reliable methods; not commercially available
Pneumocystis carinii		No reliable serologic test available

*IFA, indirect fluorescent antibody; ELISA, enzyme-linked immunosorbent assay; CF, complement fixation; IHA, indirect hemagglutination.

fection in both humans and swine have been reviewed by Despommier.[42] The CIE test yields a yes-or-no result and offers the advantages of being rapid (1 hour) and specific. It is not as sensitive as ELISA and cannot be correlated with the clinical state of infection or with BF test titers. Counterimmunoelectrophoresis will yield positive results in more than 95% of the patients with *T. spiralis* larvae in their muscles. Commercial CIE kits are available.

The ELISA test has been widely used in the serodiagnosis of swine[43] as well as human trichinellosis. During infection in man, the titer rises with the onset of clinical symptoms but does not subside in any predictable or systematic fashion.

The use of immuno-affinity column chromatography for the isolation of diagnostically relevant antigens[44] has led to an increase in both the sensitivity and the specificity of the ELISA test. It is hoped that this approach will have general application to other parasitic infections systems which are still in need of reliable serologic tests.

Toxocara canis

Infection of the human host with *Toxocara canis* occurs throughout the world. This dog ascarid nematode has an aberrant life cycle—it wanders about the tissues, seeking to complete its migration but always failing to do so. As a result, damage to various organs such as the eye, liver, and brain occurs. In addition, the patient may have signs and symptoms mimicking many other clinical disease states. The diagnosis of *T. canis* infection is very difficult, and until recently no diagnostic serologic test was available. Because involvement of the eye can closely resemble retinoblastoma, enucleation was commonly done in affected patients. An ELISA test has been developed based on the finding that the third-stage larva of *T. canis* secretes antigens into the host that elicit humoral antibodies of several classes.[45] The discovery of a method for detecting secretions from unhatched larvae in vitro was critical in the development of this assay.[46] The use of this test in evaluating patients for visceral and ocular larva migrans has been recently reviewed by Schantz et al.[47] The ELISA test is highly specific and does not cross-react with sera obtained from patients infected with many commonly occurring parasites. A titer of 1:32 or greater is considered positive. The sensitivity is sufficiently high to eliminate various nonparasitic entities that commonly show false positive reactions in other kinds of parasitic serologic tests (e.g., elevated isoagglutinins of the A and B type).[47] Hence, about 88% of all patients harboring *T. canis* larvae will be positive on the ELISA test. In treated patients titers may drop, but they usually remain above the cutoff point for negativity.

The predictive value of ELISA for visceral larva migrans appears to be higher than for ocular larva migrans.[48] It has been suggested that a comparatively low titer (e.g., 1:8) be used as the cutoff point for ruling out ocular larva migrans, since the predictive value is about 85% for positive sera at this titer and about 93% for negative sera.[45]

To date, no other reliable test for *T. canis* has been devised. There are no commercially available kits for the test.

Larval Tapeworm Infections

Many cestodes that infect animals in the adult stage can also infect humans in the larval stage. Included within this group are *Taenia solium* (causative agent of cysticercus cellulosae), *Echinococcus granulosus* (causative agent of hydatid disease), and a number of less prevalent *Taenia* species *(T. multiceps, T. serialis,* and *T. brauni).* In each case, infection of the human host results from ingestion of the egg. After hatching, the larva locates in any of various organs, including brain, liver, and eye. In no case are organisms shed into the blood or feces, so that indirect diagnostic methods—radiograms and serologies—are the only methods available to the clinician.

The serodiagnosis of larval tapeworm infections depends on immunoelectrophoresis (IEP)[49, 50] and the IHA test.[51] A specific precipitin arc, designated arc 5, if present on IEP, is diagnostic for the family Taeniidae. All of the tapeworms listed above belong to this family. Regrettably, IEP does not lead to specific diagnosis of the infection, since worm-specific reagents are not available. Nonetheless, if the patient has an extensive clinical history of infection, an accurate diagnosis of either *Taenia* sp. or *Echinococcus* sp. can be made, based on the size and location of the cyst.

When a patient from a geographic area endemic for *E. granulosus* (i.e., any sheep-raising area of the world outside of Iceland) presents with a large space-filling lesion, then IHA and IEP may be used together. There are some data to suggest that sera from patients who have been cured of hydatid disease show a gradual decline in IHA titer, and this index may be of value in long-term patient evaluation.[52] This evidence derives partly from the observation that some patients in whom remnants of hydatid cysts have been found are often negative on serologic testing.[3]

Other Helminths

On a worldwide basis, filariasis in all its forms constitutes a major health problem, especially in tropical and subtropical environments. The most significant disease-producing infections are caused by *Wuchereria bancrofti*, *Brugia malayi*, *Onchocerca volvulus*, and *Loa loa*. All of these helminths are vector-borne and reside in the tissues, the first two in the lymphatic vessels and the second two in the subcutaneous tissues. Diagnosis is made by identifying microfilariae in either blood or skin snip preparations. However, light infections or immature ones are difficult or impossible to diagnose in this fashion. Immunologic tests rely on the fact that most filarial helminth species possess common cross-reacting antigens.[53, 54] Because of

TABLE 12–2.—SEROLOGIC TESTS FOR HELMINTHIC INFECTIONS*

ORGANISM	TEST	COMMENT
Trichinella spiralis	ELISA	Most sensitive; widely used in serodiagnosis; not commercially available
	CIE	Rapid and specific; does not correlate with clinical status; commercially available
	BF	Sensitive and specific; not commercially available
Toxocara canis	ELISA	Highly specific for VLM and OLM; not commercially available
Taenia sp.	IEP	Arc 5 is diagnostic for family Taeniidae; not commercially available
	IHA	Test is of ancillary value; not commercially available
Filariasis sp.		No definitive serologic test available
Strongyloides sp.		No serologic test available

*ELISA, enzyme-linked immunosorbent assay; CIE, counterimmunoelectrophoresis; BF, bentonite flocculation; IEP, immunoelectrophoresis; IHA, indirect hemagglutination; VLM, visceral larva migrans; OLM, ocular larva migrans.

this characteristic, and because many species of filariae often occur in the same endemic region, definitive diagnosis by serology is not yet a reality.

Strongyloides stercoralis is a nematode whose life cycle includes the possibility of multiplication within the same host. This can occur if the patient is suffering from any of a wide variety of immunosuppressive events or has an intestinal blockage that delays evacuation of the large bowel. Infestation in its most serious form can lead to death, and numerous examples may be found in the clinical literature of patients dying of this infection following organ transplantation or cancer chemotherapy.[55] No serologic test has been developed for this important nematode infection, although one is critically needed. Stool examinations, even if done consecutively for several days in a row, are usually negative in light infections.

A summary of serologic tests for helminth infections is found in Table 12–2.

REFERENCES

1. Ambroise-Thomas P., Desgeorges P.T., Monget D.: Diagnostic immunoenzymologique (ELISA) des maladies parasitaires par uns microméthode modifiée: II. Résultats pour la toxoplasmose l'amibiase, la trichinose, l'hydatidose et l'aspergillose. *Bull. WHO* 56:797–804, 1978.
2. Houba V.: *Immunological Investigation of Tropical Parasitic Diseases.* Edinburgh, Churchill Livingstone, 1980.
3. Kagan I.G.: Serodiagnosis of parasitic diseases, in Sennet E.H., Balows A., Hausler W.J., et al. (eds.): *Manual of Clinical Microbiology,* ed. 3. Washington, D.C., American Society for Microbiology, 1980, p. 724.
4. Ridley M.J., Ridley D.S.: Serum antibodies and jejunal histology in giardiasis associated with malabsorption. *J. Clin. Pathol.* 29:30, 1976.
5. Owen R.L.: The immune response in clinical and experimental giardiasis. *Trans. R. Soc. Trop. Med. Hyg.* 74:443, 1980.
6. Karim, K.A., Ludlam G.B.: The relationship and significance of antibody titers as determined by various serological methods in glandular and ocular toxoplasmosis. *J. Clin. Pathol.* 28:42, 1975.
7. Khoury P.B., Soulsby E.J.L.: *Ascaris suum:* Immune response in the guinea pig. I. Lymphoid cell responses during primary infections. *Exp. Parasitol.* 41:141, 1977a.
8. Khoury P.B., Soulsby E.J.L.: *Ascaris suum:* Lymphoid cell responses during secondary infections in the guinea pig. *Exp. Parasitol.* 41:432, 1977b.
9. Scott R.J.: Toxoplasmosis. *Trop. Dis. Bull.* 75:805, 1978.
10. Hutchinson W.M., Work K.: Coccidian-like nature of *Toxoplasma gondii. Br. Med. J.* 17:142, 1970.
11. Frenkel J.K., Dubez J.P., Miller N.L.: *Toxoplasma gondii* in cats: Fecal stages identified as coccidian oocysts. *Science* 167:893, 1970.
12. Remington J.S., Miller M.J., Brownlee I.: IgM antibodies in acute toxoplasmosis: I. Diagnostic significance in congenital cases and a method for their rapid demonstration. *Pediatrics* 41:1082, 1968.
13. Duermeyer W., Wielaard F., Gruijthuijsen H., et al.: Enzyme-linked immu-

nosorbent assay for detection of immunoglobulin M antibodies against *Toxoplasma gondii. J. Clin. Microbiol.* 12:780, 1980.

14. Noat Y., Guptill D.R., Remington J.S.: Duration of IgM antibodies to *Toxoplasma gondii* after acute acquired toxoplasmosis. *J. Infect. Dis.* 145:770, 1982.

15. Mahajan R.C., Chhabra M.B., Ganguly M.B., et al.: Fluorescent antibody tests in immunodiagnosis of toxoplasmosis. *Indian J. Med. Res.* 66:29, 1977.

16. Vietzke W.M., Gelderman A.H., Grimley P.M., et al.: Toxoplasmosis complicating malignancy: Experience at the National Cancer Institute. *Cancer* 21:816, 1968.

17. Conley F.K., Jenkins K.A., Remington J.S.: *Toxoplasma gondii* infection of the central nervous system. *Hum. Pathol.* 12:690, 1981.

18. Desmonts G., Ben Rashid M.S.: Le toxoplasme, la mere et l'enfant. *Arch. Fr. Pediatr.* 22:1183, 1965.

19. Desmonts G., Couvier J.: Congenital toxoplasmosis: A prospective study of 378 pregnancies. *N. Engl. J. Med.* 290:1110, 1974.

20. Farid Z., Hassan A., Trabolsi B., et al.: Hepatic amoebiasis: Diagnostic counter-immunoelectrophoresis and metronidazole (Flagyl) therapy. *Am. J. Trop. Med. Hyg.* 26:822, 1977.

21. Healy G.R.: The use of and limitations to the indirect hemagglutination test in the diagnosis of intestinal amoebiasis. *Health Lab. Sci.* 5:174, 1968.

22. Yap E.H., Singh M., Ho B., et al.: An evaluation of the indirect hemagglutination test using axenically-grown *Entamoeba histolytica* as antigen. *Singapore Med. J.* 16:31, 1975.

23. Tosswill J.H.C., Ridley D.S., Warhurst D.C.: Counter immunoelectrophoresis as a rapid screening test for amoebic abscess. *J. Clin. Pathol.* 33:33, 1980.

24. Martuschelli Q.A., Hernandez Gonzalez A., Zuniga Telleria V.: Evolucion de la reaccion de contraimmunoelectroforesis en ninos con amibiasis intestinal aguda. *Rev. Invest. Salud Publica* 37:93, 1977.

25. Mohapatra T.M., Sanyal S.C., Sen P.C., et al.: Evaluation of gel diffusion precipitation test in invasive amoebiasis. *Indian J. Med. Res.* 67:754, 1978.

26. Bos H.J., Von der Ezk A.A., Steerenberg P.A.: Applications of ELISA in the serodiagnosis of amoebiasis. *Trans. R. Soc. Trop. Med. Hyg.* 69:440, 1975.

27. Yang J., Kennedy M.T.: Evaluation of enzyme-linked immunosorbent assay for the serodiagnosis of amoebiasis. *J. Clin. Microbiol.* 10:778, 1979.

28. Mahajan R.C., Ganguly N.K.: Amoebic antigen in immunodiagnosis and prognosis of amoebic liver abscess. *Trans. R. Soc. Trop. Med. Hyg.* 74:300, 1980.

29. Root D.M., Cole F.X., Williamson J.A.: The development and standardization of an ELISA (enzyme-linked immunosorbent assay) method for the detection of *Entamoeba histolytica* antigens in fecal samples. *Arch. Invest. Med. (Mex.)* 9(suppl. 1):203, 1978.

30. Bezjak B.: Evaluation of a new technique for sampling duodenal contents in parasitological diagnosis. *Am. J. Dig. Dis.* 17:848, 1972.

31. Visvervara G.S., Smith P.D., Healy G.R., et al.: An immunofluorescence test to detect serum antibodies to *Giardia lamblia. Ann. Intern. Med.* 93:802, 1980.

32. Fife E.H. Jr.: *Trypansoma* (Schizotrypanum) *cruzi*, in Kreir J. (ed.): *Parasitic Protozoa.* New York, Academic Press, 1977, p. 160.

33. Meuwissen J.H., Leewenberg A.D.: A micro-complement fixation test applied to infection with *Pneumocystis carinii. Trop. Geogr. Med.* 24:282, 1972.

34. Kagan I.G., Norman L.: Serology of pneumocystosis. *Natl. Cancer Inst. Monogr.* 43:121, 1976.

35. Meyers J.D., Pifer L.L., Sale G.E., et al.: The value of *Pneumocystis carinii* antibody and antigen detection for diagnosis of *Pneumocystis carinii* pneumonitis after marrow transplantation. *Am. Rev. Respir. Dis.* 120:1283, 1979.

36. Masur H., Michelis M.A., Greene J.B., et al.: An outbreak of community-acquired *Pneumocystis carinii* pneumonia. *N. Engl. J. Med.* 306:1431, 1981.

37. Wright K.A.: *Trichinella spiralis:* An intracellular parasite in the intestinal phase. *J. Parasitol.* 65:441, 1979.

38. Despommier, D.D.: Musculature, in Kennedy C.R. (ed.): *Ecological Aspects of Parsitology.* Amsterdam, Elsevier North-Holland, 1976, p. 269.

39. Despommier D.D., Müller M., Jenks B., et al.: Immunodiagnosis of human trichinosis using counter-immunoelectrophoresis and agar gel diffusion techniques. *Am. J. Trop. Med. Hyg.* 23:41, 1974.

40. Ruitenberg E.J., Van Knapen F.: The enzyme-linked immunosorbent assay and its application to parasitic infections. *J. Infect. Dis.* 136:267, 1977.

41. Kagan I.G.: Evaluation of routine serologic testing for parasitic diseases. *Am. J. Public Health* 55:1820, 1965.

42. Despommier D.D.: Serodiagnosis of *Trichinella spiralis,* in Walls K. (ed.): *Serology of Parasitic Infections.* New York, Marcel-Dekker, to be published.

43. Ruitenberg E.J., Steerenberg P.A., Brosi B.J.M., et al.: Serodiagnosis of *Trichinella spiralis* infections in pigs by enzyme-linked immunosorbent assays. *Bull. WHO* 51:108, 1974.

44. Despommier D.D., Laccetti A.: *Trichinella spiralis:* Partial characterization of antigens isolated by immuno-affinity chromatography from the large particle fraction of the muscle larvae. *J. Parasitol.* 67:332, 1981.

45. Hogarth-Scott R.S., Feery B.J.: The specificity of nematode allergens in the diagnosis of human visceral larva migrans. *Aust. J. Exp. Biol. Med. Sci.* 54:317, 1976.

46. Cypess R.H., Karol M.H., Zician J.L., et al.: Larva-specific antibodies in patients with visceral larva migrans. *J. Infect. Dis.* 135:633, 1977.

47. Schantz P.M., Glickman L.T.: Toxocariasis, in Walls K. (ed.): *Serology of Parasitic Infections.* New York, Marcel-Dekker, to be published.

48. Schantz P.M., Myer D., Glickman L.T.: Clinical serologic, and epidemiologic characteristics of ocular toxocariasis. *Am. J. Trop. Med. Hyg.* 28:24, 1979.

49. Capron A., Yarzabal L.A., Vernes A.: Le diagnostic immunologique de l'echinococcose humaine. *Pathol. Biol.* (Paris) 18:357, 1970.

50. Flisse A., Larralde C.: Immunoserology of cysticercosis, in Walls K. (ed.): *Serology of Parasitic Diseases.* New York, Marcel-Dekker, to be published.

51. Kagan I.G.: A review of serologic tests for the diagnosis of hydatid disease. *Bull. WHO* 39:25, 1968.

52. Ambroise-Thomas P., Truong T.K.: L'immuno-fluorescence dans le diagnostic serologique et le controle post-opèrative de l'hydatidose humaine: I. Matériel et méthods. *Cah. Med. Lyar.* 46:2955, 1970.

53. Capron A., Gentilini M., Vernes A.: Le diagnostic immunologique des filarioses: Possibilités nouvelles offertes par l'immunoéléctrophorèse. *Pathol. Biol.* (Paris) 16:1039, 1968.

54. Ambroise-Thomas P.: Filariasis, in Walls K. (ed.): *Serology of Parasitic Diseases.* New York, Marcel-Dekker, to be published.

55. Cuni L.J., Rosner F., Charvla S.K.: Fatal strongyloidiasis in immunosuppressed patients. *NY State J. Med.* 77:2109, 1977.

13

Immunodeficiency Disorders

C. Cunningham-Rundles, M.D., Ph.D.

W. F. Cunningham-Rundles, M.D.

THE IMMUNE SYSTEM is composed of various cells and numerous molecular factors that interact to form a defense network against a range of bacterial, viral, fungal, and neoplastic challenges. The activities of the immune system are both specific and nonspecific. Examples of specific activities are antibody production or sensitization of specific cells; examples of nonspecific factors are complement components and nonsensitized cells.

The division of immune system functions into two kinds—cell-mediated immunity and humoral immunity—provides a simple basis both for classifying the factors of immunity and for understanding the developmental origin of these components. This distinction also provides a rationale for the laboratory evaluation of immunodeficiency states, since the tests used in clinical practice analyze humoral and cellular functions separately.[1, 2]

The basic elements of the cell-mediated and humoral immunity systems are the T (thymic-derived) and the B (bone marrow–derived) lymphocytes. T and B lymphocytes go through different developmental stages, have distinctive surface morphologies, and perform quite separate immune functions. Adequate cell-mediated immunity is required in all types of delayed hypersensitivity because the local appearance of antigen causes the accumulation of specifically presensitized T cells. Two well-known examples of cell-mediated, delayed hypersensitivity are the tuberculin reaction and contact dermatitis: both monocytes and lymphocytes previously sensitized to tuberculin proteins, or to specific antigens such as poison ivy, accumulate in the area of antigen rechallenge. This kind of immunity is of particular importance in host defense against intracellular bacteria, mycobacteria, viruses, and protozoa. In contrast, humoral immunity and the production of specific antibodies by B lymphocytes are necessary for adequate defense against most bacterial infections.

DEVELOPMENT OF THE IMMUNE SYSTEM

As illustrated in Figure 13–1, both common lymphoid stem cells (LSC) and cells of the monocyte-macrophage series arise from the hematopoietic stem cells (HSC) present in the embryonic yolk sac.[3] The LSC that migrate to the thymus differentiate into T lymphocytes, and those that migrate first into the fetal liver and then into the bone marrow differentiate into B lymphocytes. T and B lymphocytes then continue their separate differentiation steps either within these organs or after further migration into other tissues. In this way, subpopulations of both T and B lymphocytes, each with specific functions, appear.

T and B lymphocytes cannot be distinguished by light microscopy; however, under the electron microscope, B lymphocytes may appear to have more villi on their surfaces. T and B lymphocytes can, however, be easily distinguished on special tests by the presence of distinctive antigenic features on their surfaces. For example, T cells bear receptors for sheep red blood cells (RBCs) and B cells bear various classes of immunoglobulin.[1, 2]

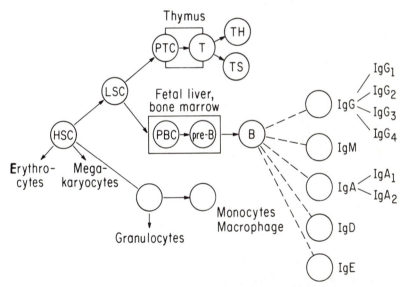

Fig 13–1.—The hematopoietic stem cell *(HSC)* gives rise to the lymphoid stem cell *(LSC)* and the granulocyte and monocyte-macrophage precursors, as well as cells of the erythrocyte and megakaryocyte lineage. The LSC is the precursor of pre-T cells *(PTC)* and pre-B cells *(PBC)*. The more mature T cells then become functionally differentiated to provide cells with helper *(TH)* or suppressor *(TS)* capabilities. Pre-B cells mature to provide cells that can secrete all classes of immunoglobulin.

In addition to these differences, other surface antigenic markers provide distinctive features for different developmental stages of T and B lymphocytes. These markers can be distinguished by the use of cell rosette assays (described in Chap. 3) and by the use of specific antisera that recognize selected cell surface proteins. Table 13–1 lists some of the different markers that appear on T and B lymphocytes. These markers provide important diagnostic information to the clinical immunologist investigating patients with suspected immunodeficiency disease, since characteristic abnormalities in the proportions of cells bearing these markers are used to classify immunodeficiency diseases.

CLINICAL INDICATIONS OF IMMUNODEFICIENCY DISEASE

In general, an evaluation of immune status is recommended for all patients who have repeated, documented infections, particularly if the infections are serious or systemic or if unusual organisms are involved. Such evaluations are particularly important if there is a family history of known immunodeficiency disease.

Specific immune defects not infrequently lead to characteristic illnesses. For example, patients with T cell defects have a propensity to infections with fungi, viruses, and intracellular organisms, while individuals with B cell defects usually have recurrent pyogenic infections, particularly those caused by encapsulated organisms. The infectious agents most frequently encountered in patients with T or B cell defects are listed in Table 13–2.

In addition to the isolation of these organisms from an individual suspected of having an immunologic defect, there are a number of clinical syndromes or disease states that indicate to the clinical immunologist that

TABLE 13–1.—Surface Marker
Differences for T and B Cells

	T CELL	B CELL
Surface immunoglobulin	(+)	+
Fc receptors	(+)	+
Complement receptors		
C1q	+	+
C3b	−	+
C3d	−	+
Sheep RBC receptor	+	−
Specific T cell markers		
OKT$_1$–OKT$_{10}$ Markers	+	−
Leu 1–6 Markers	+	−

TABLE 13–2.—COMMON
INFECTIOUS AGENTS IN T AND B
CELL DEFECTS

T CELL DEFECT
Mycobacteria
Candida albicans
Pneumocystis carinii
Cytomegalovirus
Toxoplasmosis
Measles
Varicella-zoster virus
B CELL DEFECT
Pneumococci
Streptococci
Hemophilus influenzae
Staphylococci
ECHO virus
Giardiasis

an immunologic workup should be considered. These conditions, and the underlying defect which each suggests, are listed in Table 13–3.

CLASSIFICATION OF IMMUNODEFICIENCY DISEASE

Genetic disorders of primary immunodeficiency are generally grouped by disease states affecting T cells, B cells, both T and B cells, macrophages, or the complement system. Disorders affecting T cells or macrophages will result in defective cell-mediated immunity; disorders affecting B cells will produce humoral immunodeficiencies. The range of abnormalities produced can be better understood by consulting Figure 13–2, which illustrates how a lesion affecting an early stem cell can produce a wide range of defects, such as the syndrome of reticular dysgenesis, and a lesion involving only one branch of the cellular or humoral (T or B cell) limbs of the immune system can produce a much more restricted abnormality, such as selective IgA deficiency. The specific lesions that produce complement component deficiencies are not yet understood. (For general discussions of these abnormalities and the diseases that result, see Gatti[2] and the WHO report.[4])

PRIMARY IMMUNODEFICIENCY SYNDROMES

Cellular and Humoral Immune Systems

Tables 13–4, 13–5, and 13–6 list the key features of the immunodeficiency diseases, which are grouped according to the immune systems in-

TABLE 13–3.—CLINICAL INDICATIONS OF IMMUNODEFICIENCY DISEASE

	T CELL DEFECT	B CELL DEFECT	PHAGOCYTIC DEFECT	COMPLEMENT DEFECT
Systemic illness following virus or BCG vaccination	✓			
Chronic, drug-resistant, oral candidiasis after age 6 mo.	✓			
Chronic mucocutaneous candidiasis	✓			
Cartilage hair hypoplasia	✓			
Intrauterine graft-vs.-host disease	✓			
Graft-vs.-host disease after blood transfusion	✓			
Hypocalcemia in newborn period (especially with cardiac abnormalities)	✓			
Reduced lymphocyte count (often small lymphocytes)	✓			
Recurrent bacterial pneumonia, sepsis, and/or meningitis		✓		✓ (C3, C5, C8)
Nodular lymphoid hyperplasia		✓		
Recurrent giardiasis		✓		
Clinical features of Wiskott-Aldrich syndrome (thrombocytopenia, eczema)	✓	✓		
Clinical features of ataxia-telangiectasia (conjunctival or peri-auricular telangiectasia, ataxia, recurrent sinopulmonary infections)	✓	✓		
Pneumocystis carinii pneumonia	✓	✓		

Intractable eczema	✓			
Intractable seborrheic dermatitis		✓		
Recurrent pyogenic infections			✓	
Recurrent gram-negative infections			✓	
Recurrent *Neisseria* infections			✓	✓ (C5)
Skin infections, eczema, coarse facies			✓	✓ (C5) ✓ (C6–8)
Skin infections, eczema, coarse facies, craniosynostosis			✓	✓ (C5–8)
Skin infections, coarse facies, red hair, cold abscesses			✓	
Chronic osteomyelitis, draining lymph nodes, brain or liver		(Chronic granulomatous disease)		
Lupus-like syndrome	✓		✓	C1r, C1s, C2, C4 ✓
Family history of known immunodeficiency	✓			
Presence of unusual or rapidly growing tumor (Kaposi's sarcoma), lymphoreticular malignancy			✓	
Presence of autoimmune disease, particularly hemolytic anemia, idiopathic thrombocytopenia				✓

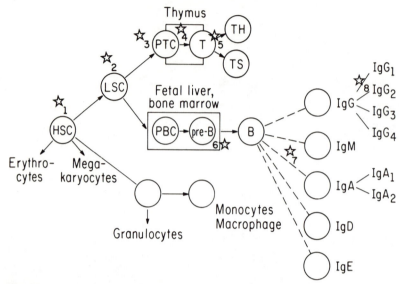

Fig 13–2.—The immunodeficiency syndromes can be visualized as resulting from specific blocks or lesions in the maturation steps shown in Figure 13–1.— For example, a lesion at the level of the HSC (starred 1) can result in reticular dysgenesis; lesion 2 can result in severe combined immunodeficiency; lesions 3 and 4, specific T cell abnormalities such as the DiGeorge syndrome; lesion 5, a deficit of helper or suppressor cells; lesion 6, X-linked agammaglobulinemia; lesion 7, selective IgA deficiency; and lesion 8, IgG2 subclass deficiency.

volved. The more commonly encountered of these diseases are further described below.

Thymic Hypoplasia (DiGeorge Syndrome)

Thymic hypoplasia is a classic example of a pure T cell defect. Clinically, the disease syndrome is characterized by neonatal tetany, unusual facies, increased susceptibility to infection, and occasional cardiac abnormalities.[5] Presumably because of a developmental lesion involving the third and fourth pharyngeal pouches, thymic abnormalities or hypoplasia are to be expected. T cell numbers and functions are depressed or absent; the chest x-ray film shows no thymic shadow. Impaired production of antibody synthesis can also occur, possibly due to defects of helper T cells.

X-linked Agammaglobulinemia (Bruton's Agammaglobulinemia)

X-linked agammaglobulinemia is an example of a pure B cell defect: B cells, plasma cells, and consequently antibody production are absent.[6]

TABLE 13–4.—T CELL DEFICIENCY*

DESIGNATION	FUNCTIONAL DEFICIENCIES	CELLULAR ABNORMALITIES	INHERITANCE	MAIN ASSOCIATED FEATURES
Thymic hypoplasia (DiGeorge syndrome)	CMI and ↓ Ab	T lymphocyte numbers and functions	Usually not familial	Hypoparathyroidism; abnormal facies; cardiovascular abnormalities
Purine nucleoside phosphorylase deficiency	CMI ± Ab	T lymphocyte numbers and functions	AR	Hypoplastic anemia
Miscellaneous T cell deficiencies	CMI ± Ab	T lymphocyte numbers and functions	Unknown or familial	
Nezelof syndrome	CMI ± Ab	T lymphocyte numbers and functions	AR, X-linked	
Bare lymphocytic syndrome	CMI ± Ab	T lymphocyte numbers and functions	Familial?	Lack of surface antigens on lymphocytes
Short-limbed dwarfism	CMI	T lymphocyte numbers and functions	Familial?	Cartilage hair hypoplasia

*CMI, cell-mediated immunity; Ab, antibody production; AR, autosomal recessive.

TABLE 13–5.—B CELL DEFICIENCY PREDOMINANT*

DESIGNATION	FUNCTIONAL DEFICIENCIES	CELLULAR ABNORMALITIES	INHERITANCE	MAIN ASSOCIATED FEATURES
X-linked agammaglobulinemia	Ab	No peripheral B cells	X-linked	
Transcobalamin II deficiency	Ab and phagocytosis	↓ Plasma cells	AR	Pancytopenia with megaloblastic anemia; intestinal villous atrophy
Selective IgA deficiency	IgA Ab	↓ IgA-bearing lymphocytes and plasma cells	Unknown > AR > AD	Autoantibody production; autoimmune disease
Selective deficiency of one other Ig class or subclass	Ab	↓ Plasma cells	Unknown	
Secretory piece deficiency	Secretory IgA Ab	↓ Intestinal IgA plasma cells	Unknown	One case reported with severe gastrointestinal disease
Ig deficiencies with increased IgM	Ab	↓ IgG and IgA plasma cells; ↑ IgM plasma cells; ↑ B lymphocytes	X-linked or AR or unknown	
Transient hypogammaglobulinemia of infancy	Ab	↓ Plasma cells	Unknown	Frequent, sometimes severe infections in first 2 years
Antibody deficiency with normal or hyperglobulinemia	Impaired Ab for some antigens (mainly primary response)	B lymphocytes	AR in some	Often severe sinopulmonary disease
Kappa chain deficiency	Ab	↓ Bκ lymphocytes	Unknown or familial	
Varied ID (common and largely unclassified); predominant Ig deficiency	Ab ± CMI	± ↓ B lymphocytes	Unknown or familial	

*CMI, cell-mediated immunity; Ab, antibody production; AR, autosomal recessive; AD, autosomal dominant.

TABLE 13–6.—COMBINED T AND B CELL DEFICIENCY*

DESIGNATION	FUNCTIONAL DEFICIENCIES	CELLULAR ABNORMALITIES	INHERITANCE	MAIN ASSOCIATED FEATURES
SCID				
Reticular dysgenesis	CMI, Ab, phagocytes	↓ T, B, and phagocytes	AR	
"Swiss type"	CMI, Ab	↓ T and B	AR	
ADA deficiency	CMI, Ab	↓ T ± B	AR	± Chondrocyte abnormalities
With B lymphocytes	CMI, Ab	↓ T (B lymphocytes without or with normal isotype diversity)	X-linked or AR	
Wiskott-Aldrich syndrome	Ab to certain antigens (mainly polysaccharides) and CMI (progressive)	↓ T and B (progressive)	X-linked	Thrombocytopenia; eczema
ID with ataxia-telangiectasia	CMI and Ab (partial)	↓ T and plasma cells (mainly IgA, IgE ± IgG)	AR	Cerebellar ataxia; telangiectasia; ovarian dysgenesis; chromosomal abnormalities
ID with thymoma	Ab and impaired CMI (variable)	↓ pre-B and B, ± ↓ T	None	Thymoma; eosinopenia; erythroblastopenia; aplastic anemia
Short-limbed dwarfism	CMI, Ab	↓ T	AR	Cartilage hair hypoplasia
Mucocutaneous candidiasis	CMI ± Ab			

*SCID, severe combined immunodeficiency disease; ID, immunodeficiency disease; ADA, adenosine deaminase; CMI, cell-mediated immunity; Ab, antibody production; AR, autosomal recessive.

Since pre-B cells (B cells with cytoplasmic IgM) are found in the bone marrow and spleen of patients with this disease, the specific developmental defect appears to be at the level of the pre-B cell. The essential abnormality is the failure of the pre-B cell to mature into an antibody-secreting plasma cell. The inheritance is X-linked; a few cases in females have been reported. Patients with X-linked agammaglobulinemia have a particular propensity to infection with encapsulated bacteria, predominantly *Pneumococcus* sp. and *Hemophilus influenzae*. A paucity of lymphoid tissue (tonsils and adenoids in particular) is characteristic. Since cell-mediated immunity is spared, viral infections (except, for unknown reasons, ECHO virus), and fungal infections elicit normal responses. Treatment is with γ-globulin given intramuscularly (0.05–0.2 mg/kg/2 weeks) or intravenously (100–200 mg/kg/3 weeks).

Selective IgA Deficiency

One of the most common of the immune deficiency disorders present in 1 in 500 to 1 in 1,000 blood donors, this humoral abnormality reflects a deficiency or absence of serum and secretory IgA and low numbers of circulating IgA-bearing B lymphocytes. By definition, IgG and IgM levels are normal, although IgG2 subclass deficiency can be found in 18% of affected patients.[7] Clinically, patients have frequent respiratory tract and gastrointestinal tract infections, and there is a higher incidence of autoimmune diseases such as systemic lupus erythematosus (SLE), rheumatoid arthritis, and hemolytic anemia. Anti-IgA antibodies are found in approximately 8% of patients; this can lead to anaphylactic reactions to blood transfusions.

Common Varied Immunodeficiency (Adult-Onset or Acquired Hypogammaglobulinemia)

This syndrome is an extremely heterogeneous entity which usually includes depressed serum IgG, IgA, or IgM levels over a wide range. Although it is classified as a humoral immunodeficiency, about 60% of patients have evidence of T cell defects (low lymphocyte proliferative capacity in response to mitogens and antigens and low levels of thymic hormones). Clinically, the disease is characterized by frequent (and often severe) sinopulmonary and gastrointestinal infections; lymphoid hyperplasia and sometimes splenomegaly are found in about 20% of patients, and autoimmune disease (particularly hemolytic anemia, thrombocytopenia, neutropenia and rheumatoid arthritis) in about 10%. Treatment is with intramuscular or intravenous γ-globulin (see above).

Transient Hypogammaglobulinemia of Infancy

This is a generally self-limited disorder characterized by low levels of serum immunoglobulins for age and can occur in infants aged 5 months to 2 years. These infants, which are often premature, may have relatively severe and frequent respiratory tract infections. The disorder is presumed to be an exaggeration of the normal physiologic hypogammaglobulinemia of infancy; the levels of immunoglobulin slowly rise into the normal range for age. No treatment is indicated except antibiotics for existing infections.

Severe Combined Immunodeficiency (Swiss-Type Agammaglobulinemia)

Potentially the most severe of the congenital primary immunodeficiency diseases, severe combined immunodeficiency (SCID) is a collection of disorders characterized by the combined absence of cellular and humoral immunity.[8, 9] If phagocytic abnormalities are present as well, the syndrome is called reticular dysgenesis and the presumed developmental defect is at the level of the HSC (see Fig 13–2). Both X-linked and autosomal recessive types have been described, and a deficiency of adenosine deaminase (ADA) may be found in some patients. Clinically, the disease is characterized by overwhelming infections beginning in the first few months of life; typical organisms include *Candida, Pneumocystis carinii,* varicella, measles, and cytomegalovirus. Laboratory evaluations usually show the absence of cellular and humoral immune systems and lymphopenia, peripheral lymphoid depletion, lack of thymic shadow, phagocytic defects (possible), and low or even normal immunoglobulin levels. When immunoglobulin levels are normal, the disease is known as the Nezelof syndrome.[10] Treatment of this lethal disorder is by bone marrow transplantation from a histocompatible family member. When ADA levels are low, infusions of normal (irradiated) RBCs may restore cellular immunity to normal.[11]

Wiskott-Aldrich Syndrome (T Cell Immunodeficiency with Eczema and Thrombocytopenia)

This syndrome is characterized by an inability to form antibodies to polysaccharide antigens and by impaired cell-mediated immunity. The inheritance is X-linked. Clinically, patients have bleeding episodes (due to thrombocytopenia), eczema, and recurrent serious bacterial infections. Laboratory findings include normal levels of IgG, usually increased levels of IgA and IgE, low levels of IgM, and low or absent serum isohemagglutinins. Impaired delayed hypersensitivity and a tendency to develop malignancies are important characteristics. (For a review, see Belohradsky et al.[12])

Immunodeficiency with Ataxia-Telangiectasia

This is a combined cell-mediated and humoral immune deficiency which can include IgA deficiency (70%–80%), IgE deficiency (80%–90%), and lymphocyte abnormalities (60%). Clinically, patients have ataxia (usually appearing in infancy) and telangiectases over the bulbar conjunctivae and around the ears. With time, the ataxia can progress to severe disability; severe sinopulmonary infections leading to bronchiectasis are common. Ovarian or testicular atrophy usually occurs, and growth hormone production may be impaired. Patients with this syndrome have a greatly increased tendency to lymphoid malignancies. An important underlying feature of this disease is a defect in DNA repair.[13] Inheritance is autosomal recessive. No treatment is known.

Mucocutaneous Candidiasis

In this disease, no immunologic parameter is consistently abnormal. The cause of the disease remains unknown, although numerous defects of cell-mediated immunity, primarily decreased lymphocyte transformation, lymphokine production, and reduced chemotaxis, have frequently been demonstrated. Clinically, patients have persistent *Candida* infection of the skin, nails, and mucous membranes, starting in the first year of life. Various lymphocyte functional abnormalities have been described but are not always present. Endocrinopathies are often associated; hypothyroidism, diabetes mellitus, and hypoadrenal states are the most common. Thymomas are found in some patients. (For a review, see Blizzard and Gibbs.[14]) Autoantibody formation is often found. Treatment is by antimicrobial therapy; transfer factor may also be effective.

The Phagocytic System

The genetic defects involving phagocytes may involve the numbers or functions of circulating neutrophils and may affect the tissue macrophages of the lymphoid organs in the reticuloendothelial system. These syndromes can be inherited as autosomal recessive or X-linked traits; most cases are sporadic, without a family history. Abnormalities of the phagocytic system can be caused by defective movement toward the bacterium, attachment to the bacterial cell wall, endocytosis, or intracellular killing of the organism. Intracellular killing depends on the release of oxygen metabolites and halide incorporation. Table 13–7 summarizes characteristics of phagocytic deficiencies that can affect neutrophils, monocytes, and macrophages. The best-known defects are described in detail below.

Chronic Granulomatous Disease

Chronic granulomatous disease is a rare disorder of granulocytes and monocytes in which ingested, catalase-positive organisms are not killed but are released intact. Chemotaxis and ingestion are normal and the exact molecular basis of the killing defect is not yet known although the screening test widely used reveals the inability of phagocytic cells to reduce nitroblue tetrazolium dye, presumably because of an abnormality in the production of superoxide anion and hydrogen peroxide.[15, 16] Neutrophils of patients with chronic granulomatous disease are able to kill catalase-negative organisms such as pneumococci, β-hemolytic streptococci, and *H. influenzae;* catalase-positive organisms *(S. aureus, E. coli,* molds, etc.) are not killed[17] and thereby lead to abscess formation. Clinically, patients have recurrent pyogenic infections, particularly liver and brain abscesses and osteomyelitis, and suppurative draining adenitis. The X-linked form affects males; a rarer autosomal recessive form affects females. The only treatments available are antibiotics and surgical drainage when necessary.

The Chédiak-Higashi Syndrome

The Chédiak-Higashi syndrome is a disorder of leukocytes that is characterized by granulocytopenia, oculocutaneous albinism, photophobia, nystagmus, and the presence of giant granules in leukocytes.[18] The neutrophils and monocytes move poorly and display defective intracellular killing of bacteria, presumably due to a failure of lysosomal degranulation. There may be additional abnormalities of the enzyme granules (elastase, for example, has been found to be absent[19]). Phagocytosis is normal. Recent reports have demonstrated that vitamin C might improve the biochemical abnormality that underlies a similar syndrome found in mice,[20] but this therapy may not help affected humans.[21]

Cyclic Neutropenia

In this syndrome, neutropenia occurs at intervals of 15–35 days due to an intrinsic defect in the bone marrow. Monocytosis is often observed in the neutropenic stages, and the immediate reason for the cycling is a periodic decline in the production of premyelocytes and myeloblasts.[22] Clinically, patients have fever, mouth ulcers, or abscesses during the neutropenic intervals. It is not unusual for the neutropenic periods to become

TABLE 13–7.—PHAGOCYTIC DEFICIENCIES

DESIGNATION	FUNCTIONAL DEFECT	CELLULAR ABNORMALITIES	INHERITANCE	MAIN ASSOCIATED FEATURES
Chronic granulomatous disease	→ Bacterial killing	Neutrophils, monocytes	X-linked, AR*	Osteomyelitis, liver and brain abscesses; mothers may have cutaneous lupus erythematosus
Myeloperoxidase deficiency	→ Bacterial killing	Neutrophils	AR	
Leukocyte G6PD deficiency	→ Bacterial killing	Neutrophils	?	
Leukocyte pyruvate kinase deficiency	→ Bacterial killing	Neutrophils	?	
Chédiak-Higashi syndrome	→ Mobility + bacterial killing	Neutrophils, monocytes	?	Albinism; giant granules in phagocytes
Actin-binding deficiency	→ Mobility	Neutrophils	AR	
Shwachman's disease	→ Mobility	Neutrophils	AR	Pancreatic insufficiency; bone abnormalities
Job's syndrome; Buckley's disease; hyper-IgE	→ Mobility	Neutrophils		Eczema
Neutropenia: benign, cyclic	→ Mobility	Neutrophils		

*AR, autosomal recessive.

extended so that the underlying cycles are no longer easily distinguishable.[23] The disease can be autosomal dominant or sporadic in inheritance. No treatment is known, but antibiotics may be given during the neutropenic periods.

The Complement System

The clinical abnormalities resulting from a deficiency of one or more complement components are particularly diverse (see Chap. 6).[24] A lack of C3, for example, precludes ingestion of bacterial particles by macrophages and leads to overwhelming bacterial infections, while a lack of C2 can be found in healthy individuals or accompany a lupus-like clinical syndrome. Table 13–8 lists the currently known syndromes and a few of the important clinical features of each. Some abnormalities of the complement system are described below.

C1 ESTERASE INHIBITOR DEFICIENCY.—A deficiency of a functional C1 esterase inhibitor leads to familial angioedema, a syndrome in which circumscribed, transient, nonpitting and nonpruritic swelling of the face, neck, soft tissue about the larynx, hands, or feet occurs.[25] The syndrome is apparently due to the lack of a functional inhibitor of C1 activation, which leads to the consumption of C2 and C4. Trauma, menses, or stress can trigger attacks. C1 esterase inhibitor deficiency is inherited as an autosomal dominant trait; it also occurs, rarely, as an acquired defect, usually in a

TABLE 13–8.—COMPLEMENT DEFICIENCIES*

DEFECTIVE COMPONENT	INHERITANCE	HLA LINKAGE	SYMPTOMS
C1q	. . .	−	(Present in severe hypogammaglobulinemia)
C1r	AR	−	SLE, arthritis, nephritis, vasculitis, bacterial meningitis, bronchitis; ANA negative
C1s	?	−	SLE, ANA positive
C1 inhibitor	AD	−	Hereditary angioedema
C2	AR	+	No symptoms or SLE or discoid lupus, vasculitis, nephritis
C3 inhibitor	1/10,000 blood donors	−	Recurrent pyogenic infections
C4	AR	+	Recurrent infections
C5	AR	−	SLE syndrome, recurrent infections
C6	AR	?	Neisserial infection, SLE
C7	AR	−	Ankylosing spondylitis
C8	AR	−	SLE
C9	?	?	None

*AR, autosomal recessive; AD, autosomal dominant; ANA, antinuclear antibody; SLE, systemic lupus erythematosus.

patient with a systemic disease such as lymphoma or SLE. In either the acquired or the genetically inherited forms, the C1 esterase inhibitor itself may be present but nonfunctional (25% of cases) or not present (75%). Treatment is with an attenuated androgen, danazol.[26]

C2 DEFICIENCY.—C2 deficiency may be the commonest of the complement deficiencies, occurring in 1 in 10,000 blood donors. The deficiency may occur without any symptoms,[24] but in some patients it is accompanied by SLE, polymyositis, anaphylactoid purpura, or other connective tissue diseases.

C3 DEFICIENCY.—This is a rare abnormality. It may be due to reduced production of C3 or increased catabolism. Since C3 is important to the functioning of the classic and the alternative complement pathway, a deficiency leads to severe pyogenic infections.[27]

C5 DEFICIENCY.—Along with C6 and C7, C5 is part of a chemotactic complex that attaches to cell membranes and permits lysis by C8 and C9.[24] C5 deficiency leads to a chemotactic defect that manifests as a susceptibility to recurrent bacterial infections.

IMMUNOLOGIC TESTS: METHODS AND INTERPRETATION

General Approach

A thorough history and complete physical examination are essential starting points in the immunologic workup. It is important to ascertain a specific history of disease, the presence of congenital defects, a family history of infections, and culture results. On physical examination, particular care should be given to height and weight relative to age, the lymphoid system, sinopulmonary function, skin, joints, and nails.

Laboratory investigations should include a complete blood cell count and, in infants, a chest x-ray for assessment of thymic shadow. A lateral neck x-ray may be important to determine the presence or absence of adenoidal tissue. Any evidence of ongoing infection should be documented by cultures.

Specific Immunologic Assessment

Valuable screening tests for immunologic deficiency disease are available at selected commercial laboratories, although further assessment is usually necessary in a research laboratory or facility. The immunologic evaluation can be divided into four parts:
1. Analysis of the T cell system (cellular immunity).
2. Analysis of the B cell system (humoral immunity).

3. Analysis of the phagocytic system.
4. Analysis of the complement system.
Each of these is discussed separately below.

The T Cell System

A scheme for the evaluation of the T cell system is given in Table 13–9. The first and simplest T cell system parameters are (1) the absolute number of circulating lymphocytes (most of which are T lymphocytes), and (2) the skin reactivity to common antigens to which the subject has been exposed (recall antigens). The skin test solutions usually used are extracts of *Candida*, purified protein derivative, mumps, streptokinase/streptodornase (SK/SD, extracts of streptococci), and tetanus. Prior sensitization is needed for the subject to respond. The absolute number of T lymphocytes should exceed 1,500 (the usual range in our laboratories is 1,860–3,410/µl). For skin testing, a minimum of three tests are usually performed. Adults and children over age 12 usually respond to mumps, SK/SD, and *Candida*, although an occasional normal individual will not respond to these antigens. SK/SD is not commercially available at present.

The second parameter of T cell immunity to examine is the numbers of T cells in the peripheral blood: this is done by the sheep RBC rosette method (E rosette), which takes advantage of the fact that sheep RBCs adhere to human T cells. This method is technically relatively simple, although care must be taken at each step.[28] In all probability, this method of T cell enumeration will be superseded by a fluorescent-labeled monoclonal antisera to mature T cells. Such reagents are now used in research laboratories, but they are still too expensive for routine use. A deficiency of T cell numbers is seen in the DiGeorge syndrome, SCID, and in isolated T cell deficiencies.

The third parameter of T cell immunity to assess is T cell function. As described in Chapter 3, the stimulation of T cells with various agents causes these cells to enlarge and undergo mitosis. The resulting blast-like cells can be enumerated directly on microscopy or can be quantitatively assessed by measuring the amount of incorporated isotope. The agents that cause this effect are nonspecific stimulators, called mitogens, and specific antigenic stimulators, such as extracts of bacterial or fungal organisms. Examples of mitogens are phytohemagglutinin (PHA), concanavalin A (Con A), and pokeweed mitogen (PWM); examples of antigens are extracts of *C. albicans*, *Escherichia coli*, *S. aureus*, and purified protein derivative. Prior exposure is mandatory to elicit a response to these antigens. Abnormalities in T cell function are seen in SCID, DiGeorge syndrome, T cell defects,

TABLE 13–9.—T CELL TESTING: CELLULAR IMMUNITY*

TEST PROCEDURE	SPECIMEN	LABORATORY	NORMAL RANGE
Absolute lymphocyte count	Citrated blood	Commercial	20%–40% of WBC; 1,860–3,410/µl
Skin testing PPD, *Candida*, SK/SD, mumps, tetanus	. . .	(Office procedure)	Some are usually positive (> 8 mm)
Lymphocyte surface markers T lymphocyte markers (E rosette)	Heparinized blood	Commercial or research	60%–93% of lymphocytes
Lymphocyte functions Mitogen stimulation	Heparinized blood	Commercial or research	
Phytohemagglutinin			> 20,000 cpm
Concanavalin A			> 12,000 cpm
Pokeweed mitogen			> 5,000 cpm
Antigen stimulation	Heparinized blood	Research	
Candida			> 4,000 cpm
E. coli			> 3,000 cpm
S. aureus			> 3,000 cpm
PPD			Negative
Mixed lymphocyte culture	Heparinized blood	Research	> 7,000 cpm
Natural killer cell analysis	Heparinized blood	Research	> 15% target lysis
T cell subsets	Heparinized blood	Research	
Helper cells			39% ± 11%
Suppressor cells			24% ± 7.5%

*PPD, purified protein derivative; SK/SD, streptokinase-streptodornase; cpm, counts per minute.

common varied immunodeficiency, ataxia-telangiectasia, and Wiskott-Aldrich syndrome.

Another test of T cell function is the mixed lymphocyte culture (MLC); in this test the patient's T cells are exposed to a mixture of lymphoid cells of unrelated individuals. Blast transformation ensues, and the degree of transformation is assessed directly on microscopy or by measuring the amount of isotope incorporated. Patients with T cell deficiencies have impaired lymphocyte transformation responses to mitogens and antigens; usually there is relative impairment in the MLC response. This test is believed to reflect an in vitro model of the graft rejection response, and if the MLC response is reduced, it indicates that this T cell function is likely to be defective. Clinically, a poor MLC response means that if the patient requires blood or blood products, these substances should be irradiated to prevent any lymphocytes present from dividing and producing graft-vs.-host disease. This is most important in SCID and in severe T cell defects.

Another important test of lymphocyte function is an assessment of natural killer (NK) cell activity. This tests the capacity of a mononuclear cell population to lyse a tumor target cell and seems to reflect the host's intrinsic resistance to tumor growth. NK cell function does not require prior sensitization. NK cell defects are present in Chédiak-Higashi syndrome[29] and sporadically in other genetic immunodeficiency diseases.

Subsets of human T cells have quite distinct functions that can also be separately tested.[30] Two major activities, helper and suppressor functions, are analyzed initially by determining whether an appropriate number of each of these cell populations is present in the peripheral blood. The complete T cell subset analysis is now accomplished by the use of specific monoclonal antibody fluorescence techniques, using new sera directed at selected surface antigens. Examples of such are the reagents OKT_1–OKT_{10} (Ortho Pharmaceuticals) and Leu 1–6 (Becton-Dickinson Corp.). From a functional point of view, helper and suppressor activities are generally assessed by the capacity of a test T cell population to enhance or suppress immunoglobulin production in the in vitro plaque assay. Patients with common varied immunodeficiency may exhibit abnormalities of helper or suppressor activity.[31, 32]

Specific Evaluations of Humoral Immunity

Humoral immunity is assessed by testing for (1) the presence of IgG, IgA, and IgM, (2) the presence of B lymphocytes in the peripheral blood, and (3) the production of specific antibodies (Table 13–10). Quantitation of immunoglobulin levels alone is not a sufficient test of humoral immune response, since antibody production can be abnormal even if the immuno-

TABLE 13–10.—B CELL TESTING: HUMORAL IMMUNITY

TEST PROCEDURE	SPECIMEN	LABORATORY	NORMAL RANGE
Immunoglobulins			
Serum electrophoresis	Serum	Commercial	
Immunoelectrophoresis	Serum	Commercial	
Quantitative IgG, IgA, IgM	Serum	Commercial	For adults: IgG, 800–1,800 mg/dl; IgA, 90–450 mg/dl; IgM, 80–300 mg/dl
Immunoglobulin IgG subclasses	Serum	Research	As established in laboratory
Antibody testing (antigens previously encountered)			
Isohemagglutinins	Serum	Commercial	One titer positive if blood group O, A, or B
Diphtheria			
Tetanus			
Streptococcus			
Epstein-Barr virus			
Herpes simplex	Serum	Commercial or research	Positive if immunized
Herpes zoster			
Rubella			
Measles			
Influenza A and B			
B lymphocyte numbers			
Immunoglobulin isotypes IgG, IgA, IgM, IgD, κ, λ	Heparinized blood	Research; some commercial	3%–20% of lymphocytes
Fc receptor			6%–30% of lymphocytes
C3 receptors (C3b, C3d)			~10%–35% of lymphocytes
Ia antigens			~3%–25% of lymphocytes
Active immunization			
Pneumococcal vaccine		Research	Rise in titer 1 month after immunization
Killed polio virus		Commercial	
Diphtheria/tetanus toxoid		Commercial	

globulin levels are normal. In the latter instance (termed antibody deficiency syndrome) intact heterogeneous immunoglobulins are produced, but these proteins apparently have little or no binding affinity for antigens. The ultimate effect of both immunoglobulin and antibody deficiency syndromes is to predispose patients to pyogenic infections, most frequently of the sinopulmonary passages and the gastrointestinal tract.

The initial step in assessing humoral immunity is to determine whether IgG, IgA, and IgM are all present in normal amounts. Serum protein electrophoresis, available at most commercial laboratories, can be used to exclude more severe cases of hypogammaglobulinemia, but partial IgG deficiency and IgA and IgM deficiencies will be missed by this method. Immunoelectrophoresis is a more specific method of detecting deficiencies, but immunoglobulins are not quantitated. Quantitation is obtained by single radial immunodiffusion or automated nephelometry. By both methods, immunoglobulin concentrations of the test sera are compared with standard solutions containing defined concentrations. The Mancini method of single radial immunodiffusion can detect as little as 10 μg/ml.[33] The normal values for children and adults are given in Table 13–11. IgG subclasses (IgG1–IgG4) can be detected by similar methods or by rocket electrophoresis.

The antibody activity of immunoglobulins is assessed by tests designed to detect increases of specific antibodies as a response to active immunization, as a response to a "natural" immunogen, or as a response to a previously encountered antigen. Active immunization can be performed with diphtheria/tetanus toxoids or pneumococcal polysaccharide vaccines. (Live vaccines such as BCG, smallpox, poliomyelitis, measles, rubella, and mumps are absolutely contraindicated when immunodeficiency is suspected.) Killed poliomyelitis vaccine can be used. Blood samples are drawn just before and 2 to 4 weeks after these active immunizations to ascertain whether antibody has been formed. Natural immunogens are the isohemagglutins (anti-A and -B blood group substances); blood banks can determine whether any of these antibodies (which are mainly IgM) are present in patients whose blood type is A, B, or O. In addition, antibodies to previously encountered disease organisms can be determined by many commercial laboratories. Examples are ASLO titer, antibody to Epstein-Barr virus, herpes simplex, herpes zoster, rubella, measles, and influenza.

It is next important to ascertain whether B lymphocytes, cells that bear immunoglobulins and other markers listed in Table 13–1, are present in the peripheral blood.[30] The methods used for cell surface immunoglobulin detection are fraught with difficulties, since complexes and aggregates in the anti-immunoglobulin reagents used can give false positive results by binding to the immunoglobulin Fc receptors of B cells rather than to specific surface immunoglobulins.[34] This is prevented by using pepsin-treated

TABLE 13–11.—NORMAL RANGE OF
IMMUNOGLOBULINS FOR AGE*

AGE	IgG (MG/DL)†	IgA (MG/DL)†	IgM (MG/DL)†
Birth	800–1,800	0–6	0–25
1 mo.	450–1,188	3–17	19–95
2 mo.	313–825	8–44	25–128
3 mo.	263–688	11–57	29–152
4 mo.	244–663	12–67	31–168
5 mo.	263–713	13–71	34–176
6 mo.	281–763	14–76	36–184
7 mo.	306–813	14–84	38–192
8 mo.	325–875	15–88	39–200
9 mo.	363–950	16–97	40–208
10 mo.	388–1,025	17–101	41–216
11 mo.	425–1,125	18–109	43–224
12 mo.	450–1,188	21–126	44–224
2 yr	538–1,400	26–147	54–264
3 yr	600–1,575	32–189	58–288
4 yr	625–1,650	37–231	59–288
5 yr	663–1,750	47–263	60–288
6 yr	688–1,875	53–292	60–288
7 yr	713–1,900	56–315	60–288
8 yr	725–1,938	61–336	60–288
9 yr	738–2,000	67–357	60–290
10 yr	750–2,000	71–378	60–291
11 yr	750–2,000	76–399	60–296
12 yr	750–2,000	78–420	60–299
13 yr	750–2,000	80–441	61–304

*Data from Buckley et al.[41] and Allansmith et al.[42]
†Normal ranges include ± 1 SD.

fluoresceinated antisera specific for the individual immunoglobulins IgG, IgA, IgM, and IgD, and for light chains κ and λ. In addition to surface immunoglobulin, other markers are present on the surfaces of B cells: Fc receptors for human IgG, receptors for complement components C3b and C3d, and Ia antigens. All of these markers can be used to help quantitate B cell numbers, although Fc receptors and Ia antigens are also found on "activated" T cells, and Fc receptors, Ia antigens and complement receptors are found on monocytes. Monocytes, however, because they are capable of phagocytosis, can be separately distinguished by their capacity to ingest latex particles.[34]

Patients with X-linked agammaglobulinemia do not have more than a very rare B cell in their circulation; the specific defect is generally believed to reside in the maturation of the pre-B cell into a mature B cell. However, patients with agammaglobulinemia may have traces of immunoglobulin (often IgM) in the circulation, so either the defect is not absolutely complete, or this immunoglobulin is biochemically different from normally secreted immunoglobulin. About 10% of patients with common varied immunodeficiency and all patients with thymoma and agammaglobulinemia have extremely few or no peripheral B cells in the circulation. Again, some immunoglobulin (usually IgG and IgM) may be present in the peripheral blood of such patients.

Specific Evaluation of the Phagocytic System

Foremost among tests of granulocyte function is the absolute neutrophil count (Table 13–12). Neutropenia is a relatively common disorder that may accompany the collagen-vascular diseases, drug reactions, or hypersplenism, or it may have no apparent associations. In many cases there is no particular propensity to increased infection, although in cyclic neutropenia, acute mouth or throat infections are common during the neutropenic intervals.

An important aspect of neutrophil function is chemotaxis, or the migration of neutrophils to specific attractants. The method used involves the Boyden chamber:[35] the patient's neutrophils are placed in one compartment and are allowed to migrate toward an attractant solution in a second chamber; the two chambers are separated by a millipore filter. The number of neutrophils that migrate to different depths of the filter in a given time can be assessed. Chemotaxis of phagocytes is abnormal in Chédiak-Higashi disease, actin-binding protein deficiency, Shwachman's disease, and some cases of hyper-IgE syndrome.

A second important function of neutrophils is phagocytosis. The test for phagocytosis is usually performed by measuring the rate of ingestion and killing of a test bacterium, such as *S. aureus*. Convenient *Candida* killing tests have also been devised. Rare instances of patients whose neutrophils fail to ingest and kill only selected organisms ("lacunar immunodeficiencies") have also been described; if repeated infections with one organism occur, it may be necessary to specifically test the patient's neutrophils with the same organism. Nitroblue tetrazolium dye reduction[28] is a specific test useful in the detection of patients with chronic granulomatous disease who have defective intracellular killing of catalase-positive bacteria.

Specific Evaluation of the Complement System

Complement system abnormalities are evaluated by functional and/or immunochemical measurements of various components of the alternative or classical pathways (Table 13–13). In general, quantitation of total hemolytic complement and of components C3 and C4 provides a useful screening assessment of this system. Deficiencies of C2 and C4 are most frequently seen in association with collagen-vascular disease; deficiencies of

TABLE 13–12.—Phagocytic Cell Testing

CELL TYPE	TEST	SPECIMEN	LABORATORY	NORMAL RANGES
Neutrophil	Absolute count	Citrated blood	Commercial	3,000–5,500 μl
	Nitroblue tetrazolium dye reduction	Heparinized blood	Commercial	Positive
	Chemotaxis	Heparinized blood	Research	Positive
	Phagocytosis	Heparinized blood	Research	Positive
	Bacterial killing	Heparinized blood	Research	Positive
Monocyte/macrophage	Chemotaxis	Heparinized blood	Research	Positive
	Phagocytosis	Heparinized blood	Research	Positive
	Bacterial killing	Heparinized blood	Research	Positive

TABLE 13–13.—FUNCTIONAL AND IMMUNOCHEMICAL ASSAYS OF COMPLEMENT
SYSTEM COMPONENTS AND PATHWAYS

FACTOR	SPECIMEN	LABORATORY	NORMAL RANGE
Total hemolytic complement (CH_{50})	Plasma or serum	Commercial	50–120 units, $\pm$ 15
C3	Plasma or serum	Commercial	70–176 mg/dl, $\pm$ 10
C4	Plasma or serum	Commercial	
C1 esterase inhibitor	Plasma or serum	Commercial	
Other components C1, C2, C5, C6–C9	Plasma or serum	Research	As established in laboratory
Immune complexes			
C1q binding	Plasma or serum	Research, commercial	< 10–20 µg/ml equivalent
Raji cell radioimmunoassay	Plasma or serum	Research, commercial	of heat aggregated IgG
C3 solid phase assay	Plasma or serum	Research	

C3 are quite rare. Since both the classical and the alternative pathways depend on C3, overwhelming, usually fatal infections occur when C3 levels are inadequate. Levels of C1q are often low in untreated or inadequately treated cases of hypogammaglobulinemia or agammaglobulinemia. After gammaglobulin therapy is initiated, C1q levels usually rise to the normal range, possibly due to stabilization of the C1q molecule.[37]

Circulating immune complexes, present in numerous diseases, can fix C3 or C1q, or both, and thereby trigger complement depletion by the classical or alternative pathways. In these circumstances, levels of total hemolytic complement and of components C2–C8 may be reduced. Measurement of circulating immune complexes is performed by a variety of assays, all of which refer to a standard curve formed by the use of heat-aggregated IgG. Examples include C1q binding,[38] C3 solid-phase assay,[39] and the Raji cell radioimmunoassay.[40] Among the immunodeficiency disease syndromes, immune complexes are commonly found in selective IgA deficiency, Wiskott-Aldrich syndrome, mucocutaneous candidiasis, and ataxia-telangiectasia. (See Chap. 6 for a more detailed discussion of immune complex assays.)

COMMENT

Since the normal immune system is composed of a number of interacting components, a complete immunologic evaluation necessarily requires many kinds of laboratory investigations. How far a clinician proceeds in such evaluation ultimately depends on clinical judgment: if a patient becomes ill too frequently or if unusual organisms are involved, an immunologic workup is required. It is not always easy to decide if a child or adult is sick more often than his peers, and a simplified immunologic evaluation (absolute blood cell counts, immunoglobulin quantitations [including IgE], total hemolytic complement, C3 and C4, and skin testing) is often of value. If results of these tests are abnormal or if the further occurrence of infections increases the suspicion that an immune defect is present, an immunologic consultation is advisable.

REFERENCES

1. Cooper M.D., Faulk W.P., Fudenberg H.H., et al.: Meeting report of Second International Workshop on primary immunodeficiency disease in man. *Clin. Immunol. Immunopathol.* 2:416, 1974.
2. Gatti R.A.: On the classification of patients with primary immunodeficiency disorders. *Clin. Immunol. Immunopathol.* 3:243, 1974.
3. Metcalf D., Moore M.A.S.: General description of blood cells and haemopoietic organs, in Neuberger A., Tatum E.L. (eds.): *Hematopoietic Cells.* Amsterdam, Elsevier North-Holland, 1971, pp. 3–11.

4. World Health Organization: *Immunodeficiency*. Technical Report Series 630. Geneva, Switzerland, WHO, 1978.

5. DiGeorge A.M.: Congenital absence of the thymus and its immunologic consequences: Concurrence with congenital hypoparathyroidism, in Bergsma D. (ed.): *Immunologic Deficiency Diseases in Man*. The National Foundation–March of Dimes, New York, 1968, pp. 116–123.

6. Bruton O.C.: The discovery of agammaglobulinemia, in Bergsma D. (ed.): *Immune Deficiency Diseases in Man*. The National Foundation–March of Dimes, 1968, New York, pp. 54–55.

7. Oxelius V., Laurell A.B., Lindquist B., et al.: IgG subclasses in selective IgA deficiency. *N. Engl. J. Med*. 304:1476, 1981.

8. Glanzmann E., Riniker P.: Essentielle lymphocytophthise: Ein neues Krankheitsbild aus der Sauglingspathologie. *Ann. Paediatr. (Basel)* 175:1, 1950.

9. Hitzig W.H., Biró Z., Bosch H., et al.: Agammaglobulinämie und Alymphocytose mit Schwund de Lymphatischen Gewebes. *Helv. Paediatr. Acta* 13:551, 1958.

10. Nezelof C., Kammet M.C., Lortholary P., et al.: L'hypoplasie hereditaire du thymus: Sa place et sa responsabilité dans une observation d'aplasie lymphocytaire normoplasmocytaire et normoglobulinemique du nourrisson. *Arch. Fr. Pédiatr*. 21:897, 1964.

11. Polmar S.H., Stern R.C., Schwartz A.L., et al.: Enzyme replacement therapy for adenosine deaminase deficiency and severe combined immunodeficiency. *N. Engl. J. Med*. 295:1337, 1976.

12. Belohradsky B.H., Griscelli C., Fudenberg H.H., et al.: Das Wiskott-Aldrich syndrom. *Ergeb. Inn. Med. Kinderheilkd*. 41:85, 1978.

13. Taylor A.M.R., Harnden D.G., Arlett C.F., et al.: Ataxia telangiectasia: A human mutation with abnormal radiation sensitivity. *Nature* 258:427, 1975.

14. Blizzard R.M., Gibbs J.H.: Candidiasis: Studies pertaining to its association with endocrinopathies and pernicious anaemia. *Pediatrics* 42:231, 1968.

15. Baehner R.L., Nathan D.G.: Leukocyte oxidase: Defective activity in chronic granulomatous disease. *Science* 155:835, 1967.

16. Klebanoff S.J., White L.R.: Iodination defect in the leukocytes of a patient with chronic granulomatous disease of childhood. *N. Engl. J. Med*. 280:460, 1969.

17. Quie P.G., White J.G., Holmes B., et al.: In vitro bactericidal capacity of human polymorphonuclear leukocytes: Diminished activity in chronic granulomatous disease of childhood. *J. Clin. Invest*. 46:668, 1967.

18. Blume R.S., Wolff S.M.: The Chédiak-Higashi syndrome: Studies in four patients and a review of the literature. *Medicine* 51:247, 1972.

19. Vassalli J.D., Granelli-Piperno A., Griscelli C., et al.: Specific protease deficiency in polymorphonuclear leukocytes of Chédiak-Higashi syndrome and beige mice. *J. Exp. Med*. 147:1285, 1978.

20. Boxer L.A., Watanabe A.M., Rister M., et al.: Correction of leukocyte function in Chédiak-Higashi syndrome by ascorbate. *N. Engl. J. Med*. 295:1041, 1976.

21. Gallin J.I., Elin R.J., Hubert R.T., et al.: Efficacy of ascorbic acid in Chédiak-Higashi syndrome (CHS): Studies in humans and mice. *Blood* 53:226, 1979.

22. Fullerton H.W., Duguid H.L.D.: A case of cyclical agranulocytosis with marked improvement following splenectomy. *Blood* 4:269, 1949.

23. Morley A.A., Carew J.P., Baikie A.G.: Familial cyclical neutropenia. *Br. J. Haematol*. 13:719, 1976.

24. Lachman P.S.: Genetic deficiencies of the complement system. *Boll. Ist Sieroter Milan* 53 (suppl):195, 1974.

25. Donaldson V.M., Evans R.R.: A biochemical abnormality in hereditary angioneurotic edema: Absence of serum inhibition of C1 esterase. *Am. J. Med.* 35:37, 1963.

26. Gelfand J.A., Sherins R.J., Alling D.W., et al.: Treatment of hereditary angioedema with danazole. *N. Engl. J. Med.* 295:1444, 1976.

27. Alper C.A., Colten H.R., Rosen F.S., et al.: Homozygous deficiency of C3 in a patient with repeated infections. *Lancet* 2:1979, 1972.

28. Rose N.R., Friedman E. (eds.): *Manual of Clinical Immunology.* Washington, D.C., American Society for Microbiology, 1976.

29. Klein M., Roder J., Haliotis T., et al.: Chédiak-Higashi genes in humans. *J. Exp. Med.* 151:1049, 1980.

30. Greaves M.F., Owen J.J.T., Raff M.C.: *T and B- Lymphocytes, Origins, Properties and Roles in Immune Responses.* New York, American Elsevier Publishing Co., 1974.

31. Waldman T.A., Durin M., Broder S., et al.: Role of suppressor T cells in pathogenesis of common variable immunodeficiency. *Lancet* 2:609, 1974.

32. Reinheiz E.L., Cooper M.D., Schlossman S.F., et al.: Abnormalities of T cell maturation and regulation in human beings with immunodeficiency disease. *J. Clin. Invest.* 68:699, 1981.

33. Mancini G., et al.: Immunochemical quantitation of antigens by single radial immunodiffusion. *Immunochemistry* 2:235, 1965.

34. Fudenberg H.H., et al. (eds): *Basic and Clinical Immunology.* Los Altos, Calif., Lange Medical Publications, 1976.

35. Boyden S.: The chemotactic effect of mixtures of antibodies and antigens on polymorphonuclear leukocytes. *J. Exp. Med.* 115:453, 1962.

36. Rapp H.J., Borsos T.: *Molecular Basis of Complement Action.* New York, Appleton-Century-Crofts, 1970.

37. Atkinson J.P., Fisher R.I., Reinhardt R., et al.: Reduced concentration of first component of complement of hypogammaglobulinemia: Correction by infusion of gammaglobulin. *Clin. Immunol. Immunopathol.* 9:350, 1978.

38. Zubler R.H., et al.: Circulating and intra-articular immune complexes in patients with rheumatoid arthritis. *J. Clin. Invest.* 57:1308, 1976.

39. Periera A.B., Theofilopoulos A.N., Dixon F.J.: Detection and partial characterization of circulatory immune complex with solid phase anti-C3. *J. Immunol.* 125:763, 1980.

40. Theofilopoulos A.N., et al.: The Raji cell radioimmune assay for detecting immune complexes in human sera. *J. Clin. Invest.* 57:169, 1976.

41. Buckley R.M., Dees S.C., O'Fallon W.M.: Serum immunoglobulins: Levels in normal children and uncomplicated childhood allergy. *Pediatrics* 41:600, 1968.

42. Allansmith M., McClellan B.M., Butterworth M., et al.: The development of immunoglobulin levels in man. *J. Pediatr.* 72:272, 1968.

14

Tumor Immunity

Sudhir Gupta, M.D.

THIS CHAPTER is divided into two parts, the first dealing with leukemias and lymphomas and the second with serum tumor antigens. The complexity of the classification of leukemias, coupled with difficulties in differentiation of cells by light microscopy, has led to the development of methods to further aid in characterizing lymphoproliferative diseases. Among such methods are cytochemical techniques, cytogenetic techniques, and techniques for the detection of cell surface markers. Following a review of the acute leukemias, the application of these methods in acute and chronic leukemias and lymphomas will be described. The measurement of a cellular enzyme, terminal deoxynucleotidyl transferase (TdT), will also be discussed. Finally, tumor-associated antigens and the potential usefulness of monoclonal antibody-defined antigens will be reviewed.

LEUKEMIAS AND LYMPHOMAS

Classification of Acute Leukemias

A uniform classification system for the acute leukemias and uniform nomenclature should permit more accurate definition of clinical cases and provide a reference standard for the application of newly developed surface markers, defining specific cell types, to cases of acute leukemia. A French-American-British cooperative group has proposed a classification of acute leukemias whereby acute lymphoblastic leukemia (ALL) is subdivided into three groups, L1, L2, and L3 (Table 14–1), and acute myeloid leukemia (AML) is subdivided into six types, M1–M6 (Table 14–2).[1] L1 ALL is the type of acute leukemia common in childhood. L2 ALL is less common in childhood and is sometimes designated "undifferentiated leukemia." B cell markers have been found in most patients with L3 ALL; however, in about 25% of patients T cell markers have been found. Of the AMLs, M1 represents myeloblastic leukemia without differentiation, M2 represents myelo-

TABLE 14–1.—FRENCH-AMERICAN-BRITISH CLASSIFICATION
OF ACUTE LYMPHOBLASTIC LEUKEMIA

FEATURES	L1	L2	L3
Cell size	Small	Large, heterogeneous	Large, homogeneous
Nuclear shape	Regular	Irregular	Regular-oval-round
Nuclear chromatin	Homogeneous	Variable	Homogeneous; finely stippled
Nucleoli	Absent/small	One or more, often large	Prominent, one or more vesicular
Cytoplasm	Scanty	Variable	Moderately abundant
Basophilia	Slight	Variable	Very deep
Cytoplasmic vacuolation	Variable	Variable	Often prominent

TABLE 14–2.—ACUTE MYELOID LEUKEMIAS

TYPE	DESIGNATION	COMMENT
Myeloblastic leukemia	M1	Without differentiation
Myeloblastic leukemia with maturation	M2	At or beyond promyelocytic stage
Hypergranular promyelocytic leukemia	M3	Auer rods in characteristic cells
Myelomonocytic leukemia	M4	Granulocytic and monocytic differentiation present
Monocytic leukemia	M5	Two subtypes
Erythroleukemia	M6	Erythropoietic component >50% in bone marrow

blastic leukemia with maturation (maturation at or beyond the promyelocytic stage), and M3 represents hypergranular promyelocytic leukemia (cells containing bundles of Auer rods randomly distributed in the cytoplasm are almost invariably present in the bone marrow and sometimes in the peripheral blood). It is necessary to distinguish M2 cases with a high proportion of promyelocytes from M3 cases. In M2 AML the cytoplasmic granulation is usually less heavy and does not obscure the basophilic cytoplasm, as happens in M3. M4 represents myelomonocytic leukemia: both granulocytic and monocytic differentiation are present in varying proportions in the bone marrow and peripheral blood. M4 resembles M2 in all respects except that the proportion of promonocytes and monocytes exceeds 20% of the nucleated cells in the bone marrow, peripheral blood, or both. In M5 or monocytic leukemia two subtypes occur: (1) a poorly differentiated monoblastic leukemia that is characterized by large blasts in the bone marrow and sometimes in the peripheral blood, and (2) a differentiated monoblastic leukemia in which monoblasts, promonocytes, and monocytes are found; the proportion of monocytes in the peripheral blood is higher than in the bone marrow, in which the predominant cell is the promonocyte. M6 AML is erythroleukemia: the erythropoietic component usually exceeds 50% of all the nucleated cells in the bone marrow, and the erythroblasts show bizarre morphological features, especially multiple lobulation of the nucleus.

Cytochemistry of Leukemic Cells

In cytochemistry, special histochemical stains are applied to individual cells to determine their biochemical composition and thereby aid in identification. Families of cytochemical stains that are of varying diagnostic significance will be discussed with regard to leukemic cells. These stains are (1) the peroxidases, of which only myeloperoxidase (MPO) is cytochemically significant, (2) naphthol AS-acetate (NASA) esterase, with or without sodium fluoride, (3) leukocyte acid phosphatase, (4) α-naphthyl acetate (ANAE), (5) periodic acid Schiff (PAS), (6) N-acetyl-β-glucosaminidase, (7) leukocyte alkaline phosphatase (LAP), (8) β-glucuronidase, and (9) Sudan black.

AML, Acute Myelomonocytic Leukemia (AMML), and Acute Monocytic Leukemia (AMOL)

The peroxidase reaction distinguishes undifferentiated leukemia from poorly differentiated myeloblastic leukemia: the presence of 3% or more peroxidase-positive cells justifies removal from the undifferentiated leukemia category. Myeloperoxidase stains primary granules of myeloblasts and often the rough endoplasmic reticulum and Golgi membranes. The MPO-positive granules in promonocytes are as a rule smaller than in myeloblasts and promyelocytes. The MPO reaction is particularly useful in demonstrating granulocytic differentiation leukemias with mixed lymphoblasts and myeloblasts. Auer rods are strongly MPO positive.[2] Although the reaction is variable, almost all cases of AMML show peroxidase activity. Sudan black, a phospholipid stain, is positive in granulocytic precursors. Sudan black and peroxidase staining usually parallel each other, but occasionally Sudan black staining is more prominent.

Esterase (NASA) and acid phosphatase reactions are early characteristics of monoblasts, while the MPO reaction is a relatively late differentiation characteristic.[3] ANAE is a more consistently positive stain than NASA in patients with chronic granulocytic leukemia (CGL) in blastic crisis with predominant monocytic differentiation.[4] The addition of sodium fluoride has no effect on the positivity of esterase in AML but AMML cases show partial inhibition; therefore, this technique may aid in differentiating these two leukemias. Acid phosphatase is positive in leukemia of monocytic differentiation, although to a varying degree. The most reliable results are obtained by combining the acid phosphatase and esterase techniques.

Although most cases of AML are PAS negative, approximately one third are positive, some showing coarse granules. About one half of cases of AMML are PAS positive, varying from a single glycogen granule to a fine to globular pattern. Almost 80% of cases of AMOL show PAS positivity with aggregated blocks or a ring pattern. N-acetyl-β-glucosaminidase reactivity correlates with an increasing monocytic component.

CGL

A low LAP level is found in most cases of CGL. The LAP level may be used in differentiating CGL from polycythemia vera, myelosclerosis, and leukemoid reactions, in which the LAP is high. A low LAP is also found in patients with agnogenic myeloid metaplasia, infectious mononucleosis, infectious hepatitis, sarcoidosis, megaloblastic leukemia, congenital hypophosphatasia, and paroxysmal nocturnal hemoglobinuria. Successful treatment of CGL is not always associated with an increase in LAP over previous levels. Using cytochemical staining with MPO, platelet peroxidase, esterases and LAP, TdT enzyme estimation, and immunologic markers (discussed below), it is possible to differentiate leukemia of distinct cell lineage during a blastic crisis of CGL.

ALL

In most cases of ALL varying percentages of the blasts give positive PAS reactions. When present, PAS is not diffuse but is seen as course granules against a negative cytoplasmic background. It is this pattern of reactivity rather than the percentage of positive blast cells that is diagnostic. As previously noted, PAS positivity is also found in cases of non-ALL, and so this assay must be interpreted with caution.

Most blast cells of T cell ALL have strong acid phosphatase activity characteristically localized on electron microscopy in the membranes of the Golgi apparatus and in lysosomal granules in its vicinity.[5, 6]

Specimens from approximately 25%–30% of patients with common ALL that could be of pre-T cell type show positive acid phosphatase reactions. Therefore, acid phosphatase may facilitate the recognition of T cell ALL.

Chronic Lymphocytic Leukemia (CLL)

β-glucuronidase levels are low in patients with B cell CLL.[7] Most lymphocytes from these patients show no β-glucuronidase activity. A close correlation is observed between β-glucuronidase activity and acid phosphatase activity, and therefore acid phosphatase activity is low (<25%) or absent in lymphocytes of B cell CLL. In contrast, in CLL of T cell origin, a rare disorder, all patients have a high content of β-glucuronidase and acid phosphatase in more than 90% of the peripheral blood lymphocytes. Therefore, these two enzymes may be useful in identifying a subgroup of patients with T cell CLL.

Hairy Cell Leukemia

These leukemic cells are characterized by high acid phosphatase activity, although the intensity varies from patient to patient and from cell to cell. The enzyme activity is characteristically resistant to inhibition by tartaric acid,[8] and tartarate resistance is usually observed only in hairy cells with strong acid phosphatase activity.[9] The weak or moderate reactivity of lymphocytes and the strong reactivity of monocytes are both totally inhibited by tartaric acid. The peroxidases, Sudan black, and chloracetate esterase stains (characteristic reactions of granulocytes) are all negative in hairy cell leukemia. The PAS reaction is usually weakly positive.

The cytochemical characteristics of the various cells described above are summarized in Table 14–3. These characteristics can help differentiate acute leukemias: (1) Myeloblasts stain with peroxidase and Sudan black but frequently do not stain well with PAS. (2) Lymphoblasts show large coarse granules with PAS staining but do not stain with peroxidase. (3) Fluoride will inhibit the esterase activity of monoblasts.

In chronic leukemia, an LAP determination in mature neutrophils may

TABLE 14–3.—CYTOCHEMICAL CHARACTERISTICS OF LEUKEMIC CELLS*

STAIN	CHARACTERISTICS
Myeloperoxidase	Positive in AMML; helps separate undifferentiated from myeloblastic leukemia
Esterase (NASA)	Positive in early monoblastic leukemia; with sodium fluoride, helps differentiate AML from AMML
Leukocyte acid phosphatase	Positive in early monoblastic and monocytic leukemia, T cell ALL, T cell CLL, hairy cell leukemia
α-Naphthyl acetate	Positive in CGL in blast crises with predominant monocytic differentiation
Periodic acid Schiff	May differentiate ALL from non-ALL (see text)
N-acetyl-β-glucosaminidase	Positive with increasing monocytic component of AMOL
Leukocyte alkaline phosphatase	Positive in polycythemia vera, myelosclerosis, leukemoid reactions; low levels in CGL
β-Glucuronidase	Positive in T cell CLL; low in B cell CLL
Sudan black	Negative in hairy cell leukemia; positive with myeloblasts

*AMML, acute myelomonocytic leukemia; AML, acute myeloblastic leukemia; ALL, acute lymphoblastic leukemia; CLL, chronic lymphocytic leukemia. CGL, chronic granulocytic leukemia; AMOL, acute monoblastic leukemia.

be important in the diagnosis since it is almost always low in CGL but elevated in leukemoid reactions and other myeloproliferative disorders. T cell CLL is characterized by high content of β-glucuronidase and acid phosphatase.

Cytogenetics of Leukemias and Lymphomas

Karyotyping may be done on direct preparations from bone marrow. This study may reveal chromosomal abnormalities that will aid in the characterization of some leukemias and lymphomas. This has been facilitated by the quinacrine fluorescent banding technique.

CGL

The Philadelphia chromosome (Ph[1]), a unique chromosomal abnormality, is found in about 85% of patients with CGL. Chromosomal banding techniques have shown that the translocation involves the long arms of chromosomes 9 and 22 in approximately 93% or more Ph[1]-positive cases.[10] An absent Y chromosome has also been reported in patients with Ph[1]-positive CGL.

Ph[1]-negative CGL patients have other chromosomal abnormalities, including a missing Y chromosome,[11] trisomy 8,[12] and trisomy 13.[13] Patients with Ph[1]-negative CGL and a missing Y chromosome have a long survival time and better response to treatment.[14]

In general, Ph[1]-negative patients have a more rapidly fatal course that lasts about 18 months, as opposed to 45 months in Ph[1]-positive CGL. Ph[1]-negative patients tend to be older.

In the acute phase of Ph[1]-positive CGL, 70%–80% of patients develop other chromosomal abnormalities, most commonly an additional Ph[1] chromosome and trisomy 8.[15, 16] Approximately 30% of patients in blastic crisis develop an isochromosome of the long arm of chromosome 17.[15, 16] In general, change in the original karyotype in patients with CGL is a grave sign and usually suggests an imminent blastic crisis.

AML

Approximately 30% of patients with AML demonstrate nonrandom chromosomal abnormalities in the bone marrow. Chromosome 8 is most frequently affected, with trisomy occurring in most instances and reciprocal translocation (8q−, 21q+) in a significant proportion of patients.[16] Translocation involving chromosomes 6 and 9 has also been described. The other commonly involved chromosomes are 7, 21, 17, X, Y, and 5. The mean survival time in patients with a normal karyotype is 8 months, and in patients with both normal and abnormal karyotypes, 2–3 months. Patients with an abnormal karyotype have a mean survival of 1 month.[14]

CLL

In B cell CLL there are usually no chromosomal abnormalities; however, in patients with T cell CLL, translocation of chromosome 14 has been described.[17] The 14q + chromosome is perhaps the most common and significant genetic marker of lymphoid malignancies.

ALL

O'Shimura and Sandberg[18] observed partial deletion of a long arm of chromosome 6 in a series of patients with ALL. This chromosomal abnormality may well prove to be specific to ALL, since it has not been reported for AML. Trisomy 7 has been observed in approximately 7% of patients with ALL. As a rule, trisomy 7 is infrequently observed in T cell ALL; however, it is found in most cases of Japanese adult T cell leukemia.[19] The other conditions in which trisomy 7 have been observed include Hodgkin's disease, lymphosarcoma, nonendemic Burkitt's lymphoma, and multiple myeloma.

In summary, the finding of the Ph^1 chromosome is important in confirming the diagnosis of CGL. About one half of patients with acute leukemia have normal karyotypes; however, one third of patients with AML and one half of patients with ALL have abnormal karyotypes. In patients with AML, karyotype abnormalities are nonrandom and may be of prognostic significance.

Malignant Lymphomas

The malignant lymphomas were among the first human neoplasms to be studied systematically with chromosomal techniques. Approximately one third of patients with Hodgkin's disease have structural chromosomal abnormalities and about 50% of these have numerical chromosomal abnormalities. Reeves[20] studied three patients with Hodgkin's disease and observed that each patient's cells contained a number of random rearrangements. He stated that he could differentiate Hodgkin's disease from other malignant lymphomas on the basis of numerical chromosomal changes. Approximately 50% of patients with Hodgkin's disease have 50–80 chromosomes as the usual number, whereas patients with other lymphomas have 54–56 chromosomes. The most significant chromosomal abnormality in lymphoma is of the 14q + chromosome.[21] This has been identified in virtually every instance of Burkitt's lymphoma, Hodgkin's lymphoma, and non-Hodgkin's lymphoma. It appears that a 14q+ chromosome is more common in poorly differentiated lymphoma (PDL) than in diffuse histiocytic lymphoma (DHL). It is more common in B cell lymphomas than in T cell lymphomas. Except for those involving the 14q+ chromosome, other structural rearrangements occur much more frequently in DHL than in PDL; this is particularly true for breaks in chromosomes 1, 2, 3, 6, 7, and 9. Other differences between PDL (a B cell disorder) and T cell lymphoma include more common rearrangements of arms of the 11q and 18q chromosomes in PDL. An abnormality of chromosome 11 has been seen only once in T cell lymphoma. It also appears that the number of structural rearrangements per cell is greater in DHL than in PDL. A close association of chromosome 14 with the Epstein-Barr virus (EBV) DNA and the expression of EBV nuclear antigen has been reported. Furthermore, the genes for human heavy chain immunoglobulin may be located on chromosome 14. This is an example of a gene-chromosomal relationship that may be important.

TdT

In normal hematopoietic and nonhematopoietic tissues, TdT occurs only in the thymus gland and bone marrow.[22, 23] Originally, the enzyme was considered to be a marker limited to cells of T cell lineage; however, it is now known to be more widely distributed. Leukemic cells from almost every patient with ALL of both childhood and adult onset contain TdT (see review by McCaffrey et al.[24]). Table 14–4 shows the occurrence of TdT in leukemic cells from patients with a variety of leukemias. It is evident that TdT is not restricted to patients with ALL, as approximately 5%–14% of patients with AML also have it. Leukemic cells from approximately one third of patients with chronic myelocytic leukemia in blastic crisis and approximately 50% of patients with acute undifferentiated leukemia are TdT positive. TdT-positive blasts are also present in acute leukemias that develop following chemo/radiotherapy, polycythemia vera, or myeloid metaplasia with myelofibrosis.

Approximately 5% of patients with ALL are TdT negative. Such patients usually have aggressive disease with an initial remission lasting less than 18 months. Approximately 70% of CGL patients with blast cells that are TdT positive during blastic crisis achieve remission, whereas less than 10% with TdT-negative blast cells achieve remission. Therefore, TdT has predictive value with regard to the response of CGL to treatment.[25] TdT activity in the normal bone marrow is biochemically indistinguishable from that in leukemic marrow. During remission, marrow may show high levels of TdT activity, but this finding has no relationship to a relapse of the disease. A

TABLE 14–4.—TERMINAL TRANSFERASE (TdT) IN
LEUKEMIC CELLS

DISEASE	POSITIVE*	NEGATIVE
Acute lymphoblastic leukemia	+	
Acute myeloblastic leukemia	+ s	
Acute undifferentiated leukemia	+ s	
Chronic granulocytic leukemia in blastic crisis	+ s	
Leukemia following:		
Polycythemia vera	+ s	
Chemoradiotherapy	+ s	
Myeloid metaplasia	+ s	
B cell chronic lymphocytic leukemia		−
T cell chronic lymphocytic leukemia		−
Chronic granulocytic leukemia		−
Sézary syndrome		−
Hairy cell leukemia		−

*s = subgroup of patients.

more recent study,[26] however, has demonstrated that a progressive increase in marrow TdT activity is associated with subsequent relapse in patients with acute lymphoblastic leukemia or lymphoma.

Markers of Acute Leukemias

ALL

Analysis of leukemic cell phenotypes using cell surface antigens/receptors have indicated that immunologic cell surface markers may be highly discriminating with respect to cellular identity in the hematopoietic system. Thus, these markers can be very helpful in the classification of leukemias and lymphomas. Using a variety of markers already described in chapter 3, ALL can be subdivided into four categories: (1) B cell ALL, (2) T cell (or thymic) ALL, (3) common ALL, and (4) "null" or unclassified ALL. It is also known that heterogeneity exists within each of these groups (Table 14–5).

B CELL ALL.—B cell ALL is a rare variant that, unlike all other ALLs, consists of relatively mature B lymphocytes rather than immature lymphoid progenitors.[27] Lymphocytes in B cell ALL bear surface immunoglobulins with κ or λ light chains and are Ia antigen positive. The lymphocytes are commonly ALL antigen negative and T cell antigen negative, do not form rosettes with sheep RBCs, and lack TdT, acid phosphatase, and hexosaminidase. B cell ALL presents with intestinal lymphadenopathy and carries the worst prognosis among all ALLs.[28]

TABLE 14–5.—CELL SURFACE MARKERS

B CELL MARKERS
   Surface immunoglobulin
   Ia- peptide coded by HLA locus; also found on macrophages
     and activated T cells
   Complement component receptors (C3b, C3d, C4b)
T CELL MARKERS
   TH_2
   IgG Fc (Tγ); IgM Fc (Tμ); IgA Fc (Tα)
   OKT_1—All T cells
   OKT_3—All T cells
   OKT_4—Helper T cells
   OKT_5—Suppressor T cells
   OKT_6—Thymocytes
   OKT_8—Suppressor T cells
   OKT_9—Early thymocytes
   OKT_{10}—Thymocytes
CALL ANTIGEN (common ALLA)
   Antigen found on cells of some patients with ALL

T CELL ALL.—T cell ALL is a heterogeneous group.[29] Using conventional markers, it can be subdivided into a common variant (90%) that is negative for common ALL antigen (ALLA) and a relatively minor group (10%) which is common ALLA positive.[27] Common ALLA is present in 80% of non-T cell ALLs and 60% of all ALLs. The expression "common" is used because this is the most common leukemia antigen. Acid phosphatase and rosette formation with sheep RBCs give variable results.

Approximately 60% of cases of T cell ALL are found in an early thymocyte or prothymocyte state (stage I), since most of the leukemic blasts react with antibody to surface markers for immature cells (OKT_{10} or OKT_9 and OKT_{10}). In only about 15% of cases of T cell ALL do cells react with OKT_6 antibody, suggesting origin from a more mature thymus cell population (stage II). The cells react variously to OKT_4, OKT_8, and OKT_9 antibodies. Rare cases of a mature thymocyte variety (stage III), in which cells react to OKT_3 antibodies as well as OKT_4 or OKT_8 phenotypes, have been reported. It should be pointed out that application of these monoclonal antibodies alone may not be sufficient to establish T cell lineage of a leukemia. For example, T cell ALL of the stage I type reacts with OKT_{10} antibody; however, OKT_{10} antigen is also expressed on non-T cells and myeloid leukemia cells. Therefore, additional markers may be necessary to confirm the lineage. The use of anti-Ia antibody will distinguish between T cell ALL and non-T cell ALL and AML, and the use of common ALLA will further distinguish between non-T cell ALL and AML.

T cell ALL has also been subclassified using TH_2 heteroantisera.[30] Approximately 20% of cases of T cell ALL are TH_2 positive. This group corresponds to the one reacting with OKT_6 monoclonal antibody (stage II). Patients with TH_2-positive T cell ALL tend to have a more prolonged disease-free survival period. Leukemic blasts from T cell ALL have also been shown to express receptors for IgM Fc, IgG Fc, or IgA Fc.[31, 32] Patients with T cell ALL with Fc receptors have a prolonged survival compared to patients whose leukemic T cells do not express Fc receptors for immunoglobulin isotypes.[33]

COMMON ALL.—Approximately 25% of patients with common ALL have more than 10% lymphoblasts with cytoplasmic μ chains but no detectable immunoglobulin light chains or cells with surface immunoglobulins; the entity is therefore called pre-B cell ALL. The pre-B cell variant of common ALL is usually TdT positive. A subgroup of pre-B cell ALL are Ia positive. Approximately 4%–5% of pre-B cell ALL patients lack common ALLA. Fc receptors and C3 receptors are usually lacking from leukemic cells. There is no significant difference in the remission rate and short-term remission duration between patients with pre-B cell ALL or common ALL and patients with "unclassified" ALL.[34]

NULL CELL ALL.—The subgroup of ALL about which least is known is the "unclassified" or "null" group. No definite marker is available for this subgroup. Approximately 90% of leukemic cells are Ia positive and hexosaminidase positive. Although the cells lack common ALLA they may acquire it during a relapse; therefore, this subgroup could be related to common ALL.

B cell ALL carries the worst prognosis of all the ALL, followed by T cell ALL, unclassified ALL, pre-B cell ALL, and common ALL. When corrected for white blood cell count, the difference in prognosis between T cell ALL and common ALL disappears, patients with high count common ALL faring as badly as patients with high count T cell ALL.

The phenotypes of ALL are summarized in Table 14–6.

Blastic Crisis of CGL

Leukemic cells in approximately one third of adults with CGL in blastic crisis have common ALLA (common ALL leukemia), thus demonstrating a selective lymphoid transformation.[35, 36] Recently, it has been shown that some patients in this common ALL group have leukemic blasts containing a cytoplasmic μ chain of immunoglobulin, which identifies them as having pre-B cell leukemia.[35, 36]

This latter finding suggests that the Ph^1 chromosome penetrates into the B cell lineage and originates in a common progenitor of lymphoid and granulocytic cells. Ph^1-positive CGL in children, however, is very rare. Greaves[27] has observed a blastic crisis of Ph^1-positive CGL in childhood in four patients. Three had a phenotype of common ALL, and one had a nonlymphoid (TdT negative, common ALL negative) or myeloid phenotype. Lymphoid transformation has also been reported in Ph[1]-negative CGL patients in blastic crisis, which also may show a phenotype of CALL (TdT positive, common ALL positive) or null-unclassified ALL (TdT positive, common ALL negative). The overall prognosis of CGL patients in blastic crisis is poor; however, those with a lymphoid phenotype have a much higher incidence of initial clinical response to ALL treatment.[36] There is no significant difference in prognosis between patients with common ALL and patients with pre-B cell phenotypes.

Surface Markers of Acute Nonlymphoid Leukemias

The diagnosis of AMOL and AML is largely based on clinical, morphological, and cytochemical features. Leukemic blasts from AMOL have receptors for IgG Fc and C3 complement receptors but lack surface immunoglobulin.[37, 38] Occasionally, cytophilic IgG is found[38]; however, trypsinization of leukemic cells would differentiate between cytophilic IgG and IgG that is synthesized by cells (in B cell malignant proliferation). They do not form rosettes with sheep RBCs.

Only a few leukemic blasts in AML have IgG Fc receptors or C3 receptors. They also lack surface Ig and do not form rosettes with sheep RBCs. Recently, a monoclonal antibody has been developed that reacts with an antigen (MY-1) expressed on peripheral blood granulocytes, granulopoietic precursors, and various myeloid leukemic cell types.[39]

Markers of Chronic Leukemias

CLL

CLL is usually a malignant expansion of B lymphocytes. The lymphocytes are small and more than 90% of patients demonstrate surface immunoglobulin on leukemic lymphocytes. The remaining 10% lack demonstrable surface immunoglobulin. The surface immunoglobulin is punctate in distribution, with no tendency to polar cap formation. Surface immunoglobulins are predominantly of the IgM class, and in approximately 50% of cases both surface IgM and IgD are present. In occasional cases surface IgGs have been observed.[40] The ratio of patients in whom leukemic cells express κ or λ light chain is 2:1, similar to that found in normals. Complement receptors are present in a majority of patients. Interestingly, C3d and not C3b receptors are present; in normal subjects more B cells express C3b than C3d.[41] These cells express Ia antigen, and a large proportion of B cells form rosettes with mouse RBCs.[42] This feature of mouse RBC rosette for-

TABLE 14–6.—Markers of Acute Lymphocytic Leukemia*

LEUKEMIA	E ROSETTE	T ANTIGEN†	COMMON ALLA	IA	SIG	CIG	TDT	HEX-1	AP
T cell ALL (90%)	+	+	−	−	−	−	+	−	+
(10%)	±	+	+	−	−	−	+	−	±
Common ALL	−	−	+	+	−	−	+	+	−
Pre-B cell ALL	−	−	+	+	−	+	+	±	−
B cell ALL	−	−	−	±	+	−	−	−	−
Null or unclassified ALL	−	−	−	±	−	−	±	±	−

*Hex-1, hexosaminidase "intermediate" isoenzyme; AP, acid phosphatase; SIg, surface immunoglobulin; TdT, terminal deoxynucleotidyl transferase; CIg, cytoplasmic μ chain; common ALLA, common ALL antigen; E rosette, receptor for sheep RBCs.
†Different T cell antigens defined with monoclonal antibodies are present on different leukemic blasts.

TABLE 14–7.—Markers of Chronic Lymphocytic Leukemia (CLL)*

	E ROSETTE	T ANTIGEN†	COMMON ALLA	IA	SIG	CIG	MOUSE RBC	IGM FC	IGG FC	IGA FC	C3B	C3D
B cell CLL	−	−	−	+	+	−	+	+	+	+	−	+
T cell CLL	+	+	−	−	−	−	−	−	+	−	−	−

*For abbreviations, see Table 14-6.
†T cell antigens defined with monoclonal antibodies of OKT series.

mation distinguishes B cell CLL from B cell lymphoma in a leukemic phase.[43] CLL cells do not bind to nonimmune sheep RBCs or react with T cell antibodies. B cells also express receptors for IgM, IgG, or IgA Fc in variable proportions.[44]

An increased proportion of normal T cells in B cell CLL have IgG Fc receptors (Tγ) and a decreased or normal proportion have IgM (Tμ) or IgA (Tα) Fc receptors.[45] An increase in the proportion of OKT$_8$-positive and a decrease in OKT$_4$-positive T cell subsets have also been observed.[46] T cell CLL is rare in the United States, being found predominantly in Japan. A summary of markers in CLL is given in Table 14–7.

Japanese Adult T Cell Leukemia

Japanese adult T cell leukemia is a unique T cell leukemia, the clinical features of which include both visceral and skin infiltration of leukemic cells and a subacute or chronic course. Patients have been shown to have powerful suppressor cell activity against B cell differentiation to plasma cells or against the proliferative response of normal T cells to alloantigens.[47, 48] In all patients tested by Hattori et al., the surface phenotype of the leukemic cells was OKT$_1$ positive, OKT$_3$ positive, and OKT$_{10}$ positive, with OKT$_6$, OKT$_8$, and OKT$_5$ antigens lacking.[49] This finding provides strong evidence that in pathologic states, there are phenotypically different T cells that do not perform the same functions as T cell subsets from healthy controls.

Hairy Cell Leukemia

Different investigators have considered hairy cell leukemia as a malignant expression of monocytes or lymphocytes or as a hybrid cell growth with properties of both monocytes and lymphocytes. More recent investigations have clearly demonstrated that these cells are of lymphocytic origin, although they have some features of monocytes. Cells from most patients express surface immunoglobulin. Four distinct patterns are observed according to the presence or absence of surface immunoglobulin.[50] Group I comprehends a very small group of patterns in which leukemic cells do not express immunoglobulin; group II hairy cells have surface IgM and IgD together; group III hairy cells have surface IgG; and in group IV, the most common grouping, the hairy cells possess multiple heavy chains of immunoglobulin. Hairy cells are predominantly κ chain positive. A subpopulation of hairy cells react with monoclonal antibodies B$_{A-1}$(reacts with B cells), OKM$_1$ (reacts with E rosette–positive T cells, monocytes and granulocytes), and 7.2 (anti-Ia antibody). Hairy cells fail to react with monoclonal antibodies directed against T cell antigens exclusively (9-6, OKT$_3$, J-5). Receptors for the Fc portion of IgM, IgG, and IgA have been reported on hairy cells.[51] Receptors for C3 are present on variable proportions of hairy cells.[52] In a few cases intracytoplasmic IgM and light chains are present.[53] Hairy cells lack TdT activity.

Markers of Non-Hodgkin's Lymphomas

There is some confusion as to the classification of non-Hodgkin's soft tissue lymphomas. Analysis of lymph node lymphocytes in suspension is complicated by the frequent occurrence of apparently normal cells mixed with the malignant cells in the partially involved nodes. It is therefore necessary to evaluate the nature of cell types using cytocentrifuged preparations or preparations passed through millipore filters as well as the use of markers on frozen sections.[53] Surface marker analysis has shown that nodular lymphomas represent a monoclonal expansion of follicular B cells.

In all patients, lymphoma cells bear surface immunoglobulin, predominantly IgM alone (in a small proportion, both IgM and IgD). The surface κ-λ light chain ratio is 2:1.[54] Most of the lymphocytes express both C4b and C3d receptors, and some express C4b, which is attached predominantly to cells at the periphery of nodules.[55] Only a few cells form rosettes with mouse RBCs. Diffuse, poorly differentiated lymphocytic lymphomas in adults are a monoclonal expansion of B lymphocytes expressing surface immunoglobulin, almost exclusively IgM, with a κ-λ ratio of 2:1. Complement receptors are present in 60% of patients. Diffuse, poorly differentiated lymphomas in children are either of the T cell or null cell type. Recently, Ritz et al.[56] reported the presence of common ALLA in nodular, poorly differentiated lymphocytic lymphomas and in approximately 40% of patients with T cell lymphoblastic lymphoma. Nodular lymphomas in the leukemic phase consist of B cells,[57] and diffuse lymphomas in the leukemic phase may consist of T, B, or null cells. It has been observed that lymphomas of T cell or null cell types have a greater tendency to become leukemic than those of B-lymphocytic type.

In diffuse histiocytic lymphoma, both small and large cells appear to share the same membrane markers as B lymphocytes, i.e., surface immunoglobulin, Fc receptors, and C3 receptors.

In Burkitt's lymphoma, almost all cells bear surface IgM, which fluoresces brightly and gives a dotted appearance.[58] Common ALLA is present on most cells in Burkitt's lymphoma. Burkitt's lymphoma may represent a childhood counterpart of nodular lymphomas in adults.

Analysis of T cell lymphoma with monoclonal antibodies demonstrates the immature T or thymocyte nature of the tumor cells.[59] Almost all T lymphoma cells react with OKT_{10} antibody and a majority lack OKT_3 antigen (marker for mature T cells). OKT_4 and OKT_8 antigens coexist in more than 50% of patients. Some 40%–50% of cells from patients with T cell lymphoma also react with OKT_6.

Sézary Syndrome and Mycosis Fungoides

The Sézary syndrome and mycosis fungoides are rare malignant disorders that have been grouped with cutaneous T cell lymphomas. In mycosis fungoides the malignant cells are confined to skin and lymphoid tissues, whereas in the Sézary syndrome malignant cells also circulate in the peripheral blood. The malignant cells appear to be mature T cells. They form rosettes with sheep RBCs, react with monoclonal antibodies OKT_1, OKT_3, and OKT_4, and do not react with OKT_5 and OKT_8 antibodies. Therefore, the malignant T cells are helper cells in phenotypic expression[60] and on functional assay.[61] Variable proportions of the malignant T cells have receptors for IgM Fc but lack receptors for IgG Fc.[62] C3 receptors and surface immunoglobulins are lacking.

The clinical usefulness of cell surface markers is currently limited by the relatively small number of laboratories with facilities and properly trained personnel to carry out such tests. Nevertheless, these assays should prove to be helpful since more precise differentiations of lymphoid tumor types can aid in determining treatment and judging prognosis.

TUMOR ANTIGENS

Tumor-Associated Antigens

Certain tumor cells express surface antigens that are not present on cells in the tissue from which the tumor was initially derived. Such antigens have been called tumor-associated antigens. The serologic measurement of some tumor-associated antigens has been found to be clinically useful. Because these measurements are not very sensitive or specific, they are mainly of value in judging prognosis and response to therapy in certain malignant diseases.

α-Fetoprotein (AFP)

Gene products that have normal expression on certain fetal tissues may be reexpressed in tumors. These have been designated oncofetal or carcinoembryonal gene products. AFP is perhaps the best characterized oncofetal protein. In humans, AFP is synthesized by the fetal yolk sac, liver, and, to a small extent, by the fetal gastrointestinal tract. It is found in amniotic fluid, in the serum of newborns, and in pregnant women.

Patients with primary liver cancer often have elevated serum AFP levels.[63] The levels may vary from near normal to several milligrams per milliliter of serum. In adults, up to 80% of primary hepatocellular carcinomas are associated with AFP production, although about 20%–30% of hepatocellular carcinomas are not associated with an abnormal serum AFP level.[64] Some of these tumors may be AFP producers that do not secrete AFP into the serum. Hepatoblastomas are consistently AFP positive. Cholangiocellular tumors also produce AFP.[64] Elevated AFP levels have been reported in gastric and pancreatic cancer without hepatic metastasis. AFP levels may also be elevated in liver diseases other than primary cancer of the liver; these include metastatic liver cancer, acute and chronic hepatitis, and cirrhosis. Recovery from acute hepatitis is accompanied by a fall in AFP. Repeated determinations over a period of time increase the diagnostic reliability of the AFP determination. Normalizing or fluctuating values suggest a benign disease, whereas rising levels are characteristic of malignancy. Serum AFP levels above 500 ng/ml are associated with liver cancer about 40 times more often than with other liver disease.[64] A prolonged elevation of serum AFP in humans has been correlated with tumor burden. AFP determination is unlikely to be useful as a routine screening test because of the relative infrequency of AFP-producing tumors. Tyrosinemia, leading to development of primary hepatic cancer, is associated with an elevated AFP level.[65]

AFP levels are also elevated in germ cell tumors, which have been subdivided into three groups: (1) endodermal sinus tumors, (2) choriocarcinoma, and (3) teratoma. Endodermal sinus tumors are yolk sac tumors and in their purest form occur most often in the ovaries of young women and children and in the testes of children. The tumor is rare in adult testes. Approximately 36%–86% of patients with germ cell tumors have elevated AFP values.

After therapeutic intervention, the decline in the serum AFP level is indicative of the completeness of the removal of the tumor. The rate of decline of the AFP level may also be important. If the tumor is not completely removed, a prolonged half-life (> 6 days) of serum AFP can be expected. Subsequent elevation of AFP is an indication of tumor recurrence, and often occurs before clinical evidence of recurrence. By utilizing such information, therapy can be started at a very early stage of recurrence and a rapid and prolonged remission may be achieved. Table 14–8 lists other nonmalignant conditions in which AFP levels are elevated in serum or in the amniotic fluid of pregnant women.

Carcinoembryonic Antigen (CEA)

CEA was discovered in 1965 and was then defined as a tumor-specific antigen of the human gastrointestinal tract.[66] Although the CEA test cannot

TABLE 14–8.—NONMALIGNANT CONDITIONS
WITH INCREASED α-FETOPROTEIN LEVELS

Ataxia telangiectasia
Hereditary tyrosinemia
Neonatal hepatitis
Trophoblastic disease—vesicular mole
Neural tube defects
Congenital nephrosis
Meckel's syndrome (a congenital neural tube defect)
Turner's syndrome
Exomphalos (umbilical hernia)
Multiple pregnancy

be considered useful for screening the general population for early colon cancer, CEA levels can be used as an adjunct in the diagnosis of patients with colon carcinoma.[67] Values obtained by different assay methods, however, cannot be used interchangeably. There is a definite association between the CEA level and the stage of malignancy. Approximately 50% of patients with colon cancer have CEA levels above 10 mg/ml; CEA levels of this magnitude are found in less than 5% of patients with nonmalignant diseases. About one third of colon carcinoma patients, however, have normal circulating levels of CEA.[68]

The use of CEA levels as an indicator of malignant change in ulcerative colitis is controversial. In general, increased CEA levels are associated with villous adenomata and large polyps; however, levels do not correlate well with the early detection of malignant transformation.[69] When serial measurements are done in patients with ulcerative colitis, patients who demonstrate progressive elevation of CEA in the absence of acute exacerbations of the colitis often develop malignant transformation of the colonic epithelium.[70] It should also be emphasized that CEA levels should not be used to rule out the presence of a malignancy. The concurrent use of CEA and barium enema produces a higher rate of cancer detection than either test alone.

The best clinical use of the CEA assay is in assessing the prognosis of patients with colorectal carcinoma. The preoperative concentration of circulating CEA in sera from patients with colon carcinoma correlates well with the extent of disease.[70] Serial CEA determinations have also provided an excellent indication of "curative" resection and may serve as an index of tumor regrowth 3–24 months before the recurrence of clinical symptoms and before any other laboratory abnormalities are found.[70] In a proportion of patients an unexplained transient rise in CEA levels is observed in the postoperative period. These levels return to baseline without any evidence of recurrence of tumor. Such transient rises in CEA levels can be caused by heavy smoking, liver dysfunction, or transfusion of CEA-positive blood. It is therefore suggested that liver function be measured simultaneously. CEA levels may also be elevated in patients with renal failure.

The frequency of a positive CEA test and absolute CEA levels increase with an increase in tumor burden. Therefore, a positive CEA test may be seen in not 20% but 90% in patients with progressively severe colon carcinoma.[71]

A correlation between tumor burden and CEA levels is also observed in carcinomas other than those of the colon or rectum. Reynoso et al.[72] reported that 15 of 25 patients with metastatic breast carcinoma had elevated CEA levels, whereas 9 of 10 patients with localized disease had normal CEA levels. Similar data have been reported for lung carcinomas.[73] Determination of CEA levels improves the rate of detection of hepatic metastasis from colorectal carcinoma when used with the hepatic scan. It appears that CEA-producing tumors metastasize earlier and have a poorer prognosis than those that are CEA negative.

Preoperative plasma levels of CEA also serve as an important indication of the probability of postoperative tumor recurrence. There is an inverse relationship between the probability of postoperative recurrence of tumor and preoperative CEA levels. In breast cancer, normal levels are associated with a 24-month recurrence rate of 20% whereas elevated levels are associated with a recurrence rate of 65%.[74] These observations are similar to those for colorectal carcinoma.

The most sensitive and reliable prognostic indicator in the therapeutic management of patients with colorectal carcinoma is the finding of serial, rather than single, elevated levels of CEA, even when a single level is above 20 ng/ml. The CEA assay has also been used as an indication in the management of pancreatic cancer, lung cancer, breast cancer, and neuroblastoma, with similar results achieved as for colorectal carcinoma.

CEA levels have been used to monitor chemotherapy and radiotherapy. Vider et al.[76] reported good correlation between CEA levels and clinical progress in 73% of patients undergoing radiation therapy and in 65% of those treated with chemotherapy. Similar correlations have been observed in patients with breast cancer undergoing hormonal and drug therapy.

Prostate-Specific Antigen

Recently a prostate-specific antigen (PA) has been identified and isolated.[77] It is distinct from prostatic acid phosphatase. Both primary and secondary prostatic tumors express PA, whereas tumors of nonprostatic origin do not react with anti-PA antibody.[78] PA is localized within the prostatic ductal epithelial cells. Cell lines of malignant prostastic origin retain

PA and release the antigen in vitro into culture fluid and in vivo into the circulation of athymic mice bearing prostate tumors.[79] Recently an enzyme-linked immunoassay has been developed to quantitate circulating PA with a sensitivity of 100 pg of PA per 1 ml of serum. In a large series, patients with metastatic prostatic carcinoma who failed to respond to hormonal treatment were randomly assigned to various chemotherapy protocols.[80] Pretreatment levels of PA were found to be of prognostic significance: the lower the PA levels, the longer the survival, regardless of treatment regimen. Serum PA can also be used to detect disease progression in patients with localized disease who have had curative therapy. During follow-up, persistent and increasing levels of PA have been demonstrated in patients who developed metastases. These data suggest that a progressive increase in PA levels indicates recurrent disease with high likelihood.

Monoclonal Antibody-Defined Antigens

As noted previously, certain tumor cells express surface antigens that are not present on cells in the tissue from which the tumor was initially derived. Monoclonal antibodies have been developed against a number of these tumor-specific antigens. The potential uses of such monoclonal antibodies are (1) isolation of tumor-associated antigens, (2) detection of the expression of portions of a gene in bacterial colonies or phage plaques with a part of the tumor-antigen gene incorporated, (3) diagnosis of tumor and detection of metastasis, (4) specific delivery of covalently bound cytotoxic drugs to tumor cells, and (5) cytolysis of tumor cells. Monoclonal antibodies have been developed against tumor-specific antigens from malignant melanoma,[81, 82] human colorectal carcinoma,[83] human neuroblastoma,[84] and renal adenocarcinoma.[85]

Ueda et al.[85] have developed 17 monoclonal antibodies representing defined antigen systems related to HLA and blood group antigens. Six of these are glycoproteins. These antigen systems can be further classified into three groups on the basis of their distribution on different cell types: (1) those with the characteristics of restricted differentiation, (2) more broadly differentiated antigens, and (3) antigens expressed by every human cell type tested. There is a possibility of identifying a subset of renal carcinomas using antigens from group 1 (gp 120). More broadly reacting antibodies may be useful in studying other tumors (e.g., for distinguishing astrocytomas from melanomas).

Monoclonal antibodies react with a single antigenic determinant, and because of structural homology, it is possible for the same or very similar antigenic determinants to appear on two different molecules. Thus, unless the identity of an antigen is determined biochemically, the reactivity of a monoclonal antibody with two different cell types does not necessarily indicate that the same gene product is expressed on both.

It should also be emphasized that none of the monoclonal antibodies so far described strictly recognizes tumor-specific antigen. Although claims have been made for the tumor specificity of mouse antibodies reacting with human tumor cells, none of these reports has provided good serologic evidence.

REFERENCES

1. Bennett J.M., Catovsky D., Daniel M.T., et al.: Proposal for the classification of the acute leukemias. *Br. J. Haematol.* 33, 451, 1976.
2. Bennett J.M., Reed C.E.: Acute leukemia cytochemical prolife: Diagnostic and clinical implications. *Blood Cells* 1:101, 1975.
3. Catovsky D., O'Brien M., Cherchi M.: Cytochemistry: An aid to the diagnosis and classification of the acute leukemias. *Recent Results Cancer Res.* 64:108, 1978.
4. Catovsky D., Cardullo L.D.S., O'Brien M., et al.: Cytochemical markers of differentiation in acute leukemias. *Cancer Res.* 41:4824, 1981.
5. Catovsky D., Galetto J., Okos A., et al.: Cytochemical profile of B and T leukemic lymphocytes with special reference to acute lymphoblastic leukemia. *J. Clin. Pathol.* 27:767, 1974.
6. Catovsky D.: T cell origin of acid phosphatase-positive lymphoblasts. *Lancet* 1:327, 1976.
7. Lorbacher P., Yam L.T., Mitus W.J.: Cytochemical demonstration of beta-glucuronidase in blood and bone marrow smears. *J. Histochem. Cytochem.* 15:680, 1967.
8. Yam L.T., Li C.Y., Finkel H.E.: Leukemic reticuloendotheliosis: The role of tartrate acid phosphatase in diagnosis and splenectomy in treatment. *Arch. Intern. Med.* 130:248, 1972.
9. Catovsky D., Pettit J.E., Galton D.A.G., et al.: Leukemic reticuloendotheliosis ("hairy" cell leukemia): A distinct clinicopathological entity. *Br. J. Haematol.* 26:9, 1974.
10. Lawler S.D., O'Malley F., Lobb D.S.: Chromosome banding studies in Philadelphia chromosome positive myeloid leukemia. *Scand. J. Haematol.* 17:17, 1976.
11. Mossfeld D.K., Wendhorst E.: Ph[1] negative chronic myeloid leukemia with a missing Y chromosome. *Acta Haematol.* 52:232, 1974.
12. Hsu L.Y.F., Aiter A., Hirschhorn K.: Trisomy 8 in bone marrow cells of patients with polycythemia vera and myelogenous leukemia. *Clin. Genet.* 6:258, 1974.
13. Hsu L.Y.F., Papenhausen P., Greenberg M.L., et al.: Trisomy D in bone marrow cells in a patient with chronic myelogenous leukemia. *Acta Haematol.* 52:61, 1974.
14. Nilsson P.G., Brandt L., Mitelman F.: Prognostic implications of chromosome analyses in acute nonlymphocytic leukemia. *Leukemia Res.* 1:31, 1977.
15. Goh K.: Additional Philadelphia chromosomes in acute blastic crisis of chronic myelocytic leukemia: possible mechanism of producing additional chromosomal abnormalities. *Am. J. Med. Sci.* 267:229, 1974.

16. Rowley J.D.: Population cytogenetics of leukemia, in Hook E.B., Parter I. (eds.): *Population Cytogenetics: Studies in Humans.* New York, Academic Press, 1977, p. 1189.

17. Finan J.B., Damele R.P., Rowland S.-T. Jr., et al.: Cytogenetics of chronic T cell leukemia: Including 2 patients with a 14q+ translocation. *Virchows Arch.* [*Cell. Pathol.*] 29:121, 1978.

18. O'Shimura M., Sandberg A.A.: Chromosomal 6q anomaly in acute lymphoblastic leukemia. *Lancet* 2:1405, 1976.

19. Ueshima Y., Fukuhara S., Hattori T., et al.: Chromosome studies in adult T cell leukemia in Japan: Significance of trisomy 7. *Blood* 58:420, 1981.

20. Reeves B.R.: Cytogenetics of malignant lymphomas. *Human Genetik* 20:231, 1973.

21. Rowley J.D., Fukuhara S.: Chromosome studies in non-Hodgkin's lymphomas. *Semin. Oncol.* 7:255, 1980.

22. Chang L.M.S.: Development of terminal deoxynucleotidyl transferase activity in embryonic calf thymus gland. *Biophys. Res. Commun.* 44, 124, 1971.

23. McCaffrey R.P., Harrison T.A., Baltimore D.: Terminal deoxynucleotidyl in human bone marrow. *Blood* 44:931, 1974.

24. McCaffrey R., Lillquist A., Sallan S., et al.: Clinical unity of leukemia cell terminal transferase measurements. *Cancer Res.* 41:4814, 1981.

25. Froehlich T.W., Buchanan G.R., Cornet J.A.M., et al.: Terminal deoxynucleotidyl transferase-containing cells in peripheral blood: Implications for the surveillance of patients with lymphoblastic leukemia or lymphoma in remission. *Blood* 58:214, 1981.

26. Bradstock K.F., Pizzolo G., Papageorgiou E.S., et al.: Terminal transferase expression in relapsed acute myeloid leukemia. *Br. J. Haematol.* 49:621, 1981.

27. Greaves M.F.: Analysis of the clinical and biological significance of lymphoid phenotypes in acute leukemia. *Cancer Res.* 41:4752, 1981.

28. Wolff L.J., Richardson S.T., Nieburger R.G., et al.: Poor prognosis of children with acute lymphocytic leukemia and increased B cell markers. *J. Pediatr.* 89:956, 1976.

29. Reinherz E.L., Schlossman S.F.: Derivation of human T-cell leukemias. *Cancer Res.* 41:4767, 1981.

30. Reinherz E.L., Nadler L.M., Sallaw S.E., et al.: Subset derivation of T cell acute lymphoblastic leukemia in man. *J. Clin. Invest.* 64:392, 1979.

31. Moretta L., Mingari M.C., Movetta A., et al.: Receptors for IgM are expressed on acute lymphoblastic leukemic cells having T cell characteristics. *Clin. Immunol. Immunopathol.* 7:405, 1977.

32. Beck J.D., Haghbin M., Wollner N., et al.: Subpopulations of human T lymphocytes: VI. Analysis of cell markers in acute lymphoblastic leukemia with special reference to Fc receptor expression on E-rosette forming blasts. *Cancer* 46:45, 1980.

33. Gupta S., Fernandes G.: Natural killing and antibody-dependent cytotoxicity by T leukemic blasts from acute lymphoblastic leukemia, *Scand. J. Immunol.*, in press, 1982.

34. Vogler L.B., Crist W.M., Sarrif A.M., et al.: An analysis of clinical and laboratory features of acute lymphoblastic leukemias with emphasis on 35 children with pre-B leukemia. *Blood* 58:135, 1981.

35. Greaves M.F., Verbi W., Reeves B.R., et al.: "Pre-B" phenotypes in blast

crisis of Ph[1] positive CML: Evidence for a pluripotential stem cell "target." *Leukemia Res.* 3:181, 1979.

36. Janossy G., Woodruff R.K., Peppard M.J., et al.: Relationship of "lymphoid" phenotypes and response to chemotherapy incorporating vincristine-prednisolone in the acute phase of Ph[1] positive leukemia. *Cancer* 43:426, 1979.

37. Koziner B., McKenzie S., Straus D., et al.: Cell marker analysis in acute monocytic leukemias. *Blood* 49:895, 1977.

38. Fernandes G., Garrett T., Nair P.M.N., et al.: Studies in acute leukemias: I. Antibody-dependent and spontaneous cellular cytotoxicity by leukemic blasts from patients with acute nonlymphoid leukemia. *Blood* 45:573, 1979.

39. Civin C.I., Mirro J., Banguerigo M.L.: MY-1, a new myeloid-specific antigen identified by a mouse monoclonal antibody. *Blood* 57:842, 1981.

40. Aisenberg A.C., Wilkes B.M.: Relevance of surface markers in chronic lymphocytic leukemia to acute lymphocytic leukemia. *Cancer Res.* 41:4810, 1981.

41. Ross G.D., Polley M.J., Rabellino E.M., et al.: Two different complement receptors on human lymphocytes. *J. Exp. Med.* 138:798, 1973.

42. Gupta S., Good R.A., Siegal F.P.: Rosette formation with mouse erythrocytes: III. Studies in primary immunodeficiency and lymphoproliferative disorders. *Clin. Exp. Immunol.* 26:204, 1976.

43. Koziner B., Filippa D., Mertelsmann R., et al.: Characterization of malignant lymphomas in leukemic phase by multiple differentiation markers of mononuclear cells: Correlation with clinical features and conventional morphology. *Am. J. Med.* 63:556, 1977.

44. Gupta S., Platsoucas C.D., Good R.A.: Receptors for IgA on a subpopulation of human B lymphocytes. *Proc. Natl. Acad. Sci. USA* 76:4025, 1979.

45. Platsoucas C.D., Good R.A., Gupta S., et al.: Receptor for immunoglobulin isotypes on T and B lymphocytes from patients with untreated chronic lymphocytic leukemia. *Clin. Exp. Immunol.* 40:256, 1980.

46. Matutes E., Wechsler A., Gomez R., et al.: Unusual T-cell phenotype in advanced B-chronic lymphocytic leukemia. *Br. J. Haematol.* 49:635, 1981.

47. Uchiama T., Sagawa K., Takatsuki K., et al.: Effect of adult T cell leukemia cells on pokeweed mitogen-induced normal B cell differentiation. *Clin. Immunol. Immunopathol.* 10:24, 1978.

48. Tatsumi E., Takiuchi Y., Domae N., et al.: Suppressive activity of some leukemic T cells from adult patients in Japan. *Clin. Immunol. Immunopathol.* 15:190, 1980.

49. Hattori T., Uchiyama T., Toibana T., et al.: Surface phenotype of Japanese adult T cell leukemia cells characterized by monoclonal antibodies. *Blood* 58:645, 1981.

50. Jansen J., Schmit H.R.E., Meijer C.J.L.M., et al.: Cell markers in hairy cell leukemias, in Knapp W. (ed.): *Leukemia Markers.* New York, Academic Press, 1981, p. 179.

51. Lydyard P.M., Powell R.G., Fanger M.W., et al.: Expression of receptors for IgA in hairy cell and other B-cell leukemias. *Br. J. Haematol.* 49:643, 1981.

52. Utsinger P.D., Yount W.J., Fuller C.R., et al.: Hairy cell leukemia: B lymphocyte and phagocytic properties. *Blood* 49:19, 1977.

53. Gupta S., Good R.A.: Markers of human lymphocyte subpopulations in primary immunodeficiency and lymphoproliferative disorders. *Semin. Hematol.* 17:1, 1980.

54. Aisenberg A., Wilkes B.M.: Relevance of surface markers in chronic lymphocytic leukemia to acute lymphocytic leukemia. *Cancer Res.* 41:4810, 1981.
55. Cossman J., Jaffe E.S.: Distribution of complement receptor subtypes in non-Hodgkin's lymphomas of B-cell origin. *Blood* 58:20, 1981.
56. Ritz J., Nadler L.M., Bhan A.K., et al.: Expression of common acute lymphoblastic leukemia antigen (CALL) by lymphomas of B-cell and T-cell lineage. *Blood* 58:648, 1981.
57. Brouet J.C., Labaume S., Seligmann M.: Evaluation of T and B lymphocytic membrane markers in human non-Hodgkin's malignant lymphomata. *Br. J. Cancer* 31:121, 1975.
58. Koziner B., Kempin S., Passe S., et al.: Characterization of B cell leukemias: A tentative immunomorphological scheme. *Blood* 56:815, 1980.
59. Bernard A., Boumsell L., Reinherz E.L., et al.: Cell surface characterization of malignant T cells from lymphoblastic lymphoma using monoclonal antibodies: Evidence for phenotypic differences between malignant T cells from patients with acute lymphoblastic leukemia and lymphoblastic lymphoma. *Blood* 57:1105, 1981.
60. Boumsell L., Bernard A., Reinherz E.L., et al.: Surface antigens on malignant Sézary and T-CLL cells correspond to those of mature T cells. *Blood* 57:526, 1981.
61. Broder S., Edelson R.L., Lutzner M.A., et al.: The Sézary syndrome: A malignant proliferation of helper T cells. *J. Clin. Invest.* 58:1297, 1976.
62. Gupta S., Safai B., Good R.A.: Subpopulations of human T lymphocytes: IV. Distribution and quantitation in patients with mycosis fungoides and Sézary syndrome. *Cell. Immunol.* 39:18, 1978.
63. Abelev G.I.: Alpha-fetoprotein in oncogenesis and its association with malignant tumors. *Adv. Cancer Res.* 14:295, 1971.
64. Ruoslahti E., Pihko H., Seppala M.: Alpha-fetoprotein: Immunochemical purification and chemical properties expression in normal state and in malignant and nonmalignant liver disease. *Transplant. Rev.* 20:383, 1971.
65. Bélanger L., Bélanger M., Prive L., et al.: Tyrosinemie héréditaire el alpha-1-foetoprotéinie: I. Intéret clinique de l'alpha-foetoproteine dans la tyrosinémie héréditaire. *Pathol. Biol.* 21:449, 1973.
66. Gold P., Freedman S.O.: Demonstration of tumor specific antigen in human colon carcinomata by immunological tolerance and absorption techniques. *J. Exp. Med.* 121:439, 1965.
67. Cullen K.J., Stevens, D.P., Frost M.A., et al.: Carcinoembryonic antigen (CEA) smoking and cancer in a longitudinal population study. *Aust. NZ J. Med.* 6:279, 1976.
68. Frost M.A., Coates A.S.: Plasma carcinoembryonic antigen in an Australian hospital population. *Med. J. Aust.* 1:950, 1976.
69. Doos W.G., Wolff W.I., Shinya A., et al.: CEA levels in patients with colorectal polyps. *Cancer* 36:1996, 1975.
70. Gold P., Shuster J., Freedman S.O.: Carcinoembryonic antigen (CEA) in clinical medicine: historical perspectives, pitfalls and projections. *Cancer* 42 (3 Suppl.):1399, 1978.
71. Booth S.N., Jamieson G.C., King J.P.G., et al.: Carcinoembryonic antigen in management of colorectal carcinoma. *Br. J. Med.* 2:183, 1974.
72. Reynoso G., Chu T.M., Holyoke D., et al.: Carcinoembryonic antigen in patients with different cancers. *JAMA* 220:361, 1972.

73. Lawrence D.J.R., Stevens U., Bettelheim R., et al.: Role of plasma carcinoembryonic antigen in diagnosis of gastrointestinal, mammary and bronchial carcinoma. *Br. Med. J.* 3:605, 1972.
74. Chu T.M., Nemoto T.: Evaluation of carcinoembryonic antigen in human mammary carcinoma. *J. Natl. Cancer Inst.* 51:1119, 1973.
75. Zamcheck N.: Carcinoembryonic antigen: Quantitative variations in circulating levels in benign and malignant digestive tract disease. *Adv. Intern. Med.* 19:413, 1974.
76. Vider M., Kashmin R., Meeker W.R., et al.: Carcinoembryonic antigen (CEA) monitoring in the management of radiotherapeutic and chemotherapeutic patients. *AJR* 124:630, 1975.
77. Wang M.C., Valenzuela L.A., Murphy G.P., et al.: Purification of a human prostatic antigen. *Invest. Urol.* 17:159, 1979.
78. Nadji M., Tabei S.Z., Castro A., et al.: Prostatic specific antigen: An immunologic marker for prostatic neoplasm. *Cancer* 48:1229, 1981.
79. Papsidero L.D., Kuriyama M., Wang M.C., et al.: Prostatic antigen a marker for human prostatic epithelial cells. *J. Natl. Cancer Inst.* 66:37, 1981.
80. Kuriyama M., Wang M.C., Lee C.I., et al.: Use of human prostate-specific antigen in monitoring prostate cancer. *Cancer Res.* 41:3874, 1981.
81. Dippold W., Llyod K.O., Li L.T.C., et al.: Cell surface antigens of human malignant melanoma: Definition of 6 antigenic systems with mouse monoclonal antibodies. *Proc. Natl. Acad. Sci. USA* 77:6114, 1980.
82. Koprowski H., Steplenski Z., Herlyn D., et al.: Study of antibodies against human melanoma produced by somatic cell hybrids. *Proc. Natl. Acad. Sci. USA* 75:3405, 1978.
83. Herlyn M., Steplewski Z., Herlyn D., et al.: Colorectal carcinoma specific antigen: Detection by means of monoclonal antibodies. *Proc. Natl. Acad. Sci. USA* 76:1438, 1979.
84. Kennett R.H., Jonak Z.L., Bechtol K.B.: Monoclonal antibodies against human tumor-associated antigens, in Kennett R.H., McKearn T.J., Bechtol K.B. (eds.): *Monoclonal Antibodies.* New York, Plenum Press, 1980, p. 155.
85. Ueda R., Ogata S.I., Mernsey D.M., et al.: Cell surface antigens of human renal cancer defined with monoclonal antibodies. *Proc. Natl. Acad. Sci. USA* 78:5122, 1981.

15

Histocompatibility Antigens

Stephen D. Litwin, M.D.

HISTOCOMPATIBILITY GENE COMPLEX[1-5]

Basic Anatomy and Organization

The macroorganization of human chromosomes is conveniently presented as a linear array of discrete gene loci. The pattern of DNA bases within each locus is "read off" into mirror image RNA *(transcription)*, and eventually a discrete protein gene product is produced in the cell *(translation)*. Linear distance along the chromosome is measured in a functional unit called the *centimorgan*, which is defined as that separation between genetic markers which permits recombination to take place, during meiotic synapsis, 1% of the time. Estimates are that a 1-centimorgan stretch of chromosome can accomodate up to 1,000–2,000 discrete gene loci, or about 1,000 kilobases of DNA. Although it is accurate to emphasize the separateness of each gene locus and the individual control of each gene product protein, there are adjacent genes which can and will interact with each other. These groups are known as *gene clusters* or *supergenes* or *gene complexes*[4]; among them are the human leukocyte antigens (HLA) of man.

The general morphological details described in the preceding paragraph can now be applied to the major human histocompatibility gene complex, HLA. (H is for human; L for leukocyte—the cells on which these antigens were initially tested; and A indicates the first system of this kind). The HLA complex occupies 1–2 centimorgans on the short arm of chromosome 6. The major landmarks of the gene complex are the HLA-A, -B, -C, and -D histocompatibility gene loci, the BF, C4, and C2 complement gene loci, and the Ia alloantigen and MLC loci (related to HLA-D). HLA-A, -B, and -C loci are determined on cells *(typed)* by cytotoxic antibodies, which usually develop in pregnant women in the process of immunization with fetal antigens. There are 20 known A locus antigens, 42 B locus antigens, and 8 C markers: A current list is given in Table 15–1.[5] HLA-A and -D lie approximately 1.6 centimorgans apart, while HLA-B and -D are separated by

TABLE 15–1.—LISTING OF CURRENT RECOGNIZED HLA
SPECIFICITIES*

HLA-A	HLA-B	HLA-C	HLA-D	HLA-DR
HLA-A1	HLA-B5	HLA-Cw1	HLA-Dw1	HLA-DR1
HLA-A2	HLA-B7	HLA-Cw2	HLA-Dw2	HLA-DR2
HLA-A3	HLA-B8	HLA-Cw3	HLA-Dw3	HLA-DR3
HLA-A9	HLA-B12	HLA-Cw4	HLA-Dw4	HLA-DR4
HLA-A10	HLA-B13	HLA-Cw5	HLA-Dw5	HLA-DR5
HLA-A11	HLA-B14	HLA-Cw6	HLA-Dw6	HLA-DRw6
HLA-Aw19	HLA-B15	HLA-Cw7	HLA-Dw7	HLA-DR7
HLA-Aw23	HLA-Bw16	HLA-Cw8	HLA-Dw8	HLA-DRw8
HLA-Aw24	HLA-B17		HLA-Dw9	HLA-DRw9
HLA-A25	HLA-B18		HLA-Dw10	HLA-DRw10
HLA-A26	HLA-Bw21		HLA-Dw11	
HLA-A28	HLA-Bw22		HLA-Dw12	
HLA-A29	HLA-B27			
HLA-Aw30	HLA-Bw35			
HLA-Aw31	HLA-B37			
HLA-Aw32	HLA-Bw38			
HLA-Aw33	HLA-Bw39			
HLA-Aw34	HLA-B40			
HLA-Aw36	HLA-Bw41			
HLA-Aw43	HLA-Bw42			
	HLA-Bw44			
	HLA-Bw45			
	HLA-Bw46			
	HLA-Bw47			
	HLA-Bw48			
	HLA-Bw49			
	HLA-Bw50			
	HLA-Bw51			
	HLA-Bw52			
	HLA-Bw53			
	HLA-Bw54			
	HLA-Bw55			
	HLA-Bw56			
	HLA-Bw57			
	HLA-Bw58			
	HLA-Bw59			
	HLA-Bw60			
	HLA-Bw61			
	HLA-Bw62			
	HLA-Bw63			
	HLA-Bw4			
	HLA-Bw6			

*Table from Terasaki.[5]

half that distance. The HLA region and the ordering of the major gene loci are shown schematically in Figure 15–1 and the approximate linear distances are given in centimorgans.

Biomedical scientists have developed enormous enthusiasm about the histocompatibility genes for two reasons. First, most advanced organisms

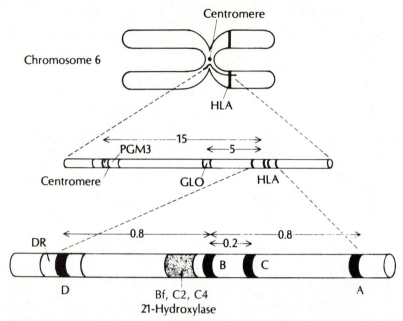

Fig 15–1.—*Top,* region on the short arm of human chromosome 6 that contains the HLA supergene. *Middle,* expanded figure showing the region adjacent to HLA, with the distances between the glyoxalase-1 *(GLO)* and phosphoglucomutase-3 *(PGM3)* enzyme markers indicated in centimorgans. *Bottom,* enlargement of the HLA area showing the HLA-A, D, B, and C markers, the Bf, C2, and C4 complement genes, and the region between HLA-B and D in which the 21-hydroxylase gene is believed located. (Schaller and Hansen.[44] Figure drawn by and reproduced courtesy of Bunji Tagawa.)

have histocompatibility gene complexes with strikingly parallel properties. This universality suggests that key functions are involved. Second, the biologic properties of histocompatibility-linked genes of all species surveyed are related to cell-to-cell surface interactions in general and to the immune response and neoplasia specifically: all these are areas of current research interest. Table 15–2 lists histocompatibility-linked genes of mouse and man that have expressed such properties to date. Perhaps the most important and widely popularized of these genes are the 25–30 immune response genes of the mouse.[3] Although similar genes have not yet been described in man, it should be kept in mind that their formal demonstration is difficult both because purposeful immunization cannot be justified and because humans are not as inbred as laboratory mice. The demonstration of genes determining mouse viral leukemogenesis has stimulated fevered efforts to establish parallel human data. On the other hand, no parallel animal model of the HLA-disease relationship in man has yet been uncovered. Finally, in both species complement components are determined by histocompatibility-linked genes as well as immune functions. The list given in Table 15–2 is abbreviated. It is designed to emphasize the fact that histocompatibility-linked genes in higher organisms have universal and critical functions closely related to immune response, neoplasia, and perhaps differentiation of tissues.

Testing Techniques

HLA-A, -B, and -C loci antigens are detected by antibody-mediated methods using reagents standardized by testing of frozen cells of established specificity. Such testing or typing is usually performed on human lymphocytes that carry a high density of HLA surface molecules, although other than white cells can be typed. Figure 15–2 depicts one widely used serologic complement fixation (CF) cytotoxicity test (see Chap. 3). The minute amounts of antibody that are required have helped expand testing facilities. These detection techniques are only as powerful as the specificity of the antibodies available for typing. The introduction of monoclonal antibodies should strengthen and sharpen existing capabilities.

The HLA-D locus is tested using a method of cellular immunity (no antibody) to recognize tissue (cell) differences. In the *mixed lymphocyte culture* (MLC), shown schematically in Figure 15–3, lymphocytes from two individuals are cultured together in vitro. One set of cells is prevented from responding by irradiation or by chemical block: its role is that of the *stimulator cell*. The untreated cells are called *responder cells;* they signal tissue histocompatibility differences by proliferation, measured as incorporation of labeled thymidine into DNA. If responder A cells are mixed with

TABLE 15–2.—HISTOCOMPATIBILITY-LINKED GENES OF BIOLOGIC SIGNIFICANCE[3]

	MOUSE	MAN	EXAMPLES
Serologically determined histocompatibility	+	+	HLA-A,B,C (man)
Lymphocyte-determined histocompatibility	+	+	HLA-D (man)
Complement components	+	+	C2, C4
Immune response genes	+	?	I region of murine H2 major
Genes that restrict interactions between immune cells	+	?	histocompatibility gene complex
Genes associated with human disease	−	+	HLA, -A, -B, -C, and -D/DR genes (man)
Resistance to viral leukemogenesis	+	−	Resistance to Gross leukemia virus (mouse)
Differentiation of lymphocyte	+	−	Tla (mouse)
Embryogenesis	+	−	T locus (mouse)

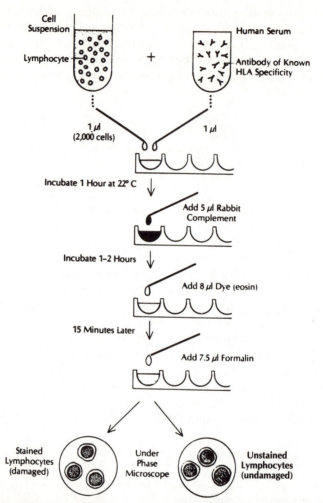

Fig 15–2.—Serologic complement fixing cytotoxicity test. HLA-A, B, or C antigens are tested for on human lymphocytes by mixing a cell suspension with a serum containing antibody of known HLA specificity in a microwell plate, adding complement, and incubating. Formalin halts the reaction and the dye stains dead or injured cells damaged by the cytotoxic reaction. Scoring is expressed as the percentage of cells killed. (Schaller and Hansen.[44] Figure drawn by and reproduced courtesy of Bunji Tagawa.)

irradiated cells of a second person Bx (stimulator), the A + Bx combination can be compared with the control combination A + Ax and the difference recorded either directly, counts per minute of radioactivity, or as a ratio of counts per minute divided by control baseline counts per minute (see Chap. 3).

A set of HLA antigens related to HLA-D were later described using antisera. The DR system, now widely employed, is closely related but may not be identical to HLA-D. Finally, Ia and various alloantigens are determined by genes close to the HLA-D locus. These antigens promise to be particularly useful in the diagnosis of certain diseases but are undergoing further analysis.

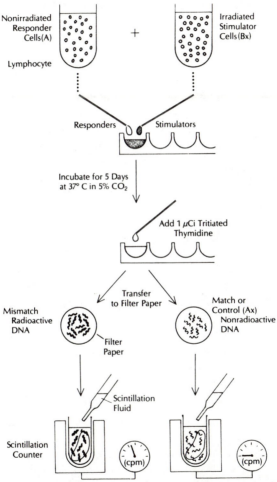

Fig 15–3.—Scheme for the mixed lymphocyte culture technique (MLC). A mixture of responder and stimulator (irradiated) cells is incubated for 5 days; radiolabeled thymidine is added; the isotope present in the experimental cells *(left)* vs. control cells is counted. This MLC reaction is determined by histocompatibility genes in man at the HLA-D locus. (Schaller and Hansen.[44] Figure drawn by and reproduced courtesy of Bunji Tagawa.)

Nomenclature and Terminology[5]

Table 15–1 lists the known, accepted HLA specificities at each locus. The small w indicates specificities that have provisional status. The overlapping specificities of early classifications have been continually refined and distinguished.

BASIC IMMUNOGENETIC CONCEPTS

HLA Polymorphism and HLA Haplotypes[1, 2]

HLA polymorphism is the most diverse encountered in any human genetic system, with most individuals being heterozygous rather than homozygous for different alleles. This means the chance of two individuals having even one similar HLA gene complex is small for all but those few HLA antigens that have a high population frequency. The problems stemming from this situation in tissue grafting, where histocompatibility differences correlate closely with results, are evident and widely appreciated.

Since the four HLA loci are contiguously positioned on chromosome 6, allelic genes at these four loci are inherited together as linked rather than as independent traits. It is possible to follow the inheritance of a series of linked genes as a unit called a *haplotype* (Fig 15–4). Each individual has two HLA haplotypes, one on each homologous chromosome. Each haplotype contains a representative of each of the four HLA loci, e.g., haplotype HLA-A7, -B27, -C6, -D3. HLA haplotypes can also be written to include HLA-linked genes, such as complement alleles, if that form is useful. One approach adopted by many laboratories has been to designate the maternal haplotypes as A and B, respectively, and the paternal haplotypes as C and D. All offspring, except for rare recombinants, therefore must be AC, AD, BC, or BD. (Don't confuse the letters in this convenient notation with the HLA-A, -B, -C, and -D loci.)

Linkage Equilibrium and Dysequilibrium

Although very little recombination takes place ($< 1\%$) within the HLA gene complex, even limited reshuffling within a chromosome, over time, will continuously reassort the linkage relationships between HLA alleles. The predicted result should be a random series of haplotypes. This phenomenon of reassortment among linked genes is known as *linkage equilibrium* and is supported by genetic theory and experiments. Although linkage equilibrium has been verified many times and is generally present, there are groups of linked genes, including many within the HLA supergene, in which equilibrium fails to occur either because of interference

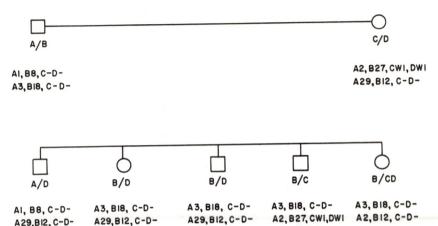

Fig 15–4.—Family kindred, typed at HLA-A, B, C, and D loci. Various haplotype combinations are inherited by the children, including a recombination in a maternal chromosome (child on far right). The A/B or C/D designations of parents and children are not haplotypes but a "shorthand" for haplotypes (see text). (Courtesy of Dausset J., Svejgaard A. (eds.): *HLA and Disease.* Baltimore, Williams and Wilkins, 1977, p. 25. Reproduced by permission.)

with free and random recombination of genes or because of selection pressure for a haplotype. This obverse phenomenon is called *linkage dysequilibrium* and the reasons underlying it are unclear (see discussion by Bodmer[4]). As a consequence, certain alleles at different loci within the HLA supergene occur together in a population at a higher than chance frequency (Table 15–3). In some instances an entire or a part of a haplotype (such as A1 and B8) that are in linkage dysequilibrium may be associated with a disease (e.g., myasthenia gravis), and it is uncertain which, if any, allele in the haplotype has the closest physiologic relationship to the disease pathology. In other cases, such as the HLA-B27-ankylosing spondylitis (AS) relationship, the higher disease risk is clearly HLA-B27 related but not haplotype related.

Genetic Association Versus Genetic Linkage

In considering the physiologic reasons for the HLA marker-disease relationship, it is useful to review the subject of genetic markers and disease states. *Genetic linkage and genetic association* are the two primary and alternative explanations usually given. The biologic connotations are enormously different.

Genetic linkage assumes that a genetic marker, be it a blood group antigen, histocompatibility antigen, enzyme polymorphism, or an electropho-

TABLE 15–3.—LINKAGE
DYSEQUILIBRIUM AMONG SELECTED
HLA-A and -B HAPLOTYPES [1,2]

HLA HAPLOTYPE	$\Delta/1,000$*
A1, B5	13.7
A1, B8	57.2‡
A1, B17	16.0
A2, B12	27.2‡
A3, B7	18.5
Aw23, B12	17.6‡
A26, Bw38	5.3
A29, B12	27.3‡
Aw30, B18	16.6‡
Aw33, B14	6.4‡

*Δ is a mathematical way of expressing linkage dysequilibrium: the higher the values the greater the dysequilibrium. Further explanation of the calculation, see Bodmer,[2] pp. 309-316.
‡0.1% significance level of χ^2.

retic mobility difference, is linked to a second and unrelated gene that initiates the disease. One example is the linkage between the Rh system and elliptocytosis. The implications of genetic linkage are that marker and disease will be inherited together in families, but that the gene products in question are probably unrelated to each other in any biologic sense. Many persons may carry the marker but not the disease, and vice versa. If the marker and disease are in genetic equilibrium (as are most genes), they will not necessarily be closely associated within populations, and persons with that marker may not have a higher disease risk. For example, although hemophilia and colorblindness are linked genes on the X chromosome, colorblindness is not a uniformly useful predicator of hemophilia in a population. (This does not preclude using colorblindness to predict hemophilia in a fetus if family data can show that the colorblindness and hemophilia genes are "coupled," i.e., on the same chromosome, in the parent.) If, on the other hand, linkage dysequilibrium exists, then the genetic marker and the disease gene remain together as an inherited unit, and within populations they will appear together at a higher-than-random frequency. This is one plausible explanation for the HLA-disease risk situation.

The second explanation, genetic association, implies that the gene involved is closely related to the cause of the disease. It is not necessary to postulate linkage. One example are the alleles of α_1-antitrypsin. When the Z allele is present, the α_1-antitrypsin gene product is decreased, and as a consequence of the absence of protease neutralization, the patient is likely to develop premature chronic pulmonary disease. The implications of genetic association are that marker and disease will be inherited together in families and found together in populations. Although some persons with the marker might not express the disease, their risk remains high and family disease incidence will be high. The genetic marker and the disease are biologically related as cause and effect.

It is obvious that genetic association and genetic linkage may be hard to distinguish, particularly if linkage dysequilibrium is present, until such time as the pathophysiology of the disease is unveiled.

PATHOPHYSIOLOGY OF HLA-GENETIC MARKER DISEASE ASSOCIATION

In the previous section I discussed basic immunogenetic concepts and introduced the question of whether the relationship between a genetic marker and disease was due to genetic linkage or to genetic association. With respect to HLA, several points must be kept in mind.

Among the several dozen HLA-associated diseases there is genetic heterogeneity, suggesting that different mechanisms may be involved. Although hemochromatosis and 21-hydroxylase deficiency are present only when the individual in question has two HLA-related disease genes (recessive inheritance), the general rule is that only one HLA disease gene is necessary to confer increased risk. For example, in the relationship between HLA-B27 and ankylosing spondylitis there is no rise in relative risk when two HLA-B27 genes are carried. To complicate the situation even further, in the relationship between C2 deficiency, HLA loci, and lupus erythematosus, one C2 deficiency gene confers an increased risk and two deficiency genes an even higher relative risk.

Many diseases associated with a higher incidence of a specific HLA marker are of unknown cause and associated with immune system aberrations. The combination of abnormal immune mechanisms, including autoimmunity in man, coupled with the discovery that the mouse major histocompatibility complex, H2, includes immune response genes has stimulated speculation on whether an abnormal HLA immune response gene is a disease mechanism. It should be realized that abnormal immunity does not completely explain diseases such as hemochromatosis, 21-hydroxylase deficiency, or diabetes mellitus, which are HLA-linked.

Many laboratories now regard genetic linkage between an HLA gene and a second disease gene as the best explanation for many HLA-disease relationships. This explanation is supported by the presence of linkage dysequilibrium between many HLA haplotypes (see Table 15–3). There is further support in the demonstration that certain diseases are related to different HLA markers in different populations (see section on psoriasis).

Finally, it should be understood that the associations we are discussing are found at all of the HLA loci. In hemochromatosis, the relationship is with the A locus, in psoriasis with the C locus. Most other diseases implicate the D or B gene loci. The inference is that there must be multiple disease susceptibility genes that are nonallelic, and it is unlikely that they all operate in the same way.

The possibilities of genetic association due to direct cause and effect between HLA gene and pathogenic state cannot be fully dismissed. Some work suggests that persons carrying HLA-B27 have a tendency to *Klebsiella* infection because the surface histocompatibility antigen serves as a bacterial receptor.[6] A role for the HLA-A2 antigen in iron transport has been suggested in hemochromatosis.

In summary, the pathophysiology underlying the HLA-disease relationship is presently obscure,[7] but it seems fair to conclude that the answer will lie in the critical biologic roles played by the several hundred or so genes in the histocompatibility region.

SELECTED HLA DISEASE ASSOCIATIONS

B27 and Seronegative Spondyloarthropathy[8]

The seronegative spondyloarthropathies include AS, Reiter's syndrome, some forms of psoriatic arthritis, the arthritis of inflammatory bowel disease, and a subset of juvenile rheumatoid arthritis (RA): they have in common the absence of rheumatoid factors, sacroileitis, with or without spondylitis, frequent peripheral arthropathy, and frequent skin, genital, ocular, and gastrointestinal manifestations.

The prototype for these problems is AS, which was also the first disease in which a dramatic increase in relative risk for persons with HLA-B27 was clearly demonstrated. Relative risk is a useful way of expressing HLA-disease risk. It is calculated by dividing the frequency of a disease in HLA-positive persons by the frequency in HLA-negative persons. If there is no increment in risk associated with a genetic marker, the ratio is 1.0. A relative risk of 3 translates into a threefold greater disease risk.

Less than 10 years ago, HLA-B27 was reported to be present in more than 85% of patients with AS, in contrast to its 4%–7% incidence in the general population. The initial observations have been repeatedly confirmed; further, it has been established that only one B27 gene is required for the relative risk to be increased and that the HLA-disease association is with B27 alone rather than an HLA haplotype. This suggests that the mode of inheritance is dominant.

Perhaps the most critical result of these observations was the consolidation of the seronegative spondyloarthropathies as a genuinely related disease group. The seronegative spondyloarthropathies, in addition to having clinical similarities, are all HLA-B27 associated (Table 15–4). In persons with Reiter's syndrome the increased prevalence of B27 holds, whether or not the individual manifests spondylitis (which is not uniformly found), making it virtually a variant of AS. On the other hand, arthritis of various types is characteristic of inflammatory bowel disease and psoriasis. Only patients in whom spondylitis develops have a higher likelihood of being HLA-B27 positive.[9] Approximately 50% of persons with acute uveitis are B27 positive. Patients who are positive have a different clinical picture characterized by conjunctivitis, spondyloarthropathy, and Reiter's syndrome-like disease; in addition they may have a more protracted course of illness.

The interdependence between *Shigella* infection, Reiter's syndrome, and B27 is illustrated in the careful documentation of an epidemic of shigellosis affecting 602 of the 1,276-man crew members of a U.S. Navy cruiser at sea.[10] Ten cases of postinfectious Reiter's syndrome appeared within 2 weeks of the enteric problems. Thirteen years later, five of those ten persons were reexamined. One HLA-B27-negative individual had minimal problems and was essentially symptom free. The remaining four men were B27 positive and had chronic active disease. It may be that B27-positive Reiter's syndrome patients do not fare as well as B27-negative patients even when the environmental trigger is the same; however, the group was too small for any firm conclusions to be drawn. The extrapolated risk of Reiter's syndrome after the episode of dysentery was as high as 19%–32% in HLA-B27-positive crewmen, while the risk to a B-27-negative crewman was quite low.

An obvious issue is raised by these data: What is the risk of AS appearing

TABLE 15–4.—HLA-B27 POSITIVITY IN ANKYLOSING SPONDYLITIS
AND RELATED DISORDERS

DISORDER	% POSITIVE FOR B27
Ankylosing spondylitis	88–96
Reiter's syndrome	80
Psoriatic spondylitis	35–75
Yersinia arthritis	66
Acute anterior uveitis	50
Salmonellosis	
With reactive arthritis	69
Without reactive arthritis	8
Förster's disease*	34
Healthy controls	4–7

*Data on percentage of B27-positive patients are limited or conflicting.

in an HLA-B27-positive person? The incidence of overt clinical disease is only a fraction of a percent, while 4%–7% of the general population are B27 positive. The attack rate, even in genetically predisposed populations must be low. A corollary problem is the male preponderance of clinical AS, since the HLA genetic markers are autosomal and thus equal in frequency in the sexes. Further findings help to interpret the data. Studies using minimal radiologic signs for AS show that the disease incidence in B27-positive persons can be as high as 20%.[11] This means that close to 2 million persons in the United States (20% of the 5% of the population who are B27 positive) have this disease, with most persons having only a minimal subclinical form. The sex incidence in these latter studies using minimal criteria was equal. Thus the clinical male dominance reflects disease severity but not disease liability or susceptibility.

Racial differences must be taken into account when interpreting HLA data. Among black Americans, only half of AS patients are B27 positive. For white Americans the figure is 90%. However, the HLA-B27 incidence in black Americans is only 2%. Thus, the relative risk for AS in B27 positive black Americans is high, but the test is not very useful for ruling out the diagnosis, since only half of patients with AS are B27 positive.

Psoriasis[12]

The association of psoriasis with HLA illustrates the point that different races may have the same disease related to a different HLA allele.

HLA-Cw6 is associated with a high incidence of psoriasis both in Japanese (53%) and in caucasians (50%), but since the normal frequency of Cw6 is much lower in Japanese, they have a higher relative risk than caucasians (Table 15–5).

Both the frequency of an HLA-disease association in a population and

TABLE 15–5.—HLA Associations
With Psoriasis[12]

HLA	FREQUENCY (%) PATIENTS/CONTROL	RELATIVE RISK
Caucasian		
Cw6	50/23	3.3
B13	23/5	5.7
B17	19/9	2.4
B37	5/2	2.6
Japanese		
Cw6	53/7	15
B13	18/1	22
B37	35/2	26
A1	30/2	21

TABLE 15–6.—DISEASES FOUND WITH AN
INCREASED FREQUENCY OF HLA-DR3, B8

Chronic active hepatitis
Myasthenia gravis
Gluten-sensitive enteropathy and dermatitis herpetiformis
Insulin-dependent diabetes mellitus
Thyrotoxicosis
Sicca syndrome (primary)
Addison's disease
Thyroiditis
Polyglandular endocrine failure

the relative risk conferred by that HLA antigen are useful data and must be considered. That HLA-disease associations may vary with the ethnic group has been used to argue strongly that genetic linkage is the proper interpretation of HLA pathophysiology, since the HLA antigen itself does not have a characteristic disease posture in all populations.

The DR3 and B8 Haplotype: A Related Disease Group?[13–15]

The HLA-A1, B8, DR3 haplotype is a striking example of a haplotype in which similarities among a group of associated problems suggest an underlying physiologic basis. These similarities are not in the target organ; rather, the diseases encountered include many with unclear etiology and autoantibody formation (Table 15–6). Immune mechanisms are suspected.

In some HLA-A1, -B8, -DR3 haplotype-related disorders, experimental data suggest differences in the immune responses, possibly attributable to histocompatibility-linked immune response genes. For example, Eddleston and William reported that in chronic active hepatitis, the HLA-B8, DR3 haplotype was found most frequently in patients with high titers of antinuclear and antismooth muscle autoantibodies.[13] In myasthenia gravis antibody formed against the acetylcholine receptor at the motor end-plate correlates with disease activity and can simulate the pathology in animal models. In gluten-sensitive enteropathy it has been suggested but not proved that the immune response to gluten is abnormal due to the DR3, B8 haplotype.

In thyrotoxicosis (see Table 15–6) The long-acting thyroid stimulator (LATS) has been found to be IgG. Animal models confirm that antibody bound to the thyroid hormone receptor can stimulate thyroid tissue to increased activity. In the myasthenia gravis model it is implied that autoantibody interferes with function; in thyrotoxicosis the opposite is suggested. It is clear that the elucidation of underlying pathophysiology requires careful attention to mechanism and rigorous proof.

DR4 and RA: Ia Alloantigens[16]

The association between RA and DR4 carries a twofold to threefold increase in relative risk. The high normal frequency of the DR4 marker (10%–40%, depending on the population) limits its diagnostic power, but several studies agree that the DR4-RA relationship is valid. The main conclusion reached, that RA has an underlying genetic propensity, was long debated[17] and now represents a valuable point of departure for future efforts. The female predominance of RA is opposite to what is seen in AS, but the basic principle may be similar. In both diseases the HLA association emphasizes the equal genetic propensity by sex, while clinical findings suggest that the actual attack rate or severity of disease is sex modified.

Long-standing arguments about the diagnostic implications of seropositive versus seronegative RA and of the overlap between RA and SLE have also been illuminated by HLA data. One study showed that seronegative RA patients lacked the expected DR4-RA relationship.[16] While RA is DR4 associated in several populations, systemic lupus erythematosus (SLE) is not, which distinguishes the two diseases. Even more convincing are studies of histocompatibility-linked Ia alloantigens (Table 15–7).[18]

Ia B cell antigens are determined by genes located close to HLA-D. Their position is analogous to the site of the immune response genes in mice, and this similarity has prompted the suggestion that they are antigens on gene products that regulate the immune response. The point is unproved but attractive.

Ia alloantigens[18, 22] are polymorphic, although their inheritance has not been as carefully defined as for the HLA genes. Ia alloantigens are valuable for several reasons: They may be even more closely correlated with individual diseases than HLA markers (see sicca syndrome in Table 15–7). They can be used to distinguish closely related conditions, such as the primary and secondary sicca syndromes and SLE and RA. They may be antigens on the actual disease gene product rather than linked to a disease gene. Table 15–7 provides data on three groups of histocompatibility-linked Ia antigens that have been particularly useful. A fourth B cell alloantigen, known as the gluten-sensitive enteropathy-associated B cell alloantigen,[20] is unrelated to HLA but is included in Table 15–7 because it is a polymorphic B cell antigen that has a genetic marker-disease association and may have a physiologic basis similar to that of Ia (HLA-linked) alloantigens.

Diabetes Mellitus[23, 24]

Insulin-dependent diabetes mellitus (IDDM) is significantly related to the D locus of HLA, with the disease gene in linkage dysequilibrium with

TABLE 15–7— B LYMPHOCYTE ALLOANTIGENS
IN SELECTED DISEASES

ALLOANTIGEN	POPULATION FREQUENCY (%)		
	Sicca Syndrome[21]		
	Normals	Primary Sicca	Secondary Sicca With RA
HLA-B8	24	59	9
DR3	31	64	9
DR4	27	28	64
Ia 172	37	100	82
350	21	59	82
715	14	68	9
	Rheumatoid Arthritis and Systemic Lupus Erythematosus[18]		
	Normals	SLE	RA
Ia 2	30	47	20
Ia 3	20	53	25
Ia 4-7-10	25	7	80
	Multiple Sclerosis[22]		
	Normals	Multiple Sclerosis	
Ag 7a	44	100	
	Gluten-Sensitive Enteropathy[20]		
	Normals	Dermatitis Herpetiformis*	Gluten-Sensitive Enteropathy*
GSE-associated ⎱ B1	0	81	79
B cell antigen ⎰ W1	0	94	100

*Includes both HLA-B8-positive and -negative subjects.

both DR3 and DR4. This finding has resolved some of the arguments surrounding the genetic basis of the insulin-dependent form of the disease but has not yet disclosed the actual mode of inheritance.[24] IDDM differs from other HLA-disease systems in two respects: first, it is not generally regarded as an "autoimmune problem" (a number of experimental observations support an immune basis for diabetes mellitus), and second, individuals carrying two susceptibility genes have higher risks, which suggests but does not prove recessive inheritance. This is reflected in the data in Table 15–8: the relative risk of a DR3/3 homozygous person is higher than that of an individual carrying a single DR3 gene. The same is true for DR4. What is perplexing about the data in Table 15–8 is the documented observation that HLA-DR3/4 persons have a greater risk than the homozygotes, which precludes a simple genetic interpretation. As can be ascertained from Table 15–8, the relative risk of IDDM underlines a strong genetic basis for the disease. The attack rate from these data, from other proband data, and from observations of identical twins may be as high as 50%, assuming an individual carries diabetes risk genes.

There is no reason to regard the DR3/3, DR4/4, and DR3/4 forms of IDDM as discrete clinical entities. However, it has been pointed out that

TABLE 15–8.—HLA AND INHERITANCE
OF INSULIN-DEPENDENT DIABETES
MELLITUS (IDDM)*[24]

DR GENOTYPE	% OF IDDM CASES	RELATIVE RISK
3/3†	10.7	97.9
3/4	41.1	173.6
4/4†	9.8	76.9
3/X	7.1	4.6
4/X	25.9	15.4
X/X	5.4	1

*X refers to a DR antigen other than DR3
or DR4; e.g., DR1, 2, 5, 6, 7, 8, 9, 10.
†Since not all haplotypes can be typed,
these genotypes in theory could also be 3/0 or
4/0, with the 0 standing for an untyped HLA
antigen(s).

DR4 patients have a tendency to earlier onset of disease. Earlier reports of significant differences with respect to anti-islet cell antibody and anti-insulin antibody have not been confirmed.

DR2 and Mulitple Sclerosis[25]

The closest HLA association in multiple sclerosis is to HLA-DR2. Fifty-six percent of all multiple sclerosis patients carry this marker, and persons in the general population who are DR2 positive have a relative risk of 4. There are other associations as well, including an Ia alloantigen.[22] Current evidence favors a dominant gene with a selection coefficient near 10% and suggests a possible second non-HLA-linked gene.[25] While the multiple sclerosis gene is DR2-associated in caucasians and Italians, it is not in Israeli Jews and in Japanese. Immune aberrations that have been reported include a high response to measles virus and variations in suppressor cell activity.

INTERPRETATION AND USE OF DATA

Interaction Between HLA Determinants and Environment

The genetic factors in diseases with prominent HLA marker-disease relationships must be interpreted differently from other familial problems. Inheritance is rarely mendelian. Rather, there is a highly significant genetic predisposition and a low attack rate. Thus, for these diseases to manifest clinically, there must be a large vulnerable population and environmental events that elicit gene expression. One example is AS, in which

5%–7% of the general population carry the HLA-B27 marker, but only 10%–20% of these show any stigmata, often mild. Persons who become seriously ill with AS constitute approximately 0.1% of the population as a whole. The strong dependence on environmental factors makes formal genetics difficult but offers special opportunities in preventive medicine. For example, it would seem wise for HLA-B27-positive individuals to avoid travel to areas where they would risk exposure to the enteric infections known to provoke spondyloarthropathy. Another application of preventive medicine is diet control in individuals with HLA haplotypes related to IDDM.

Diagnosis

HLA typing is an ancillary procedure in developing a diagnosis. It is rarely if ever pathognomonic, and HLA alleles are present in a large fraction of normal populations. Thus HLA markers will always be more common in healthy than in diseased individuals, and it is only their relative increase in the diseased population that is significant. Further, a considerable percentage of diseased individuals lack the genetic marker. At present, only HLA-B27 is widely employed as a diagnostic aid, and its widespread application has been challenged.[26]

With these caveats in mind, there are many clinical circumstances in which HLA typing is useful in clarifying disease problems or in strengthening disease classification. The sicca syndrome can be separated more readily into primary and secondary forms using HLA typing.[21, 27] Among the skin diseases, psoriasis can be somewhat distinguished from its look-alike psoriaform problems by genetic markers. Among rheumatologic problems, the diagnosis of a spondyloarthropathy complicating psoriasis or a bowel disease can be distinguished from the typical arthritis of psoriasis or from independent inflammatory arthritis (such as rheumatoid arthritis). The HLA-DR3, B8, A1 haplotype in the setting of hepatitis suggests chronic active hepatitis whose course and complications will differ from other hepatic problems. Renal diseases are beginning to be explored and the diagnostic complexities may be easier to deal with in the future. HLA typing can confirm a clinical suspicion of multiple sclerosis (relative risk is only 4), dermatitis herpetiformis, and Behçet's disease. Recent reports suggest that pulmonary fibrosis[28] and Goodpasture's syndrome[29] may be HLA associated.

Surprising familial differences emerge when psoriasis and psoriatic arthritis are analyzed.[30] When the relatives of psoriatic arthritis patients are examined, there are, as expected, many cases of psoriasis (21%) and a high incidence of psoriatic arthritis (Table 15–9). The incidence of psoriasis

Table 15–9.—Disease Incidence in First-Degree
Relatives of Persons With Psoriatic Arthritis or
Psoriasis and Non-Psoriatic Arthritis.[30]

DISEASE	INCIDENCE IN FIRST DEGREE RELATIVES (%)	INCIDENCE IN GENERAL POPULATION (%)	INCIDENCE IN SPOUSES (%)
A. Index Case Has Psoriatic Arthritis			
Psoriatic Arthritis	4.4	.09	0
Psoriasis Alone	21	1.1	2.5
Sacroileitis	7.4	1.1	1.3
B. Index Case Has Psoriasis and Other Non-Psoriatic Arthritis			
Psoriatic Arthritis	0	.09	0
Psoriasis Alone	18.1	1.1	2.5
Sacroileitis	0	1.1	0

among first-degree relatives of psoriasis patients without arthritis is again high, but very few relatives have psoriatic arthritis. Thus the familial tendency to psoriatic arthritis is, to a degree, independent of the skin disease. In other studies HLA patterns of association are different between psoriasis alone and psoriatic arthritis, which suggests these are more discrete problems than might be anticipated. The information is useful in genetic counseling. Only family members of psoriatic arthritis patients need be seriously concerned about inheriting the arthritic complications of the disease.

HLA associations have proved most disappointing in the neoplastic and infectious diseases, in which they should in theory have been most rewarding. On the other hand, they have provided exciting and useful data on rheumatologic and immunopathologic problems, for which some evidence of immune abnormalities was already available. Diabetes mellitus has also been the focus of considerable productive activity.

Future directions of research are difficult to predict. One projection is that researchers may focus on broad patterns of disease proclivity, such as the seronegative spondyloarthropathy-HLA-B27 association. These classificatory attempts assume an underlying genetic proclivity expressed in a limited number of gene-carrying individuals during their lifetime and contingent on different environmental insults for their target organs and clinical patterns. The HLA-DR3, B8 haplotype association fits the pattern of disease haplotype co-occurring with an immune response capable of bypassing normal tolerance mechanisms to establish autoreactive immunopathology.

Therapy and Prognosis

The impact of HLA typing on disease therapy and prognosis is quite limited. One study frequently cited is the work of Wooley et al.,[31] who found that rheumatoid arthritis patients receiving gold or penicillamine and who were HLA-DR3 positive had a 32-fold higher incidence of renal proteinuria but no change in incidence of skin or hematologic complications. The HLA antigens DR3 and B8 were not increased in the underlying disease. Another example is the hydralazine induced lupus-like syndrome, which is more readily induced in females, slow acetylators and (in one paper) DR4 individuals.[32]

A second area in which HLA typing has potential clinical importance is the projection of disease course: individuals who carry an HLA-associated genetic marker may have a more severe and protracted disease course if the disease becomes clinically evident. Evidence for an extended, severe disease course is meager; some of the data on Reiter's syndrome have already been cited. There is also evidence suggesting *Yersinia* arthritis is more severe in HLA-B27-positive persons.[33] Chronic active hepatitis, when present in a young female with multiple tissue autoantibodies, is frequently HLA-DR3, B8 associated,[14] and the possibility that DR3, B8 persons are "sicker" has not been settled. In myasthenia gravis the physiologic derangements of the thymus (more thymic hyperplasia and fewer tumors in DR3, B8 persons) and the titers of receptor antibody are HLA correlated.[15]

Genetic Counseling and Population Screening

The restricted use of HLA for genetic counseling is attributable to the fact that the diseases encountered are usually not severe enough to warrant any type of early intervention. It would be overkill to advise termination of pregnancy for spondylitis, knowing that the gene is expressed only in one of five persons who carry it, that the disease does not begin until adulthood, and that it is subclinical in most cases. IDDM is far more serious, but prenatal counseling is beleagured by the unclear pattern of genetic transmission and by the fact that IDDM is clinically expressed in only half of carriers. If prevention of IDDM becomes feasible in the future then the situation might change. The association of the 21-hydroxylase deficiency of congenital adrenal hyperplasia with the histocompatibility region suggests the possibility of prenatal diagnosis in families in which an affected sibling has alerted physicians to the problem. Similarly, deficiency of C2 and C4 has troublesome consequences, and early knowledge would benefit the individual.

Population screening would identify persons at increased risk for certain diseases but lacks a rational basis. Most of the diseases discussed are not treatable, and the risks to the single individual, although much greater than in the general population, remain low. The psychological burden of such a program cannot be discounted.

Paternity Testing

The prodigous polymorphism of HLA makes it an almost ideal approach to legal exclusion of paternity.

Previous testing of putative father, mother and offspring usually employed the major erythrocyte blood group antigens because of their wide availability and accuracy. ABO typing on red blood cells carried only an estimated 18% probability of paternity exclusion, Rh testing carried a 32% probability, and together these two modes could exclude approximately 44% of putative fathers. Adding the MNSs red cell antigen system raised the figure to over 60%, but if HLA is added the exclusion possibilities are above 98%. If other serum protein polymorphisms such as the IgGm markers are utilized, the exclusion rates approach 100%.

At the New York Blood Center HLA-A, HLA-B, and HLA-C is done with multiple testing reagents. The average frequency of exclusion for HLA alone is estimated at 95%.[34] This figure will vary in different laboratories. In general, HLA-C adds only limited improvement in resolution, while the HLA-DR reagents are still expensive and more difficult to obtain.

The above estimates are valid for unrelated persons. When the issue of paternity exclusion is raised for related individuals, each of the testing systems is about 50% as efficient, and there is a need to recruit multiple genetic markers to ensure accurate conclusions.

Paternity testing is judicial and pragmatic; however, the increasingly sophisticated use of genetic variations in systems such as HLA as exclusion criteria highlight the oft repeated cliche of the almost personal chemical individuality of human beings.

Tissue Transplantation[35]

HLA typing is the basis for donor-recipient matching for organ transplantation. Most laboratories still rely on HLA-A and B testing. HLA-D and DR typing may offer better results, but disparate data from various units leave the issue unresolved.[36] In renal grafts between donor-recipient pairs who share two HLA haplotypes, more than 90% of grafts survive 2 years or more; when one haplotype is shared and the other is disparate the success rate falls to 60%–70%. Unrelated donors have even lower success rates (40%–60%), depending on the reporting method. Bone marrow grafting is associated with yet more severe problems that depend on HLA identity.

SURVEY OF SELECTED HUMAN HLA-DISEASE ASSOCIATIONS

Associations of gastrointestinal, endocrine, immunopathologic, renal, rheumatic, neurologic-psychiatric, and dermatologic disorders are summarized in Table 15–10.

CONCLUSIONS

The major immunogenetic concepts of the human histocompatibility gene complex have been reviewed and the HLA association with several dozen diseases has been presented. There are both variety and complexity within the established data. Although the majority of HLA-disease associations are with rheumatologic (e.g., seronegative spondyloarthropathies, RA) or immunopathologic (e.g., sicca syndrome, myasthenia gravis, thyroiditis) problems of unknown etiology and in which immune aberrations are frequent, there are also associations with congenital adrenal hyperplasia due to 21-hydroxylase deficiency, diabetes mellitus, and hemochromatosis. The latter disrupt any universal pattern because they cannot be explained by disordered immune response genes.

It is unclear whether the HLA antigens themselves or the cell surface molecules they are on directly initiate the disease, or whether they serve as disease markers because of their linkage to disease genes clustered within or around the histocompatibility supergene complex. Most evidence, including the different racial HLA-disease associations, favors the latter.

Finally, different loci at the HLA complex have associations with different diseases. For example, diabetes mellitus, chronic active hepatitis, and rheumatoid arthritis are closest to the HLA-D locus, hemochromatosis to the A locus, and sicca syndrome to the B locus. The logical inference is that the disease genes are spread out over the histocompatibility region.

Current applications of HLA genetic typing to modern medicine are limited. HLA data can strengthen a diagnosis only when the data are skillfully applied to a disease situation. Genetic counseling based on the presence of HLA markers is relatively unexplored, and there will be little pressure to expand this field, as the diseases in question remain late in onset and limited in serious pathology. Diabetes mellitus may be an exception. Population screening is potentially attractive, but the ability to predict future disease in an individual will remain academic as long as disorders with low

TABLE 15–10.—SURVEY OF SELECTED HUMAN HLA-DISEASE ASSOCIATIONS[1, 2, 5, 42]

	HLA ASSOCIATION (Relative Risk)	COMMENTS	REFERENCE
GASTROINTESTINAL			
Gluten-sensitive enteropathy	DR3 (17) DR7 (4)	DR3, B8, A1 haplotype: DR3 and/ or DR7 in 89% of cases (caucasians)	20
Chronic active hepatitis	DR3 (2)*	DR3, B8, A1, haplotype, especially marked in young females with autoantibodies	14
Hemochromatosis	A3 (4) B14 (5)	Evidence favors recessive inheritance with high gene expressivity; haplotypes A3, Cw, Bw4, BfF, DRw6 most common	37
ENDOCRINE			
Insulin-dependent diabetes mellitus	DR3 (98) DR4 (77)	Mechanism of inheritance is unclear; DR4 is associated with earlier onset of disease	24
Thyrotoxicosis	DR3 (5.1)		38
Idiopathic Addison's disease	B8 (3.9)		39
Subacute thyroiditis	Bw35 (22.2)		40
21-Hydroxylase deficiency	Bw47 (15)	Gene is near B and DR loci; no other enzyme deficiency involved in congenital adrenal hyperplasia is known to be HLA associated	
IMMUNOPATHOLOGIC			
Sicca syndrome	B8 (3.3) primary DR4 secondary	Incidence of tissue-specific salivary antibodies is higher in secondary syndrome, while incidence of lymphoma and pseudolymphoma is the same in primary and secondary Sicca syndrome	21, 27
RENAL			
Membranous glomerulonephritis	DR3 (4)†	In one report DR3 present in 73% of cases as compared to 21% of controls; some series do	41

RHEUMATIC			
AS	B27 (87.8)	See text	8, 11
Reiter's disease	B27 (35.9)		8, 10, 11
Yersinia arthritis	B27		11
Uveitis	B27		11
Salmonellosis with spondylitis			8, 9
RA	DR4 (3)	DR4 associated with seropositivity for RA but not with disease severity	16
Juvenile-onset RA	DR5 (2)	DR5 association is with an articular form of disease	16
SLE	DR8 (2)		18, 42
NEUROLOGIC-PSYCHIATRIC			
Multiple sclerosis	DR2 (4) B7 (4)		22
Myasthenia gravis	DR3 (3)	DR3, B8, A1: HLA association correlates with thymic hyperplasia and antibody to motor end-plate	15
Depression		No association with specific HLA antigen but genetic analysis of families discloses susceptibility gene	41
DERMATOLOGIC			
Psoriasis	Cw6	Associations also with B13, B17, B37; varied associations in different races (see Table 15–5)	12
Dermatitis herpetiformis	DR3, B8	This skin disease is associated with gluten-sensitive enteropathy and IgA antibody in skin deposits	
Behcet's disease			
Ocular forms	B5 (Japan)	Ocular morbidity higher in men	43
Arthritis	B27		
Mucocutaneous forms	B12		

*DR3 is found in 37.1% of patients with chronic active hepatitis, compared with 20.9% of the general population. If only young females with autoantibodies are considered, DR3 may be found in up to 82% of cases.[14]

†Other renal diseases may also have HLA associations: Goodpasture's syndrome, which shows anti-glomerular basement membrane antibody, is associated with HLA-DR2.[29] Poststreptococcal glomerulonephritis is associated with an Ia alloantigen.

attack rates are encountered. Among the most critical needs for HLA-disease association data is to educate the biomedical community, particularly practicing doctors, on their significance. This has two major advantages: it will forestall overinterpretation of results, and at the same time it will encourage exploration of the pathophysiology of present and future diseases. More direct applications will certainly follow closely and are already on the horizon for diabetes mellitus and the seronegative spondyloarthropathies.

REFERENCES

1. Dausset J., Svejgaard A. (eds.): *HLA and Disease.* Baltimore, Williams & Wilkins Co., 1977.
2. Bodmer W.F.: The HLA system. *Br. Med. Bull.* 34:213, 1978.
3. Benacerraf B., Dorf M.E. (eds.): *The Role of the Major Histocompatibility Complex in Immunobiology.* New York, Garland Press, 1979.
4. Bodmer W.F. *HLA: A Super, Supergene. Harvey Lect.* 72:91, 1976–1977.
5. Terasaki P.I. (ed.): *Histocompatibility Testing, 1980.* Los Angeles, UCLA Tissue Typing Laboratory, 1980.
6. Saeger K., Bashir H.V., Gaeczy A.F., et al.: Evidence for a specific B-27 associated cell surface marker on lymphocytes of patients with ankylosing spondylitis. *Nature* 277:68, 1979.
7. Bodmer W.F.: Models and mechanisms for HLA and disease associations. *J. Exp. Med.* 152:353s, 1980.
8. *Twenty-Third Rheumatism Review. Arthritis Rheum.* 21:R38, 1978.
9. Russell A.S.: Arthritis, inflammatory bowel disease and histocompatibility antigens. *Ann. Intern. Med.* 86:870, 1977.
10. Calin A., Fries J.F.: An "experimental" epidemic of Reiter's syndrome revisited. *Ann. Intern. Med.* 84:564, 1976.
11. Woodrow J.C. Genetics of B27-associated diseases. *Ann. Rheum. Dis.* 38(suppl.):135, 1979.
12. Joint report on psoriasis, in Bodmer W., et al. (eds.): *Histocompatibility Testing, 1977.* Copenhagen, Munksgaard, 1978, p. 230.
13. Eddleston A.L.W.F., William S.R.: HLA and liver disease. *Br. Med. Bull.* 34:295, 1978.
14. Tait B.D., MacKay I.R., Kastelan A., et al.: Chronic liver disease including chronic active hepatitis, in Terasaki P.I. (ed.): *Histocompatibility Testing, 1980.* Los Angeles, UCLA Tissue Typing Laboratory, 1980.
15. Dawkins R.: Myasthenia gravis, in Terasaki P.I. (ed.): *Histocompatibility Testing, 1980.* Los Angeles, UCLA Tissue Typing Laboratory, 1980, p. 662.
16. Stastny P., et al.: Rheumatoid arthritis, in Terasaki P.I. (ed.): *Histocompatibility Testing, 1980.* Los Angeles, UCLA Tissue Typing Laboratory, 1980, p. 681.
17. O'Brien W.M.: The genetics of rheumatoid arthritis. *Clin. Exp. Immunol.* 2:785, 1967.
18. Gibofsky A., Winchester R., Hansen J., et al.: Contrasting patterns of newer histocompatibility determinants in patients with rheumatoid arthritis and systemic lupus erythematosus. *Arthritis Rheum.* 21:S134, 1978.
19. Marn D.L., Abelson L., Henkart P., et al.: Specific human B lymphocyte alloantigens linked to HL-A. *Proc. Natl. Acad. Sci. USA* 72:5103, 1975.
20. Mann D.L., Katz S.I., Nelson D.L., et al.: Specific B-cell antigens associated

with gluten-sensitive enteropathy and dermatitis herpetiformis. *Lancet* 1:110, 1976.

21. Moutsopoulos H., Chused T.M., Johnson A.H., et al.: B lymphocyte antigens in Sicca syndrome. *Science* 199:1441, 1978.
22. Winchester R.J., Ebers F., Fu S.M., et al.: B-cell alloantigen Ag 7a in multiple sclerosis. *Lancet* 2:814, 1975.
23. Cudworth A.G., Festenstin H.: HLA genetic heterogeneity in diabetes mellitus. *Br. Med. Bull.* 34:285, 1978.
24. Svejgaard A., Platz P., Ryder L.P.: Insulin-dependent diabetes mellitus, in Terasaki P.I. (ed.): *Histocompatibility Testing, 1980.* Los Angeles, UCLA Tissue Typing Laboratory, 1980, p. 638.
25. Jersild C.: The HLA System and multiple sclerosis, in *Birth Defects* 14:123, 1978.
26. Calin A.: HLA-B27: To type or not to type? *Ann. Intern. Med.* 92:208, 1980.
27. Moutsopoulos H.M., Mann D.L., Johnson A.H., et al.: Genetic differences between primary and secondary sicca syndrome. *N. Engl. J. Med.* 301:761, 1979.
28. Libby D.M., Gibfosky A., Fotino M., et al.: Immunogenetic and clinical findings in idiopathic pulmonary fibrosis: Association with the B-cell-alloantigen. *Clin. Res.* 28:428A, 1980.
29. Rees A.J., Peters D.K., Compston D.A.S., et al.: Strong association between HLA-DRw2 and antibody-mediated Goodpasture's syndrome. *Lancet* 1:966, 1978.
30. Moll J.N.H., Wright V.: Familial occurrence of psoriatic arthritis. *Ann. Rheum. Dis.* 32:181, 1973.
31. Wooley P.H., Griffen J., Penayi G.S., et al.: HLA-DR antigens and toxic reaction to sodium aurothiomalate and d-penicillamine in patients with rheumatoid arthritis. *N. Engl. J. Med.* 303:300, 1980.
32. Batchelor J.R., et al.: Hydralazine-induced systemic lupus erythematosus: Influence of HLA-DR and sex on susceptibility. *Lancet* 1:1107, 1980.
33. Laitinen O., Leirisalo M., Skylv G.: Relationship between HLA-B27 and clinical features in patients with *Yersinia* arthritis. *Arthritis Rheum.* 20:1121 1977.
34. Allen F.H.: Unpublished data.
35. Carpenter C.B.: HLA and renal transplantation. *N. Engl. J. Med.* 302:860, 1980.
36. Terasaki P.I. (ed.): *Histocompatibility Testing, 1980.* Los Angeles, UCLA Tissue Typing Laboratory, 1980, pp. 392–637.
37. Simon M., Bourel M., Genetet B., et al.: Idiopathic hemochromatosis: Demonstration of recessive transmission and early detection by family HLA typing. *N. Engl. J. Med.* 297:1017, 1977.
38. Farid N.R.: Grave's disease, in Farid N.R. (ed.): *HLA in Endocrine and Metabolic Disorders.* New York, Academic Press, 1981, p. 86.
39. Farid N.R.: Thyroiditis, in Farid N.R. (ed.): *HLA and Endocrine and Metabolic Disorders.* New York, Academic Press, p. 145.
40. Weitkamp L.R., Stancer H.C., Persad E., et al.: Depressive disorders and HLA: A gene on chromosome 6 that can affect behavior. *N. Engl. J. Med.* 305:1301, 1981.
41. Garavoy M.R.: Idiopathic membranous glomerulonephritis: An HLA associated disease, in Terasaki P.I. (ed.): *Histocompatibility Testing, 1980.* Los Angeles, UCLA Tissue Typing Laboratory, 1980, p. 673.

42. Dupont B.: Association between HLA and disease, in Litwin S.D., Christian C.L., Siskind G.W. (eds.): *Clinical Evaluation of Immune Function in Man.* New York, Grune & Stratton, 1976, p. 97.
43. James D.G.: Behçet's syndrome. *N. Engl. J. Med.* 301:431, 1979.
44. Schaller J.G., Hansen J.A.; HLA relationships to disease. *Hosp. Pract.* 16:41, 1981.

Index